T0235340

Lecture Notes in Computer Science 9185

Commenced Publication in 1973
Founding and Former Series Editors:
Gerhard Goos, Juris Hartmanis, and Jan van Leeuwen

More information about this series at http://www.springer.com/series/7409

Vincent G. Duffy (Ed.)

Digital Human Modeling

Applications in Health, Safety, Ergonomics
and Risk Management: Ergonomics and Health

6th International Conference, DHM 2015
Held as Part of HCI International 2015
Los Angeles, CA, USA, August 2–7, 2015
Proceedings, Part II

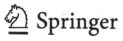 Springer

Editor
Vincent G. Duffy
Purdue University
School of Industrial Engineering
West Lafayette, IN
USA

ISSN 0302-9743   ISSN 1611-3349   (electronic)
Lecture Notes in Computer Science
ISBN 978-3-319-21069-8   ISBN 978-3-319-21070-4   (eBook)
DOI 10.1007/978-3-319-21070-4

Library of Congress Control Number: 2015942488

LNCS Sublibrary: SL3 – Information Systems and Applications, incl. Internet/Web, and HCI

Springer Cham Heidelberg New York Dordrecht London
© Springer International Publishing Switzerland 2015

Printed on acid-free paper

Springer International Publishing AG Switzerland is part of Springer Science+Business Media
(www.springer.com)

Foreword

The 17th International Conference on Human-Computer Interaction, HCI International 2015, was held in Los Angeles, CA, USA, during 2–7 August 2015. The event incorporated the 15 conferences/thematic areas listed on the following page.

A total of 4843 individuals from academia, research institutes, industry, and governmental agencies from 73 countries submitted contributions, and 1462 papers and 246 posters have been included in the proceedings. These papers address the latest research and development efforts and highlight the human aspects of design and use of computing systems. The papers thoroughly cover the entire field of Human-Computer Interaction, addressing major advances in knowledge and effective use of computers in a variety of application areas. The volumes constituting the full 28-volume set of the conference proceedings are listed on pages VII and VIII.

I would like to thank the Program Board Chairs and the members of the Program Boards of all thematic areas and affiliated conferences for their contribution to the highest scientific quality and the overall success of the HCI International 2015 conference.

This conference could not have been possible without the continuous and unwavering support and advice of the founder, Conference General Chair Emeritus and Conference Scientific Advisor, Prof. Gavriel Salvendy. For their outstanding efforts, I would like to express my appreciation to the Communications Chair and Editor of HCI International News, Dr. Abbas Moallem, and the Student Volunteer Chair, Prof. Kim-Phuong L. Vu. Finally, for their dedicated contribution towards the smooth organization of HCI International 2015, I would like to express my gratitude to Maria Pitsoulaki and George Paparoulis, General Chair Assistants.

May 2015

Constantine Stephanidis
General Chair, HCI International 2015

HCI International 2015 Thematic Areas and Affiliated Conferences

Thematic areas:

- Human-Computer Interaction (HCI 2015)
- Human Interface and the Management of Information (HIMI 2015)

Affiliated conferences:

- 12th International Conference on Engineering Psychology and Cognitive Ergonomics (EPCE 2015)
- 9th International Conference on Universal Access in Human-Computer Interaction (UAHCI 2015)
- 7th International Conference on Virtual, Augmented and Mixed Reality (VAMR 2015)
- 7th International Conference on Cross-Cultural Design (CCD 2015)
- 7th International Conference on Social Computing and Social Media (SCSM 2015)
- 9th International Conference on Augmented Cognition (AC 2015)
- 6th International Conference on Digital Human Modeling and Applications in Health, Safety, Ergonomics and Risk Management (DHM 2015)
- 4th International Conference on Design, User Experience and Usability (DUXU 2015)
- 3rd International Conference on Distributed, Ambient and Pervasive Interactions (DAPI 2015)
- 3rd International Conference on Human Aspects of Information Security, Privacy and Trust (HAS 2015)
- 2nd International Conference on HCI in Business (HCIB 2015)
- 2nd International Conference on Learning and Collaboration Technologies (LCT 2015)
- 1st International Conference on Human Aspects of IT for the Aged Population (ITAP 2015)

Conference Proceedings Volumes Full List

Digital Human Modeling and Applications in Health, Safety, Ergonomics and Risk Management

Program Board Chair: Vincent G. Duffy, USA

- Giuseppe Andreoni, Italy
- Daniel Carruth, USA
- Elsbeth De Korte, The Netherlands
- Jennifer Gaudioso, USA
- Afzal A. Godil, USA
- Ravindra Goonetilleke, Hong Kong
- Akihiko Goto, Japan
- Hiroyuki Hamada, Japan
- Satoshi Kanai, Japan
- Min Soon Kim, USA
- Noriaki Kuwahara, Japan
- Kang Li, USA
- Zhizhong Li, P.R. China
- Tim Marler, USA
- Caterina Rizzi, Italy
- Leonor Teixeira, Portugal
- Renran Tian, USA
- Anita Woll, Norway
- James Yang, USA
- Qianxiang Zhou, P.R. China

The full list with the Program Board Chairs and the members of the Program Boards of all thematic areas and affiliated conferences is available online at:

http://www.hci.international/2015/

HCI International 2016

The 18th International Conference on Human-Computer Interaction, HCI International 2016, will be held jointly with the affiliated conferences in Toronto, Canada, at the Westin Harbour Castle Hotel, 17–22 July 2016. It will cover a broad spectrum of themes related to Human-Computer Interaction, including theoretical issues, methods, tools, processes, and case studies in HCI design, as well as novel interaction techniques, interfaces, and applications. The proceedings will be published by Springer. More information will be available on the conference website: http://2016.hci.international/.

General Chair
Prof. Constantine Stephanidis
University of Crete and ICS-FORTH
Heraklion, Crete, Greece
Email: general_chair@hcii2016.org

http://2016.hci.international/

Contents – Part II

Motion Modeling and Tracking

Contents – Part I

Modeling Human Work and Activities

Anthropometry and Ergonomics

Estimation of Arbitrary Human Models from Anthropometric Dimensions

Yui Endo$^{(\boxtimes)}$, Mitsunori Tada, and Masaaki Mochimaru

Digital Human Research Center, National Institute of Advanced
Science and Technology, Tsukuba, Japan
{y.endo,m.tada,m-mochimaru}@aist.go.jp

Abstract. In this paper, we describe a novel approach for reconstructing arbitrary whole-body human models from an arbitrary sparse subset of anthropometric dimensions. Firstly, a comprehensive set of dimensions is estimated from the subset via the principal component space for the dimensions. Then, a skin surface model with the obtained comprehensive set of dimensions is constructed by deforming a whole-body human model template. The result is validated based on the error distribution of the dimensions of the obtained surface mesh for the target.

Keywords: Human modeling · Anthropometry

1 Introduction

Over the past few years, "digital style design" for various kinds of products has been widely applied due to the spread of a variety of CAD systems. On the other hand, those designs with high ergonomic assessment such as easy shape and comfortable user-interface for human grasp and operation, so called "human centered design", have been receiving much more attention as this could enhance the market competitiveness of products. Current ergonomic evaluation processes require experiments based on a large number of various human subjects and a variety of physical mockups. These create bottlenecks in the product development cycle, are time consuming, have a high cost, and result in fewer implementations of ergonomic assessment. Thus, human models, digital models of various kinds of human, have been proposed to conduct the ergonomic assessment in a virtual environment. This virtual ergonomic assessment, integrating human models with product models, has a high possibility to produce ergonomic design quickly with less cost and its implementation has been highly anticipated.

Reconstruction of functional human models with arbitrary body shapes is the first step to conducting "virtual ergonomic assessment" in the process of human-centered product design. Thus far, we have proposed a reconstruction method of the human model and its postures for arbitrary individuals, conducted by inputting the trajectories of landmark points on the skin surface obtained from a motion capture system [1]. Though the human models obtained are accurate enough for our purpose, experiments with a motion capture system are too time-consuming and too expensive to be conducted for a plurality of real subjects.

© Springer International Publishing Switzerland 2015
V.G. Duffy (Ed.): DHM 2015, Part II, LNCS 9185, pp. 3–14, 2015.
DOI: 10.1007/978-3-319-21070-4_1

In this paper, we describe a novel approach for reconstructing arbitrary whole-body human models from an arbitrary sparse set of anthropometric dimensions. Though this method adopts an approximate approach by referring to the large database for whole-body anthropometric dimensions, it can be conducted much faster than the previously-proposed method.

2 Definitions and Methods

2.1 Human Model Definition

Thus far, we have developed the human models, called "Dhaiba", achieving the ergonomic assessment of products based on the precise simulation of various types of human size, shape and function in a virtual environment. The Dhaiba models include the "DhaibaBody", whole body models, and the "DhaibaHand", hand models (Fig. 1(a) (b)) [2].

Each Dhaiba model fundamentally contains the following three model elements:

1. A skin surface model consisting of as a triangular mesh which represents the skin surface in a reference posture.
2. A link model which includes a set of the local coordinate system of each joint and their connectivity as the links.
3. Each anthropometric dimension for the Dhaiba model is defined as the distance between two landmark vertices on the skin surface model. In some cases, the

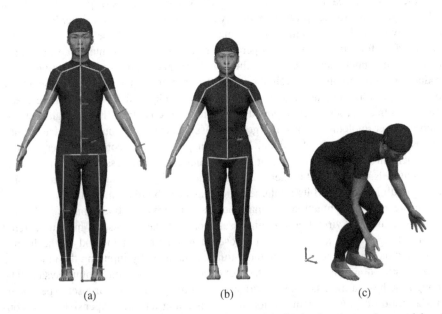

(a)   (b)   (c)

Fig. 1. The Dhaiba models. (a) The male template model, (b) the female template model and (c) the model which changed its posture.

distances along the *x/y/z*-axis in the world coordinate system are used as the definition.

The posture of the Dhaiba model is controlled by rotating the joint angles of the link model. The "Skeletal Subspace Deformation (SSD)" algorithm is used for the deformation of the skin surface model by following the joint rotation [3], so as to represent the whole-body geometry for arbitrary postures (Fig. 1(c)).

2.2   Overview of the Method

Figure 2 shows an overview of the proposed method. Firstly, the user specifies an arbitrary set of whole-body dimensions for a target, which is a subset of a comprehensive set of the dimensions. Then, the comprehensive set of the dimensions for the target is estimated from the input and a large database for the set. Finally, the human model for the target including the skin surface model and the link model is constructed by an optimization method based on the control of the "link scales".

The details are described in the following sections.

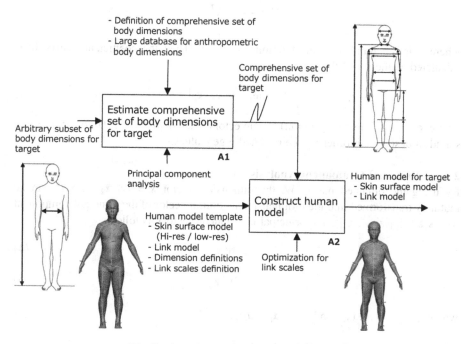

Fig. 2. Overview of the proposed method.

2.3 Estimation of the Comprehensive Set of Anthropometric Dimensions

The system performs the following steps to estimate a comprehensive set of anthropometric dimensions for the target from the arbitrary subset of the dimensions for the target.

2.3.1 Preparation

A large database for the comprehensive set of the whole-body anthropometric dimensions is prepared. A large dense matrix D is defined, where $D_{i,j}$, the (i, j)th entry of the D, represents the value of j-th dimension item for an i-th subject included in the database. Then a matrix X is calculated as the standardized matrix for the D:

$$X_{i,j} = \frac{D_{i,j} - \dot{a}_j}{\tilde{a}_j}, \tag{1}$$

where $\dot{a}_j$ and $\tilde{a}_j$ is the mean and the standard deviation for the j-th column of the D respectively. Hereafter we denote i-th row vector of the D the dimension vector $\mathbf{x}_i$. The correlation matrix C is calculated as follows:

$$C = \frac{1}{n-1} X^T X, \tag{2}$$

where n is the number of the columns of the X. Then the coefficient matrix W is calculated as the set of the eigenvectors for the C:

$$W = [\mathbf{e}_1 \quad \mathbf{e}_2 \dots \mathbf{e}_n], \tag{3}$$

where $\mathbf{e}_1, \dots, \mathbf{e}_n$ are the (column) eigenvectors related to the C. These vectors are sorted in descending order by their related eigenvalues.

2.3.2 Principal Component Analysis

By using the obtained matrix W, the dimension vector $\mathbf{x} = [x_1 \ x_2 \ \dots \ x_n]^T$ can be mutually transformed into the n-dimensional column vector of the principal component scores $\mathbf{z} = [z_1 \ z_2 \ \dots \ z_n]^T$ (the principal component vector) as follows:

$$\mathbf{z} = W\dot{\mathbf{x}}, \tag{4}$$

$$\dot{\mathbf{x}} = W^T \mathbf{z}, \tag{5}$$

where $\mathbf{x} = [\dot{x}_1 \ \dot{x}_2 \dots \dot{x}_n]^T$ and $\dot{x}_j = (x_j - \dot{a}_j)/\tilde{a}_j$.

2.3.3 Estimation of the Dimension Vector

Here, the user chooses several dimension items from the complete dimension set and specifies values for them. By using these arbitrary n_s values in $\mathbf{x}$, the first n_s principal component scores can be estimated. For instance, in the case where $n_s = 2$ and the dimension item a and b are chosen as the subset, the approximate values of z_1 and z_2 are calculated as follows:

$$\begin{bmatrix} \dot{x}_a \\ \dot{x}_b \end{bmatrix} \cong \hat{W} \begin{bmatrix} z_1 \\ z_2 \end{bmatrix}, \tag{6}$$

where

$$\hat{W} = \begin{bmatrix} (W^T)_{a,1} & (W^T)_{a,2} \\ (W^T)_{b,1} & (W^T)_{b,2} \end{bmatrix}. \tag{7}$$

Thus, the following equation is obtained:

$$\begin{bmatrix} z_1 \\ z_2 \end{bmatrix} \cong \hat{W}^{-1} \begin{bmatrix} \dot{x}_a \\ \dot{x}_b \end{bmatrix}. \tag{8}$$

So, in this case, the approximate value of complete dimension vector $\mathbf{x}$ is calculated by Eqs. (5) and (8), where the other principal component scores $z_3, \ldots, z_n$ are set to zero.

2.4 Construction of the Human Model

In this section, the Dhaiba model for the target is constructed from the Dhaiba model template, based on the dimension vector $\mathbf{x}$ obtained in the previous section.

2.4.1 The Dhaiba Model Template

Construction of the Dhaiba model template is the first step to carrying out the optimization process for constructing the Dhaiba model for the target described in the following sections.

Figure 1 (a) (b) shows the Dhaiba model templates reconstructed from a dense polygon soup obtained by a laser scanner. The Dhaiba model for the target is obtained by deforming one of the template model, so the skin surface model and the link model for the target are "homologous" with the ones for the template. That is, the following are common among all Dhaiba models respectively:

1. The number of vertices, faces and the topological structure of the skin surface models
2. The vertex index of each landmark on the skin surface models
3. The structure of the link models

2.4.2 Skin Surface Deformation Based on Link Scales

Once the Dhaiba model template is prepared, the shape of the template model can be dynamically changed by controlling the "link scales".

The link scale $s_{j,k}$ is defined as a variable for an axis k ($k \in \{+x, -x, +y, -y, +z, -z\}$) of each joint j of the link model. Based on the link scales, the origin of the local coordinate system Σ_j for each joint j is updated as follows:

$$\mathbf{o}'_j = {}^W T'_{j-1} S(j, \mathbf{o}_j) \left({}^W T_{j-1}\right)^{-1} \mathbf{o}_j, \tag{9}$$

where $\mathbf{o}_j = [o_{jx}\ o_{jy}\ o_{jz}\ 1]^T$ is the position vector of the origin of the Σ_j and $\mathbf{o}'_j$ is the updated one. ${}^W T_{j-1}$ is the 4×4 matrix which transforms the world coordinate system into the local coordinate system Σ_{j-1} ($j-1$ indicates the index of the parent joint of the j) and ${}^W T'_{j-1}$ is the updated one. The 4th column vector of ${}^W T_j$ is updated from $\mathbf{o}_j$ to $\mathbf{o}'_j$ and ${}^W T'_j$ is obtained as the result. $S(j, \mathbf{v})$ is the 4×4 scaling matrix defined as follows:

$$S(j, \mathbf{v}) = \begin{bmatrix} s_{j,x'} & & & O \\ & s_{j,y'} & & \\ & & s_{j,z'} & \\ O & & & 1 \end{bmatrix}, \quad \left(\mathbf{v} = [v_x\ v_y\ v_z\ 1]^T\right), \tag{10}$$

where

$$x' = \begin{cases} x & (v_x \geq 0) \\ -x & (v_x < 0) \end{cases}, \quad y' = \begin{cases} y & (v_y \geq 0) \\ -y & (v_y < 0) \end{cases}, \quad z' = \begin{cases} z & (v_z \geq 0) \\ -z & (v_z < 0) \end{cases}. \tag{11}$$

On the other hand, the position of each vertex v on the skin surface model of the template is updated as follows:

$$\mathbf{v}' = \sum_j w^j_v\ {}^W T'_j\ S(j, {}^j\mathbf{v}) \left({}^W T_j\right)^{-1} \mathbf{v}, \tag{12}$$

where $\mathbf{v}$ is the position vector of the v and $\mathbf{v}'$ is the updated one. w^j_v is a vertex weight of v for the link bound to the joint j, which represents the degree of the relation between each vertex on the skin surface model and each link. This weight set is also used as the parameter of the skeletal subspace deformation method (a.k.a. the linear blend skinning) [3]. For calculation of the weight set, we use the skin attachment method based on heat equilibrium [3].

Figure 3 shows an example of the relation between the link scales, the modified link model and the deformed shape of the skin surface affected by the link scales.

2.4.3   Optimization Method for Constructing the Target Human Model
By using the comprehensive set of anthropometric dimensions for the target obtained in Sect. 2.3, the system optimizes the body shape of the Dhaiba model template by controlling the link scales and obtains the Dhaiba model for the target. This nonlinear optimization problem is represented as follows:

1. The link scales for the link model of the Dhaiba model template are the variables. Based on the change of the link scales, each local coordinate system of the link model and each vertex position of the skin surface model is updated.
2. The comprehensive set of anthropometric dimensions obtained for the target should be satisfied as the constraints. As described in Sect. 2.1, each dimension is

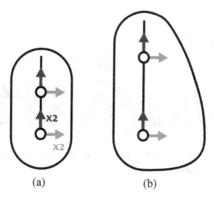

(a)   (b)

Fig. 3. The effect of link scales in the human model deformation. (a) The original shape and (b) the deformed shape. In this case, the link scales for the $+x$ (red) and the $+y$ (green) axis of the root joint are set to 2.0.

calculated as the distance between two landmark points on the skin surface model. Euclidean distance or the distance along x/y/z-axis is used as the definition of these distances. In this study, the following kinds of the dimensions are not used as the constraints: (1) dimensions which were not measured with the standard standing position and (2) ones which can not to be represented as linear distances.

3. The following energy function E is used as the objective function to be minimized:

$$E = c_S E_S + c_I E_I + c_V E_V,\qquad(13)$$

where c_S, c_I and c_V are user-specified coefficients. E_S and E_I are the energy functions defined in the correspondence optimization algorithm [4]. E_S, deformation smoothness, indicates that the transformations for adjacent triangles should be equal. E_I, deformation identity, is minimized when all transformations are equal to the identity matrix. E_V is the variance of the link scales.

3   Results and Discussion

An anthropometry database for Japanese adults collected in the national project called "size-JPN" in 2004–2006 [5] was used for the estimation of the comprehensive set of the anatomical dimensions, described in Sect. 2.3. This database includes results of the anthropometric measurements of 217 dimensions for 6,700 Japanese 18–80 year old subjects. Figure 4 shows distribution of the mean errors and the coefficients of variation of the estimated comprehensive set of dimensions. We picked up comprehensive sets of dimensions for 500 randomly chosen subjects from the database, and, by using the body height and the body mass of each set as the input, each comprehensive set of the dimensions was estimated from the method proposed in Sect. 2.3.

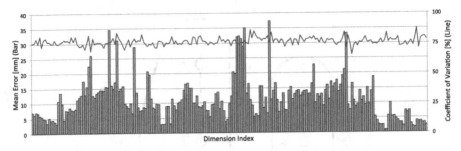

Fig. 4. Distribution of the mean errors and the coefficients of variation of the estimated comprehensive set of dimensions.

Figures 5 and 6 shows the construction result of the Dhaiba models for several targets and their error distribution of the dimensions of the obtained models. The process described in Sects. 2.3–2.4 was done in 6–7 s for each target.

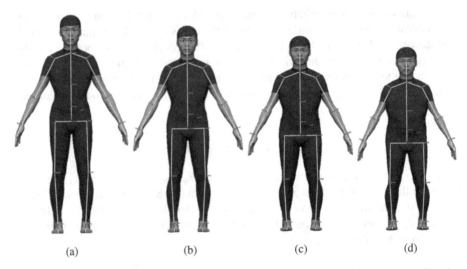

Fig. 5. Constructed Dhaiba models for several targets. Height and weight were specified for each construction as the input. Specified height was (a) 1800 mm, (b) 1700 mm, (c) 1600 mm and (d) 1500 mm. Specified weight was 67.93 kg, mean value of Japanese 30–34 year old males.

The method deforms the target mesh to satisfy the dimension constraints while keeping the details of the mesh shape, so the initial shape of the template model has a major effect on the result. Therefore constructing the appropriate template models is one of the critical issues for obtaining good results. In addition, there is a wide variety of individual whole-body shapes, so, though we currently use single template model for any target, we need to prepare several kinds of the template models and select an appropriate model suitable for the target shape.

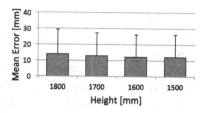

Fig. 6. Mean errors and their standard deviations of the dimensions of the obtained models for the estimated dimensions (the input of the method described in Sect. 2.4).

4 Conclusions

In this paper, we proposed a novel approach for reconstructing arbitrary whole-body human models from an arbitrary sparse subset of anthropometric dimensions. The comprehensive set of dimensions was estimated from the subset via the principal component space for the dimensions. The skin surface model with the obtained comprehensive set of dimensions is constructed by the optimization of the shape of the whole-body human model template based on the link scales control.

Annex A. Comprehensive Set List of Anatomical Dimensions

Table 1 shows the comprehensive set list of the anatomical dimensions which we used for the proposed method in Sect. 2.3.

Table 1. The comprehensive set list of the anatomical dimensions. H: height, L: length. * means the dimension is used as the optimization constraints described in Sect. 2.4.3.

Stature, p (body H, p)*	Right shoulder angle of slope 1 (acromion)	Side neck to anterior waist L via nipple
Body mass (weight)	Right shoulder angle of slope 2	Nipple to anterior waist L
Total head H*	Left shoulder angle of slope	Shoulder to anterior waist L
Pupil to vertex H*	Right nipple to fossa jugularis distance*	Fossa jugularis to anterior waist L, p
Tragion to vertex H*	Left nipple to fossa jugularis distance*	Waist to hip L
Stomion to vertex H*	Bust base angle	Outside leg L
Stomion to tragion H*	Thigh L*	Posterior waist to hip L (belt waist)
Gnathion to glabella H*	Lower leg L*	Posterior waist to hip L (horizontal waist)
Face L*	Neck breadth*	Gluteal arc

(Continued)

Table 1. (*Continued*)

Stature, p (body H, p)*	Right shoulder angle of slope 1 (acromion)	Side neck to anterior waist L via nipple
Gnathion to pupil H*	Shoulder (biacromial) breadth*	Gluteal arc, putting leg up
Gnathion to stomion H*	Shoulder (bideltoid) breadth*	Total crotch L
Head L*	Anterior biaxillary breadth*	Upper posterior arm L, elbow flexion
Head breadth*	Elbow-to-elbow breadth	Total posterior arm L, elbow flexion
Bitragion breadth*	Angulus inside by scapulae horizontal distance*	Total posterior arm L
Bizygomatic breadth*	Angulus inside by scapulae linear distance*	Cervicale to wrist L via shoulder and elbow
Interpupillary breadth*	Angulus inferior by scapulae horizontal distance*	Side neck to shoulder L
Head circumference	Angulus inferior by scapulae linear distance*	Posterior shoulder L
Sagittal arc	Nipple to nipple breadth*	Posterior chest L
Bitragion arc	Bicristal breadth*	Anterior shoulder L
Stature (body H)*	Biiliospinale anterius breadth*	Anterior chest L
Eye (pupil) H*	Chest breadth*	Sitting H
Eye (lateral canthus) H*	Bust breadth*	Eye (lateral canthus) H, sitting
Gnathion H*	Waist breadth*	Gnathion H, sitting
Cervicale H*	Abdominal breadth*	Cervicale H, sitting
Side neck H*	Hip breadth (peak of buttock)*	Shoulder H, sitting
Fossa jugularis H*	Hip breadth (maximum lower body)*	Elbow H, sitting
Shoulder H*	Armscye width*	Dactylion H, over head, sitting
Anterior axillary H*	Chest depth*	Abdominal extension H, sitting
Radiale H	Thorax depth at the nipple (bust depth)*	Trochanterion H, sitting
Dactylion H	Waist depth*	Thigh clearance, sitting
Elbow H	Abdominal depth*	Thigh H, sitting
Fist (grip axis) H	Hip depth*	Knee H, sitting
Dactylion H, over head	Hip depth, p	Knee joint H, sitting
Angulus inside by scapulae H*	Thigh depth*	Lower leg L (popliteal H), sitting
Angulus inferior scapulae H*	Knee depth*	Sitting surface H
Mesosternale H*	Calf depth*	Buttock-knee L, sitting
Nipple H*	Neck circumference	

(*Continued*)

Table 1. (*Continued*)

Stature, p (body H, p)*	Right shoulder angle of slope 1 (acromion)	Side neck to anterior waist L via nipple
		Buttock-popliteal L (seat depth), sitting
Waist H*	Neck base circumference	Buttock-trochanterion L, sitting
Posterior waist H*	Chest circumference	Buttock-abdomen depth, sitting
Anterior waist H*	Chest circumference at nipple level (bust circumference)	Hip breadth, sitting
Omphalion H*	Waist circumference 1 (horizontal waist)	Abdominal depth, sitting
Lower waist H*	Waist circumference 2 (belt waist)	Lower limb L, sitting
Iliocristale H*	Lower waist circumference	Hand L*
Abdominal extension H*	Iliocristale circumference	Palm L perpendicular*
Iliac spine H*	Abdominal extension circumference	Index finger L*
Trochanterion H*	Hip circumference	Hand breadth, diagonal*
Peak of buttock H*	Hip circumference, p	Hand breadth at metacarpals*
Maximum lower body breadth H*	Armscye circumference	Index finger breadth, proximal*
Gluteal furrow H*	Upper arm circumference	Index finger breadth, distal*
Crotch H*	Elbow circumference	Hand circumference
Maximum thigh circumference H*	Forearm circumference	Fist circumference
Mid-patellar H*	Wrist circumference	Foot L 1*
Knee joint H*	Inguinal circumference	Foot L 2*
Tibial H*	Thigh circumference	Tibial instep L*
Maximum calf circumference H*	Knee circumference	Fibular instep L*
Ankle H*	Calf circumference	Foot breadth 1, diagonal*
Span	Ankle circumference	Foot breadth 2*
Upper limb L*	Drop	Heel breadth*
Upper arm L*	Scye depth, p	Heel circumference
Forearm L*	Cervicale to posterior waist L, p	Instep circumference
Shoulder-elbow L	Cervicale to posterior hip L, p	Foot circumference
Forearm-fingertip L	Posterior full L, p	Instep circumference maximum H*
Elbow-grip L	Cervicale to side neck L	Foot circumference maximum H*
Arm reach from back	Cervicale to nipple L	Ball H*

(*Continued*)

Table 1. (*Continued*)

Stature, p (body H, p)*	Right shoulder angle of slope 1 (acromion)	Side neck to anterior waist L via nipple
Grip reach; forward reach	Cervicale to anterior waist L via nipple	Big toe outside angle
Wall-acromion distance	Cervicale to fossa jugularis L via side neck	Little toe outside angle
Elbow-wrist L	Side neck to fossa jugularis L	Sphyrion H*
Side neck to acromion horizontal distance*	Side neck to posterior waist L	Lateral malleolus H*
Side neck to acromion vertical distance*	Shoulder to posterior waist L	Sphyrion fibulare H*
Side neck to acromion linear distance*	Side neck to nipple L	Bimalleolar breadth*

References

1. Endo, Y., Tada, M., Mochimaru, M.: Reconstructing individual hand models from motion capture data. J. Comput. Des. Eng. **1**(1), 1–12 (2014)
2. Endo, Y., Tada, M., Mochimaru, M.: Dhaiba: development of virtual ergonomic assessment system with human models. In: Proceedings of The 3rd International Digital Human Symposium (2014)
3. Baran, I., Popovic, J.: Automatic rigging and animation of 3D characters. ACM Trans. Graph. **26**(3), 72:1–72:8 (2007)
4. Sumner, R.W., Popović, J.: Deformation transfer for triangle meshes. ACM Trans. Graph. **23**(3), 399–405 (2004)
5. Size-JPN project. http://www.hql.jp/database/size2004/ (in Japanese)

Optimisation of Product's Hand-Handle Interface Material Parameters for Improved Ergonomics

Gregor Harih[1(✉)], Matej Borovinšek[2], and Zoran Ren[2]

[1] Laboratory for Intelligent CAD Systems, Faculty of Mechanical Engineering,
University of Maribor, Smetanova ulica 17, 2000 Maribor, Slovenia
gregor.harih@um.si
[2] Laboratory for Advanced Computational Engineering, Faculty of Mechanical Engineering,
University of Maribor, Smetanova ulica 17, 2000 Maribor, Slovenia
{matej.borovinsek,zoran.ren}@um.si

Abstract. Most authors have focused on the sizes and the shapes of the product handles, but neglected those interface materials of the handles, which could further improve the ergonomics of the product. Therefore we utilized optimisation method to determine optimal interface material properties of a product for optimal mechanical response of the system using numerical simulations of a fingertip model grasping a product's handle. Objective function was set to find material parameters in such way that the interface material of the product stays firm during low grasping forces to provide stability of the product in hands and deforms when a critical contact pressure is reached to provide higher contact area. This increases comfort and lowers the contact pressure on the hand and thereby the risk of injury development.

Keywords: Tool handle · Material design · Optimisation · Ergonomics · Finite element analysis · Contact pressure · Grasp simulation · Hyper-elastic foams

1 Introduction

Correct design of handheld products is crucial for preventing upper extremity acute trauma disorders (ATD) and cumulative trauma disorders (CTD), such as blisters, carpal tunnel syndrome, hand-arm vibration syndrome, tendonitis, etc. [1]. In order to prevent this, authors have provided guidelines and mathematical models for determining the sizes and shapes of the product handles to maximize finger-force exertion, comfort, contact area, thus minimizing the chances to develop ATD and CTD [2–5].

The mechanical properties of the skin and subcutaneous tissue are very important during grasping tasks as they are in direct contact and the forces and moments are transferred from the product to the whole hand-arm system. It has been shown that skin and subcutaneous tissue have non-linear viscoelastic properties, where the skin is stiffer than the subcutaneous tissue [6, 7]. Both have low stiffness regions at small strains followed by a substantial increase in the stiffness when the strain increases.

A power grasp can yield a contact pressure of the fingertip of 80 kPa or over, which has been shown as excessive loading for skin and subcutaneous tissue [8]. Authors also

© Springer International Publishing Switzerland 2015
V.G. Duffy (Ed.): DHM 2015, Part II, LNCS 9185, pp. 15–25, 2015.
DOI: 10.1007/978-3-319-21070-4_2

provided rough guidelines of pressure discomfort (PDT) and also pressure-pain threshold (PPT). Values between 100 kPa and almost 200 kPa have been reported [9, 10]. Handheld products which require high grip, push, pull or torque exertion on the handle produce high contact pressures, which is known to be one of the primary factors for the ATD and also CTD development [11]. In order to maintain the desired user performance, the designer has to design tool-handles, which distributes contact pressure more evenly and do not exceed the provided limits [9].

Most authors have focused on the sizes and the shapes of the product handles, but neglected those interface materials of the handles that are in direct contact with the user's hand. Authors provided basic guidelines regarding the material choice, but did not investigate and consider the mechanical behaviour of the skin and soft tissue whilst grasping handles of different materials [12].

It has already been shown that cellular materials can be characterised to meet specific mechanical behaviour [13]. Within such context we have already proposed a composite hyper-elastic foam material that can lower the contact pressure whilst keeping the low deformation rate of the product handle material to maintain a sufficient stability rate when using the product [14].

Due to high complexity of the simulated system of the fingertip and hyper-elastic foam with non-linear materials, it is difficult to propose a foam material with optimal material properties for optimal mechanical behaviour of the system.

In this regard we utilized optimisation to find the optimal material parameters of the interface hyper-elastic foam material. The optimisation was set to determine material parameters of the interface material which stays firm during low grasping forces to provide stability of the product in hands and deforms when a critical contact pressure is reached to provide higher contact area. This lowers the contact pressure on the hand and thereby increases comfort and lowers the risk of ATD and CTD development.

2   Methods

In order to perform numerical simulations we used finite element simulation software Abaqus/CAE 6.10 from Dassault Systems (France). The optimisation procedure has been performed using an in-house developed software called OptiMax.

2.1   Finite Element Model – Geometrical and Boundary Conditions

The FE model was constructed based on existing fingertip FE models [15]. We modelled a symmetrical model to lower the needed computational power for optimisation process. The product interface material has been modelled as a flat rectangle with two sections using 1 mm protection layer of EPDM rubber and 3 mm hyper-elastic foam layer for the appropriate deformation during grasping (Fig. 1).

The displacements and rotations of the rectangle representing the interface material of the product were fixed on the lower contour. The displacement and rotations of the fingertip were fixed, except for the displacement along the vertical axis. In order to simulate the grasping, we applied displacement of the fingertip $u_p = 5$ mm, which was applied on the vertical top point of the finger bone and is directed normal to the interface material surface. The fingertip and the product interface material were meshed using 5149 and 1920 CPE8 elements, respectively.

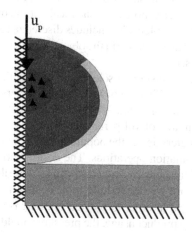

Fig. 1. Geometrical and boundary conditions

2.2 Finite Element Model – Material Properties

Fingertip bone and nail were assumed to be linear elastic with isotropic material parameters with Young´s modulus of 17 GPa and 170 MPa respectively, with a Poisson ratio of 0.3 [16]. The material parameters of skin and subcutaneous tissue were defined using the Ogden hyper-elastic material model (Table 1). Since skin and subcutaneous tissue are almost incompressible, the Poisson ratio was determined to be 0.4 [16].

Table 1. Material parameters determining hyper elasticity of skin and subcutaneous tissue

	Skin		Subcutaneous tissue	
N	μ_i	α_i	μ_i	α_i
1	−0.07594	4.941	−0.04895	5.511
2	0.01138	6.425	0.00989	6.571
3	0.06572	4.712	0.03964	5.262

Material parameters of the outer protective layer made of EPDM rubber were based on literature [14]. The material properties of the hyper-elastic foam (interface material) were not defined in advance but determined with the optimisation procedure.

2.3 Optimisation and Numerical Tests

In order to identify the interface hyper-elastic foam material with optimal material properties a single-objective optimisation problem was formulated. Since the investigated problem is highly nonlinear, more than one local optima of the objective function was expected and because the problem also includes discretized geometry with contacts, which could cause the occurrence of noise in the objective function, a non-gradient based optimisation method was used.

A genetic algorithm with elitism and selection based on the biased roulette wheel scheme was chosen for the identification of material parameters. The genetic algorithm is a well-known meta-heuristic algorithm, which follows the natural evolution process. The inputs of the algorithm are control parameters, design variables and an objective function. The control parameters define the populations size, number of generations and the rate of crossover and mutation operations. The design variables were the material parameters of the foam and the objective function will be described in the next chapters.

According to the literature we defined the limit contact pressure p_{lim} as 100 kPa, which should not be exceeded in order to prevent injuries. But if the limit pressure is reached and exceeded during product usage, the pressure should rise as slow as possible in regard to the fingertip displacement. On the other side, larger deformations of the product handle interface material decrease the users' product stability and therefore control. Figure 2 presents the typical contact pressure response when hyper-elastic foam material is used for the product handle. The response curve has a characteristic plateau region with a prominent plateau point P and a corresponding plateau slope, where the stiffness of the handle decreases and the contact pressure rises slower.

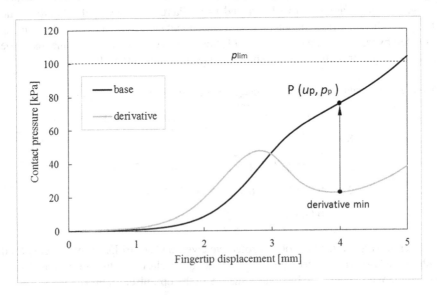

Fig. 2. Typical contact pressure vs fingertip displacement curve (black) and its derivative (grey) (Color figure online)

The plateau point is the point where the contact pressure rises the slowest so the plateau point pressure p_p should be as close to the limit contact pressure of 100 kPa as possible. At the same time the plateau angle and the fingertip displacement u_p at the plateau point should be as small as possible.

Based on these observations a single-objective function was formed. It was comprised from the difference between the plateau point pressure and the limiting pressure, plateau point angle and plateau point fingertip displacement where x represents the design variables and w represents weights of single objective functions (Eq. 1).

$$f(x) = w_1 \cdot abs\left(p_p - p_{lim}\right) + w_2 \cdot \left(u_p - 3\right) + w_3 \cdot \left(\frac{dp}{du}\right)_P \tag{1}$$

The weights were determined with preliminary simulations in such a way that the values of all objective function parts were approximately the same. They were set to $w_1 = 0.1$, $w_2 = 0.\overline{3}$ and $w_3 = 0.01$. The plateau point angle was replaced with the slope of the contact pressure curve which was determined with the derivative of the contact pressure curve at the plateau point.

In order to determine the plateau point on the contact pressure versus displacement curve, first its derivative was computed (Fig. 2). Then the last local minimum of the derivative curve was found. The fingertip displacement at derivative minimum was then taken as the plateau point fingertip displacement. Then the plateau point pressure was determined from it.

The design variables x were the material parameters of the foam material. The foam material was modelled with a hyper-foam constitutive model defined with uni-axial test data. The test data was approximated with a three-linear curve in order to reduce the number of design variables (Fig. 3). The three-linear curve is determined with four data points T_i where their coordinates correspond to the strains ε_i and stresses σ_i respectively. The first data point T_1 was fixed at $(0, 0)$ while the strain value of the fourth data point T_4 was fixed to $\varepsilon_4 = 0.9$. All five other coordinates were taken as design variables with values within interval bounds given in Table 2.

Table 2. The design space of the design variables

Design variable	Lower bound	Upper bound
ε_2 [/]	0.01	0.08
ε_3 [/]	0.21	0.58
σ_2 [MPa]	0.01	0.08
σ_3 [MPa]	0.02	0.18
σ_3 [MPa]	0.42	1.18

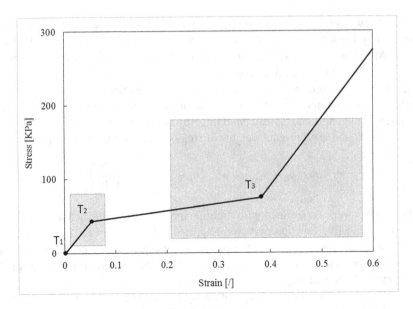

Fig. 3. The design space of the uni-axial test data of the foam material

The genetic algorithm was run using 100 samples in a generation for 50 generations. The crossover parameter was set to 0.80 and the mutation parameter to 0.05. A personal computer was used to run the optimisation procedure in parallel and a high performance cluster was used to compute the simulations. Each simulation was run on 4 cpu-cores resulting in execution time of about one minute. In total 5000 simulations were done to find the result.

3 Results

In our previous research we verified and validated the 2D FE model in regard to existing FE models and to experimental data, since it showed great correspondence between results [14].

The optimisation procedure finished after 50 generations. From the convergence curve we could observe that the best solution was quickly improved in the first five generations and then only slightly changed in the following generations. The last improvement of the solution occurred at 45th generation.

The best solution after optimisation are the following foam material parameters $\varepsilon_2 = 0.053$, $\varepsilon_3 = 0.383$, $\sigma_2 = 0.043$, $\sigma_3 = 0.075$ and $\sigma_4 = 0.796$. The deformation of the fingertip and foam with these material parameters is shown in Fig. 4. In the first stages of the simulation only skin and the soft tissue deform, where they are in contact with the foam. As the fingertip displacement increases the deformation of the foam becomes visible.

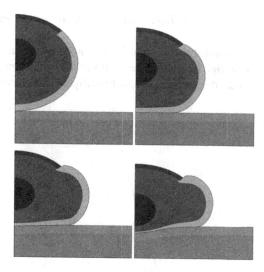

Fig. 4. The deformation of the fingertip and "foam" at the fingertip displacement of 0, 1.67, 3.33 and 5 mm.

In order to quantify the results of interface material parameter optimisation, we compared the response of the simulated system using optimised foam also to other product interface materials. Therefore we also provide the results for steel as quasi-rigid (Young's modulus of 210 Gpa and a Poisson ratio of 0.3) and a composite of EPDM rubber and PU foam as product's interface material proposed in one of our previous papers [14]. Material behaviour under uniaxial compression of the optimised

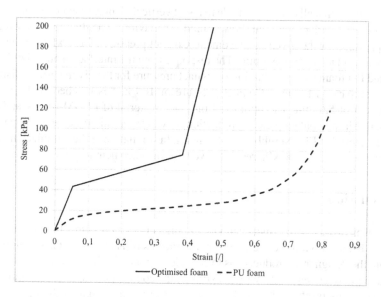

Fig. 5. Stress strain responses of PU foam and optimised foam under uniaxial compression

foam proposed in this paper and PU foam used by us in previous research can be seen in Fig. 5.

Since optimisation was performed in regard of contact pressure and displacement of fingertip and interface material, we plotted the results of the contact pressure in comparison to the combined vertical displacement of the fingertip and interface material (Fig. 6).

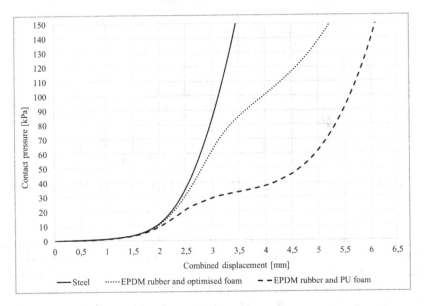

Fig. 6. Contact pressure vs combined displacement of the fingertip and interface material

Results show that all curves coincide to about vertical displacement of 1.7 mm. After that point every interface material show its unique behaviour. The steel shows the highest contact pressure for the given displacement. Contact pressure of 100 kPa is reached at the vertical displacement of 3.1 mm. The response from the interface material of EPDM rubber and PU foam shows reduction in contact pressure for the given vertical displacement in comparison to steel. Contact pressure of 100 kPa is reached at the vertical displacement of 5.6 mm. The optimized interface material of EPDM rubber and optimized foam shows contact pressure reduction, however less displacement compared to interface material of EPDM rubber and PU foam. In simulation of the optimized material the contact pressure of 100 kPa results in vertical displacement of 4 mm.

4   Discussion

Power grasps of various products can yield in high contact pressures for over 100 kPa, which has been shown to be the one of main reasons of ATD and CTD development. Therefore the designer of products has to consider ergonomics in order to develop sizes, shapes and interface materials, which distribute the contact pressures evenly and do not exceed the limits provided by the literature. Hence we investigated the peak contact pressure at the fingertip center line compared to the combined vertical displacement of the fingertip and interface material.

Results have shown that the least deformation of the fingertip and tool-handle material at any simulated contact pressure was achieved with steel as a quasi-rigid material (Fig. 6). This was to be expected, since the stress strain curve of the steel is much steeper and higher than the soft tissue, therefore almost all the deformation on the vertical axis could be addressed to the deformation of the fingertip. Since almost none deformation of the interface material was observed, we considered steel as a reference interface material to evaluate other interface materials.

From the results it is evident that all three interface materials (steel, EPDM rubber and PU foam, EPDM rubber and optimised foam) also showed almost the same contact pressure versus vertical deformation behaviour to a deformation of about 1.7 mm. This deformation can be accredited to the deformation of the fingertip, since the curve corresponds, to great extent, to the curve of steel, where almost no deformation of the product handle interface material was observed. After 1.7 mm of deformation, both composites of EPDM rubber and PU foam and EPDM rubber and optimised foam started to deform.

Due to the different stress strain behaviour and different plateau levels of both composites, the diagrams had different characteristic curves after the deformation of 1.7 mm. The lower and very prominent deformation plateau of the PU Foam accounted for "S" like shaped curve with extensive deformation of the foam when the plateau was reached. The low deformation plateau of this foam also accounts that the interface material starts to deform at around 30 kPa of contact pressure. According to literature contact pressure of 30 kPa is still safe and occurs during normal handling of products in hands. Therefore deformations of the interface material at these contact pressure are not preferred as this lowers the stability of the product in hands.

On the other hand the interface material using the optimised foam shows just slightly bigger deformations compared to the steel for the given contact pressure. The deformation plateau is reached at around 80 kPa. At this point the optimised foam starts to deform and thereby provides higher contact area and lowers the contact pressure.

According to the results, it can be seen that interface material parameters cannot be easily determined. Therefore optimisation is required, which enables the desired mechanical response of the simulated system. The optimisation was set to determine parameters in such way that the interface material did not deform at lower contact pressures, but deformed when high contact pressure was achieved, thus lowering the risk of ATD and CTD development. Using the objective function and appropriate weights the optimisation was set to produce low contact pressures and considering least additional deformation of the interface material in order to maintain high level of stability of the product when in the hand.

5 Conclusion

In this paper we have shown that due to high complexity of the simulated system of the fingertip grasping various interface materials of the product handle optimisation can be a viable method to propose a foam material with optimal material properties for optimal mechanical behaviour of the system. The success of the optimisation process is largely dependent on the correct determination of the objective function. Based on recommendations from literature and previous simulations performed by us the objective function was set to obtain optimal parameter data of the interface hyper-elastic foam material, which stays firm during low grasping forces to provide stability of the product in hands and starts to deforms only when the critical contact pressure is reached to provide higher contact area. This lowers the contact pressure on the hand, which can increase comfort and lower the risk of pressure-dependent ATD and CTD development.

Future work should further consider improving the objective function in regard of subjective responses from test users. The optimisation could also consider the thicknesses of the composite. Additionally dynamic simulations could be carried out to simulate the effect of vibration and foam damping and optimise those parameters. Three dimensional simulations should also be performed to consider a realistic geometry of a human fingertip and further improve the results.

Acknowledgements. The paper was co-produced within the framework of the operation entitled "Centre of Open innovation and Research UM (CORE@UM)." The operation is co-funded by the European Regional Development Fund and conducted within the framework of the Operational Program for Strengthening Regional Development Potentials for the period 2007–2013, development priority 1: "Competitiveness of companies and research excellence," priority axis 1.1:"Encouraging competitive potential of enterprises and research excellence," contact No. 3330-13-500032.

The paper was also produced within the framework of research programme P2-063 entitled "Design of Porous Structures", which is financed by the Slovenian Research Agency "ARRS".

References

1. Moore, A., Wells, R., Ranney, D.: Quantifying exposure in occupational manual tasks with cumulative trauma disorder potential. Ergonomics **34**(12), 1433–1453 (1991)
2. Garneau, C.J., Parkinson, M.B.: Optimization of product dimensions for discrete sizing applied to a tool handle. Int. J. Ind. Ergonom. **42**(1), 1–9 (2011)
3. Kong, Y., Lowe, B.: Optimal cylindrical handle diameter for grip force tasks. Int. J. Ind. Ergon. **35**(6), 495–507 (2005)
4. Seo, N.J., Armstrong, T.J.: Investigation of grip force, normal force, contact area, hand size, and handle size for cylindrical handles. Hum. Factors **50**(5), 734–744 (2008)
5. Oh, S., Radwin, R.G.: Pistol grip power tool handle and trigger size effects on grip exertions and operator preference. Hum. Factors **35**(3), 551–569 (1993)
6. Edwards, C., Marks, R.: Evaluation of biomechanical properties of human skin. Clin. Dermatol. **13**(4), 375–380 (1995)
7. Wu, J.Z., Cutlip, R.G., Andrew, M.E., Dong, R.G.: Simultaneous determination of the nonlinear-elastic properties of skin and subcutaneous tissue in unconfined compression tests. Skin Res. Technol. **13**(1), 34–42 (2007)
8. Gurram, R., Rakheja, S., Gouw, G.J.: A study of hand grip pressure distribution and EMG of finger flexor muscles under dynamic loads. Ergonomics **38**(4), 684–699 (1995)
9. Aldien, Y., Welcome, D., Rakheja, S., Dong, R., Boileau, P.E.: Contact pressure distribution at hand–handle interface: role of hand forces and handle size. Int. J. Ind. Ergonom. **35**(3), 267–286 (2005)

10. Fransson-Hall, C., Kilbom, Å.: Sensitivity of the hand to surface pressure. Appl. Ergon. **24**(3), 181–189 (1993)
11. Rempel, D.M., Harrison, R.J., Barnhart, S.: Work-related cumulative trauma disorders of the upper extremity. JAMA J. Am. Med. Assoc. **267**(6), 838–842 (1992)
12. Fellows, G.L., Freivalds, A.: Ergonomics evaluation of a foam rubber grip for tool handles. Appl. Ergon. **22**(4), 225–230 (1991)
13. Vesenjak, M., Borovinšek, M., Fiedler, T., Higa, Y., Ren, Z.: Structural characterisation of advanced pore morphology (APM) foam elements. Mater. Lett. **110**, 201–203 (2013)
14. Harih, G., Dolšak, B.: Recommendations for tool-handle material choice based on finite element analysis. Appl. Ergon. **45**(3), 577–585 (2014)
15. Wu, J.Z., Dong, R.G.: Analysis of the contact interactions between fingertips and objects with different surface curvatures. Proc. Inst. Mech. Eng. Part H J. Eng. Med. **219**(2), 89–103 (2005)
16. Wu, J.Z., Dong, R.G., Rakheja, S., Schopper, A.W.: Simulation of mechanical responses of fingertip to dynamic loading. Med. Eng. Phys. **24**(4), 253–264 (2002)

An Approach for Intuitive Visualization of Ergonomic Issues

Walentin Heft[1]([✉]), Michael Spitzhirn[2], Angelika C. Bullinger[2], and Paul Rosenthal[1]

[1] Visual Computing Laboratory, Department of Computer Science,
Technische Universität Chemnitz, Chemnitz, Germany
{walentin.heft,paul.rosenthal}@informatik.tu-chemnitz.de
[2] Ergonomics and Innovation Management, Department of Mechanical Engineering,
Technische Universität Chemnitz, Chemnitz, Germany
{michael.spitzhirn,angelika.bullinger-hoffmann}@mb.tu-chemnitz.de

Abstract. Ergonomics is the science of human work. One goal is the adaption of work to the human, thus to create better working conditions and to avoid health risks. Increasingly often, digital human models and corresponding evaluation methods are used. Due to the mass of data and the variety of possible analyses which come along with a simulation, the interpretation of the outcomes can take a long time. We introduce a new concept, which enables a quick and understandable visualization and navigation of critical ergonomic situations and their causes. There are filter mechanisms available for changing the level of detail. These enable a representation for specific target groups. Prior to the development of the concept, expert interviews were conducted to specify the user requirements. Each iteration step of the design process was evaluated in cooperation with ergonomics experts.

Keywords: Overview and glyph-based visualization · Ergonomics · Concept study

1 Introduction

An important property of visualization is its interactive nature. It is necessary to consider some simulation results, analyze them, and change parameters for a better understanding. Typically, a reconsideration from another viewpoint or comparison of the several outcomes has to be conducted. Furthermore, user interaction is often needed because of the mass of data which is not perceptibly at a glance. Especially in research and industry, experts use visual analytics tools to detect ergonomic problems [1]. Modest circumstances concerning ergonomics could increase working time and costs. During the beginning of professional ergonomics, ergonomists used life-size human models and prototypes, for example, to design vehicle interior. These days they are using computers and ergonomics software tools, such as digital human models (DHM), to visualize results for a fast processing and understanding. While some ergonomists

© Springer International Publishing Switzerland 2015
V.G. Duffy (Ed.): DHM 2015, Part II, LNCS 9185, pp. 26–36, 2015.
DOI: 10.1007/978-3-319-21070-4_3

still use tables in hard copy for their analysis, the following surveys show the importance of ergonomics software tools in all areas of product planning, manufacture, and usage. The results of a survey carried out by Wischniewski [2] indicate that for the majority of the sample, ergonomics tools are important today. Most of the 30 domain experts, which participated in the survey, think that these tools will take an inherent part of virtual ergonomics evaluation in the future. Another survey carried out by Muehlstedt [1] with 59 experts also emphasizes the importance of ergonomics tools. Especially the analysis function in the matter of visualization (as picture or video) next to measurement, and posture were considered to be relevant.

2 Potential Users and Requirements

In order to create an interactive visualization of ergonomics information, we had to determine potential users and their requirements. Often several target groups work on the same data base, but with different intension and from different angles. For this purpose we interviewed professionals in the field of ergonomics, the occupational health and safety department (HSE), and industrial engineering (IE) from Deutsche Bahn AG (German Railways). Six experts participated in this workshop. A further workshop was held at the Volkswagen AG with two experts. We identified the main groups of potential users and their requirements in moderated interviews. All things considered, we obtain three main areas. In the first area experts are responsible for planning and designing of work processes. This includes professionals of HSE, IE, as well as planers and designers. The latter define the final product design in collaboration with ergonomists, HSE, and the IE. They are also responsible for the implementation of the working system. The industrial engineers set, among other things, time standards. A further group of potential users are persons who actually produce the goods. Here, workers are responsible for the correct execution of the working task and they are assisted by the team leader. The team leader takes the responsibility for decision-making, monitoring, and advisory to maintain the quality and quantity goals in the production. The person has also to decide about the deployment. Hereby, the work requirements and individual productivities of the corresponding employee have to be matched [3–5]. The last area consists of the work council and management. The former is the representative of workers' interests. The management deals with economic aspects. This also includes the investment costs of workplace design.

In the following, the mentioned requirements of the participants of the workshops are explained in more detail. The respondents expressed their desire for an easier handling. In general, existing ergonomics tools are too complicated, as they told us. There is a high learning curve and a new incorporation is necessary after a few months without using the corresponding software, in particular in DHMs. In order to counter these problems, explanations, such as mouseover info boxes on all interactive elements are wanted. The second wish was a user-friendly representation of the analysis data. The design should have an eye-catching character. In their experience, most non-ergonomists aren't interested in tables. Color coding is preferred over tables. Furthermore, as the ergonomists mentioned, intuitive and sustainable graphical user interfaces are requested to demonstrate the ergonomic-critical situation in workshops, which are held for the workers. Many workers do their work already for years in the same manner. They very often lack the understanding of the necessity of the advantages the workers obtain due to ergonomic analyses of their workplaces. In addition, a prioritization is required to set a focus on major problems, such as bending. A visualization of ergonomic data should also consider that the same data has to presented in different forms, depending on whether they talk in front of the management or the workers. In result, important ergonomic issues should be visible at a glance and additional information should be provided on demand in a simple way.

3   State of the Art

Although the variety of visual metaphors is quite broad, the used approaches seem very simplistic and in many cases not human centered enough to facilitate an optimal process by ergonomists. We have recently presented an overview about the state of the art in virtual ergonomics with regard to visualization issues [6]. There are several methods to conduct ergonomic analyzes of workplaces, e.g., posture or load. We want to briefly introduce two of them, RULA and EAWS. The ergonomic tool RULA ("Rapid Upper Limb Assessment") can be utilized to investigate "the exposure of workers to risk factors associated with work related upper limb disorders" [7]. It is a gross screening method which evaluates the body posture (upper arms, lower arms, wrists, neck, trunk, and legs), based on the body angles, the applied forces and loads, the proportion of static muscle work, and the number of repetitions. The result is a rating of the working conditions, which ranges from one (no risk) to seven (high risk). In addition, a separate evaluation of the single body segments can be done. The use of the method is easy to learn [8]. With the ergonomic system EAWS ("Ergonomic Assessment Worksheet"), the biomechanical risk factors for musculoskeletal disorders can be evaluated during a working shift. The evaluation process consists of different sections, such as an assessment of additional ergonomic loads (for example caused by working on moving objects) or an assessment of static or high repetitive postures. EAWS is more complex and the method requires significant more information for a judgment than the method RULA.

As mentioned before (see Sect. 1), ergonomic investigations in companies are surprisingly often carried out by measuring or capturing data using paper-pencil methods and simple software support. For ergonomic reports, standardized sheets, such as the EAWS scoring sheet or simple diagrams, are applied as visualization. In addition, ergonomic maps or exposure registers are used for the documentation of an ergonomic evaluation of several work stations. The visualization of this kind of work is typically done using simple floor plan sketches or plain (Excel-) tables. A workstations can also receive a color coding according to the common standard DIN EN 614 (green, yellow, red) or separate evaluation points for a sharper disjunction [9].

Digital human models are becoming more and more popular [10] and usage is growing [11]. The presentation of ergonomic results with software is often bounded to lists, simple dialogs, or simple graphs. An excerpt of the most common representations of ergonomic reports in digital human models can be found in Figs. 1 and 2. The introduced tools are not able to pass the above mentioned design requirements. There is no possibility to select the depth of analysis and only information about a static pose can be displayed, instead of an overall view. The current visualization in DHM does not support the user in analyz-

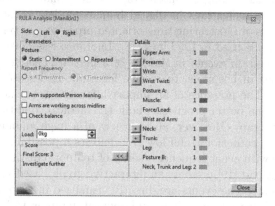

Fig. 1. Ergonomic report of RULA in the DHM "Human Builder". On the left-hand side, the ergonomists have the possibility to tune the analysis results for the corresponding body side, the final score, as well as further parameters. On the right-hand side, there are color coded fields for several body parts. The colors indicate the level of stress on the body joints (Color figure online).

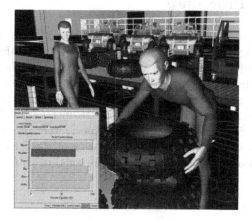

Fig. 2. Ergonomic report of RULA in the DHM "Jack" [12]. The report is displayed in a 3D scene. Here, a static pose of a male worker is considered. The analysis results are color coded for several body parts (e.g., the elbow or the shoulder), as shown in the bottom left corner.

ing ergonomic critical situations in an adequate way. The current presentation tends to demonstrate data in the absence of a context relation and without the possibility to change the depth and range of analyzing. Thus, there is room for improvement.

4   Related Work

Since time-oriented data is relevant in many practical situations, the visualization of such data has a long tradition [13] and still many recent work exists [14–16]. However, visualizations in digital human models for showing critical ergonomic situations or illustrating time-oriented processes are very limited. The concept of timelines is used in LifeLines [17]. LifeLines was developed to create an overview over certain events in the life of a person. Therefore, the authors make investigations in hospitals, to receive facts about deseases, visits to the doctor, and so on. The presence of all import information at one stage enables the doctors to make a better prognosis about the medical condition and to offer a more suitable therapy. However, an overview of a huge amount of data can still quickly lead to confusion. LifeFlow [18] delivers a possibility to counteract this circumstance with event sequences (series of temporal distinct and consecutive events). Matchpad [19] presents an interactive glyph-based visualization for realtime sport events. The events are directly visualized in an overview, during the match. SoundRiver [20] makes an audio-visual mapping to illustrate sound effects from audio sources, like movies (e.g., for hearing-impaired viewers). In this way, it symbolizes the noise of an airplane as an icon with a small aircraft, for example.

5   Evaluation Procedure

Based on the investigation of the user requirements (see Sect. 2), a first mockup was designed (see Fig. 3). We evaluated this concept with an informal survey and with the help of five ergonomic and usability experts that did not participate in the initial workshops. At the beginning of the survey, the participants were explained the aim and the single tasks of the respective parts of the mockup. After that, they had several minutes of time to internalize the visualization. Following, the interview was conducted. The experts were asked about the single components and the overall impression. On basis of the feedback and several further feedback loops, the new concept was designed in an iterative process.

6   Design Process

The initial (Fig. 3) and the final version (Fig. 4) follow Shneidermans seeking mantra "overview first, zoom and filter, then details-on-demand" [21]. Nevertheless, our user study led to significant changes, related to the initial design.

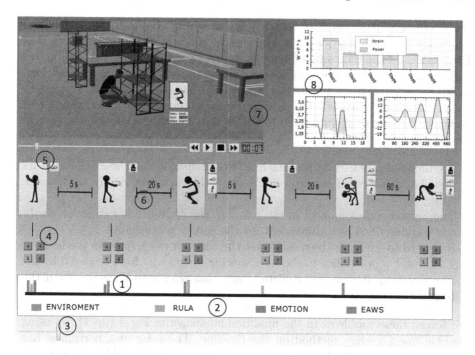

Fig. 3. Initial concept. (1) Timeline (2) Legend (3) Slider (4) Evaluation-scores (5) Pictogram with additional stress hints (6) Distance time between critical situations (7) Video sequence player (8) Further information about critical situations

The general concept shall contain a timeline for an overall view of all critical situations. We have deliberately avoided to display the overall workflow. First of all, ergonomic problem cases require a special investigation. In the initial version the design point (dp) 1 of Fig. 3 shows the timeline with vertical colored bars. The bars are located at the time, where the corresponding critical issues occurred. The colors refer to the legend beneath the timeline (Fig. 3: dp 2) and indicate the method, which delivers a poor score for an ergonomic event. The height of a bar depicts the severity of the problem. We use a slider (Fig. 3: dp 3) to specify the moment where to start with the analysis. From that point on, the following six critical ergonomic situations are displayed in more detail. The related results (Fig. 3: dp 4) are shown at a glance. Every value, in the colored boxes, represents the analysis result of the corresponding evaluation method. These colors also relate to the legend (Fig. 3: dp 2), as previously mentioned. In addition to the analysis scores, further information is necessary, such as the adverse posture of the worker as pictogram (Fig. 3: dp 5), which leads to a bad score, or hints to other reasons for this (see Fig. 3: dp 5, upper right corner). The "stickman"-pictograms are based on the depiction of poses from EAWS. An advantage is the high recognition value for ergonomists. A pictogram shall be selectable by a mouse click. This enables a deeper insight in the current problem, with further key figures and diagrams (Fig. 3: dp 8), as well as a video player (Fig. 3: dp 7) to depict the simulation sequence at the current problem time. Design point 6 of Fig. 3 indicates the time interval between two critical situations. This interactive surface contains all analysis results without an overloading of the display with information. Now, users are able to regard their data from a coarse overview to a deeper insight, if needed. This is in response to the desires of the interviewed persons. The survey results show that this initial design approach has several shortcomings:

- A number of problems at the timeline (Fig. 3: dp 1) cannot be displayed at its best; i.e., a bar could overlap other bars, if they occurred nearly at the same time.
- The permanent assignment of the colors to the appropriate evaluation methods was described as inconvenient, by the survey participants.
- It is hard to compare the results over the time for the respective method.
- There isn't a possibility to choose a specific range, e.g., from second 5 to 20.
- The duration of a single problem is not that simple to recognize from the timeline.

We solved these problems in the final design, shown in Fig. 4 (dp 1), by using a single row for every method on the timeline. The color of a horizontal bar doesn't show the method anymore, but the severity of the problem (the darker the color, the worse the ergonomic issue). Hence, problems can't overlap anymore. Furthermore, it is possible to analyze all problems, indicated by a specific method, in a row. We have added a range slider beneath the timeline (see Fig. 3: dp 2), where users can choose a scope exact to the second. These proposals were approved by all participants involved. In response to the constraints on space, not all critical situations, within a chosen range, can be displayed at a glance (respectively as pictograms), when they consist of more than 5 problems. Due to this restriction, we have added a "previous" and a "next" button (see Fig. 4: dp 6), with the quantity of the future problems, to our final concept. If a small section on the timeline contains many short trouble spots, it becomes quickly unmanageable. The respondents want a chance to choose and to enlarge this area. In the new approach, they can achieve this by specifying the considered area with the slider. This part is expanded horizontally. All problems, which are in front of and behind the range of interest are compressed and grayed out. The critical ergonomic issues of the chosen range are displayed in more detail, as previously mentioned. There is a scrollbar beneath the timelime to change the current view of the problems within the selected area; i.e., the pictograms and the corresponding single result values. The single scores of the evaluation methods are displayed in boxes above the timeline (Fig. 4: dp 3). In contrast to the first concept, we order the evaluation scores by the analysis methods (Fig. 4: dp 3). This enables a comparison of several problems over time and for one method. The adverse work postures are presented in form of pictograms (Fig. 4: dp 5) with additional indications, like the weight of an object (carried along by the worker), as mentioned above. The experts expressed the desire that the

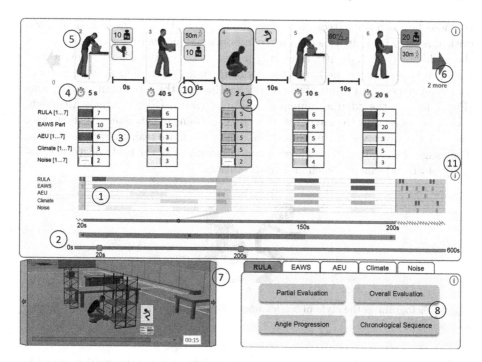

Fig. 4. Final concept. (1) Timeline (2) Sliders (3) Evaluation-scores (4) Duration of one critical issue (5) Pictogram with additional stress hints (6) Next-button shows further ergonomic problems (7) Video sequence player (8) Further information about critical situations (9) Highlighting of current selected problem (10) Distance time between critical situations (11) Mouse-over tooltip at the "i"-symbol

correlation between the timeline and a corresponding problem (the single scores and the pictogram) needs to be highlighted. We realize this wish as shown in Fig. 4 (dp 9). If the pictogram is selected, a colored background stripe appears. According to the interviews, we have swapped the lower parts of Fig. 3 (dp 1 - dp 6) with the upper parts. Now, the sections "video player" (Fig. 3: dp 7) and "detail view" (Fig. 3: dp 8) are located on the bottom. The participants consider the latter merely as additional information. The main focus lies on the overview; i.e., the timeline and the single scores including the pictograms. Therefore, we have rearranged the design and the main parts are on top. At the wish of the participants, the detail view in the first concept (Fig. 3: dp 8) is refined (Fig. 4: dp 8). The information, which is included there, may be very complex and composed of different parts, such as lists, plots, or other descriptions. These data are necessary for a more precise investigation and are requested on demand. Hence, subcategories were introduced in the new concept, in order to avoid an overloading of the graphical user interface with information which are not required in each case. In addition, the results of all analysis methods for the current issue are provided over several tabs. Therefore, an ergonomist can examine possible relations between the outcomes of several analysis methods. The duration of one critical issue (Fig. 4: dp 4) is even more important than the time interval between the problems (Fig. 4: dp 10), especially if the worker carries a heavy weight over longer distance. Hence, we have appended this time designation at the request of the ergonomists. As a result of the survey we changed the "stickman"-pictograms (Fig. 5, left) to the "digital human model"-pictograms (Fig. 5, right). Although, it is to be noted that the participants were discordant in this issue. Nevertheless, the majority approved the modification, due to the more realistic representation. The usage of this alternative allows a good assessment of the body posture, especially of 3D movements, such as trunk rotations.

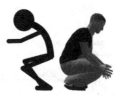

Fig. 5. Pictogram in the style of a stickman (left) and more realistic as digital human model (right)

In order to simplify the usage, some interviewees have proposed to provide mouse-over info boxes direct at the interactive parts. We deviated from this proposal, since permanently opening boxes during navigation might be cumbersome for the users. Nevertheless, we have realized this idea by adding tooltips at the right-hand edge of the display (Fig. 4: dp 11), which are accepted generally.

7   Conclusions

In this paper, we have discussed two concepts to visualize ergonomic analysis data and to explore it. The first concept (Fig. 3) was prepared on basis of several expert interviews. We have realized the requirements of the experts, such as an intuitive handling, a first overview of all critical situations, as well as the providing of deeper information on demand. An evaluation of this prototype with experts from the field of ergonomics, visualization, and usability led to significant changes in our initial concept (Fig. 3). This demonstrates the importance of our user studies. The disadvantages of the first concept were highlighted and eliminated in several iterative loops. Furthermore, we explained why we use pictograms (see Fig. 5) and why we changed the order of certain graphical elements in the final concept, as a result of the survey.

References

1. Mühlstedt, J.: Entwicklung eines Modells dynamisch-muskulärer Arbeitsbeanspruchungen auf Basis digitaler Menschmodelle. Universitätsverlag Chemnitz, Chemnitz (2012)

2. Wischniewski, S.: Delphi survey: digital ergonomics 2025 - trends and strategies for increasing product usability and designing safe, healthy and competitive socio-technical work systems (2013). http://mreed.umtri.umich.edu/DHM2013Proceedings/
3. British Standards Institute Staff. Safety of Machinery. Ergonomic Design Principles. Terminology and General Principles, B S I Standards (2006)
4. DGVU. Rolle und Aufgabe der Fachkraft für Arbeitssicherheit. http://www.dguv.de/sifa-online/Fachkraft-f%C3%BCr-Arbeitssicherheit/Rolle-und-Aufgabe/index.jsp. (20 February 2015)
5. Schlick, C.M., Bruder, R., Luczak, H.: Arbeitswissenschaft. Springer, Berlin (2010)
6. Heft, W., Spitzhirn, M., Rosenthal, P.: A survey on visualization in industrial ergonomics. In: Rosenthal, P., Laramee, R.S., Kirby, M., Kindlmann, G.L. (eds.) Proceedings of the EuroVis Workshop on Reproducibility. Verification, and Validation in Visualization, pp. 7–8. Eurographics Association, Germany (2013)
7. McAtamney, L., Corlett, E.N.: Rula: a survey method for the investigation of work-related upper limb disorders. Appl. Ergon. **24**(2), 91–99 (1993)
8. FIOH. Rula (rapid upper limb assessment). http://www.ttl.fi/en/ergonomics/methods/. 20 February 2015
9. Kugler, M., Bierwirth, M., Schaub, K., Sinn-Behrendt, A., Feith, A., Ghezel-Ahmadi, K., Bruder, R.: Förderschwerpunkt 2007: KoBRA - Kooperationsprogramm zu normativem Management von Belastungen und Risiken bei körperlicher Arbeit: Ergonomie in der Industrie - aber wie?; Handlungshilfe für den schrittweisen Aufbau eines einfachen Ergonomiemanagements. Bundesanst. für Arbeitschutz und Arbeitsmedizin, Berlin (2010)
10. Magnenat-Thalmann, N., Thalmann, D.: Handbook of Virtual Humans. Wiley, Chichester (2004)
11. Spanner-Ulmer, B., Mühlstedt, J.: Digitale Menschmodelle als Werkzeuge virtueller Ergonomie: Ergebnisse einer empirischen Studie. Industrie-Management: Zeitschrift für industrielle Geschäftsprozesse **26**(8), 69–72 (2010)
12. Siemens. Jack. http://blog.industrysoftware.automation.siemens.com/blog/2009/03/19/are-digital-humans-cool/. (20 February 2015)
13. Gantt, H.L.: Work, Wages, and Profits. Industrial management library. Engineering Magazine Company, New York (1913)
14. Aigner, W., Miksch, S., Schuman, H., Tominski, C.: Visualization of Time-Oriented Data. Human-Computer Interaction, 1st edn. Springer, London (2011)
15. Rosenthal, P., Pfeiffer, L., Müller, N.H., Ohler, P.: Visruption: intuitive and efficient visualization of temporal airline disruption data. Comput. Graph. Forum **32**(3), 81–90 (2013)
16. Zhao, J., Chevalier, F., Balakrishnan, R.: Kronominer: using multi-foci navigation for the visual exploration of time-series data. In: Proceedings of the SIGCHI Conference on Human Factors in Computing Systems, CHI 2011, pp. 1737–1746. ACM, New York (2011)
17. Plaisant, C., Milash, B., Rose, A., Widoff, S., Shneiderman, B.: Lifelines: visualizing personal histories. In: Proceedings of the SIGCHI Conference on Human Factors in Computing Systems, CHI 1996, pp. 221–227. ACM, New York (1996)
18. Wongsuphasawat, K., Gómez, J.A.G, Plaisant, C., Wang, T.D., Taieb-Maimon, M., Shneiderman, B.: Lifeflow: visualizing an overview of event sequences (video preview). In: Tan, S., Amershi, S., Begole, B., Kellogg, W.A., Tungare, M. (eds.) CHI Extended Abstracts, pp. 507–510. ACM (2011)

19. Legg, P.A., Chung, D.H.S., Parry, M.L., Jones, M.W., Long, R., Griffiths, I.W., Chen, M.: Matchpad: interactive glyph-based visualization for real-time sports performance analysis. Comp. Graph. Forum **31**(3pt4), 1255–1264 (2012)
20. Jänicke, H., Borgo, R., Mason, J.S.D., Chen, M.: Soundriver: semantically-rich sound illustration. Comput. Graph. Forum **29**(2), 357–366 (2010)
21. Shneiderman, B.: The eyes have it: a task by data type taxonomy for information visualizations. In: Proceedings of the 1996 IEEE Symposium on Visual Languages, VL 1996, pp. 336–343. IEEE Computer Society, Washington (1996)

Correlation Analysis on the Main and Basic Body Dimension for Chinese Adults

Hui-min Hu, Chao-yi Zhao, Xin Zhang, Ling-hua Ran[✉],
and Tai-jie Liu

Ergonomics Laboratory, China National Institute of Standardization, Beijing,
People's Republic of China
{huhm, zhaochy, zhangx, ranlh, liutj}@cnis.gov.cn

Abstract. In this paper, the correlations between the basic and five main body dimensions are studied based on the latest anthropometric data for the Chinese adults. Then the linear regression equations are established, which can provide technical support for optimizing anthropometric measurements. Application of this research finding in anthropometry can effectively reduce the working difficulty, shorten the working hours and cut capital investment. It can help expediting the update of the anthropometric data.

Keywords: Body dimension · Anthropometric data · Correlation · Regression equation

1 Foreword

Anthropometric data, as a kind of important fundamental data resource, are the basis of product modeling and spatial arrangement. Its applications involve almost all sectors of industrial designs. When we research human behavior in the virtual, anthropometric data is very necessary. With the social advancement and technological development, people are paying more and more attention to industrial design and the application of ergonomics, while anthropometric data are just the premises and foundation of launching industrial designs and applying ergonomics. All human related standards are established on the basis of anthropometric data, and further on applied in industrial designs [1, 2].

Anthropometric data demands stringent timeliness. According to the requirement of Anthropometry, large-scale anthropometric measurement work should be conducted every 10 years [3]. However, due to all sorts of restrictions (heavy workload, huge investment, considerable difficulty), it is hard to update the anthropometric data every 10 years. For example, China issued the Anthropometric Data of the Chinese Adults (GB 10000-88) in 19884, which was the national standard for the anthropometric data of the Chinese adults. Now, more than two decades have passed, yet no update has been made to the data. Over the past 20 plus years, China's industrial designs have always been adopting the anthropometric data released in 1988. In fact, with the improvement of the people's living standard, the Chinese people's physical characteristics have seen

© Springer International Publishing Switzerland 2015
V.G. Duffy (Ed.): DHM 2015, Part II, LNCS 9185, pp. 37–43, 2015.
DOI: 10.1007/978-3-319-21070-4_4

significant changes. Therefore, those outdated and non-timely anthropometric data are far from being able to satisfy the demands of industrial designs.

Currently, China's anthropometric data are being updated slowly, while industrial designs are in urgent need of these time-efficient anthropometric data. In light of this situation, it is necessary to find a new approach so as to facilitate the progress of updating the anthropometric data. Hence, this essay has proposed to find out the correlation between anthropometric measurements through studying the correlation of anthropometric data, in a bid to optimize the anthropometric measurements, and further on shorten the working hours, reduce the working difficulty, and cut capital investment, help collect the anthropometric data, and satisfy industrial designs' actual demands for anthropometric data.

2   The Body Dimensions Applied in the Analysis of Correlation

This article has adopted the national standard—Basic Human Body Measurements for Technological Design (GB/T 5703—1999) 5 as the major target of studies. This standard has specified the basic body dimensions needed in designing humans' working and living sites (Please refer to Table 1). There are a total of 56 anthropometric items including 41 ones at the trunk, 6 ones at the hands, 2 ones at the feet, and 6 ones at the head and face, and 1 in another category (weight).

3   Analysis of the Correlation of Anthropometric Data

According to the human being's physical characteristics, the indexes of all parts of human body are not entirely mutually independent 6. There's a close correlation between all characteristic parameters. To study the correlations between the anthropometric measurements, this research has selected the five key anthropometric items (stature, weight, chest circumference, waist circumference, and hip circumference) that influence human body's basic physical features as the independent variables of the correlation analysis, and selected the 56 basic measurements stipulated in GB/T 5703—1999 as the dependent variables.

3.1   Studies of the Relevant Parameters

This article, based on the anthropometric data of more than 3,000 Chinese adults collected by China National Institute of Standardization in 2009, attempts to study the correlation coefficient r between the anthropometric measurements of the Chinese adults, and judge the intimacy ratio of the correlations between all measurements. Correlation coefficient, also called linear correlation coefficient, is the statistical analysis index that measures the linear correlation between variables. The equation of $0 < |r| < 1$ indicates that there's linear correlation to some extent between two variables. The more $|r|$ approaches 1, the closer the linear correlation between the two variables

Table 1. List of correlation coefficient (r) between the body dimensions

No.	List of measurements	Weight	Stature	Chest circumference	Waist circumference	Hip circumference
1	Weight	1	.517**	.816**	.809**	.817**
2	Stature	.517**	1	.118**	.093**	.158**
3	Eye height	.496**	.976**	.107**	.077**	.149**
4	Shoulder height	.529**	.958**	.155**	.126**	.199**
5	Elbow height	.531**	.925**	.172**	.144**	.220**
6	Lilac spine height	.408**	.862**	.091**	.060**	.128**
7	Crotch height	.275**	.857**	−.036	−.088**	.01
8	Fist(grip axis) height	.495**	.866**	.146**	.113**	.206**
9	Tibial height	.435**	.815**	.130**	.112**	.141**
10	Sitting height	.458**	.864**	.083**	.057**	.154**
11	Eye height, sitting	.474**	.850**	.108**	.085**	.166**
12	Cervical height, sitting	.532**	.804**	.196**	.186**	.250**
13	Shoulder height, sitting	.527**	.755**	.217**	.190**	.276**
14	Elbow height, sitting	.301**	.344**	.140**	.115**	.201**
15	Lower leg length	.279**	.659**	.025	.011	-.005
16	Knee height	.539**	.849**	.207**	.184**	.248**
17	Thorax depth at the nipple	.637**	−.063**	.872**	.791**	.749**
18	Chest depth, standing	.773**	.303**	.786**	.756**	.657**
19	Body depth, standing	.727**	.094**	.815**	.864**	.723**
20	Thigh clearance	.677**	.395**	.496**	.477**	.563**
21	Abdominal depth, sitting	.720**	−0.03	.856**	.911**	.785**
22	Buttock-abdomen depth sitting	.676**	−.043*	.818**	.856**	.782**
23	Chest breadth, standing	.764**	.416**	.696**	.667**	.579**
24	Hip breadth, standing	.649**	.154**	.634**	.634**	.843**

**Correlation is significant at the 0.01 level (2-tailed)

becomes. The more $|r|$ approaches 0, the weaker the linear correlation between the two variables becomes. We can classify it into three categories: $|r| < 0.4$ represents weaker linear correlation; $0.4 \leq |r| < 0.7$ represents significant linear correlation; $0.7 \leq |r| < 1$ represents closer linear correlation.

We utilized the statistical analysis software SPSS to analyze the correlations between the anthropometric data, and obtained the correlation coefficient r between the 56 basic anthropometric measurements and the five main ones (Please refer to Table 2). As we can learn from the statistical result, there're different levels of linear correlations between the 56 basic anthropometric measurements stipulated in the national standard— *Basic Human Body Measurements for Technological Design (GB/T 5703—1999)* and the five main measurements (stature, weight, chest circumference, waist circumference, and hip circumference), and they are of great significance in statistics. The 56 basic anthropometric measurements have higher linear correlation coefficients with weight, stature and chest circumference than with hip circumference and waist circumference. The detailed analysis results are as follows:

- There're significant linear correlations between weight and circumference/width/ thickness related measurements (Correlation coefficients are basically above 0.6).
- There're comparatively closer correlations between stature and height related items, with the majority of the correlation coefficients being above 0.8. There're also

Table 2. List of correlation coefficient (r) between the body dimensions (continued)

No.	List of measurements	Weight	Stature	Chest circumference	Waist circumference	Hip circumference
25	Shoulder (biacromial) breadth	.542**	.656**	.285**	.274**	.242**
26	Shoulder (bideltoid) breadth	.790**	.552**	.624**	.609**	.555**
27	Elbow-to-elbow breadth	.665**	.166**	.698**	.682**	.633**
28	Hip breadth, sitting	.650**	.179**	.623**	.607**	.771**
29	Wall-acromion distance	.474**	.114**	.482**	.514**	.430**
30	Elbow-grip length	.472**	.702**	.207**	.201**	.213**
31	Grip reach; forward reach	.570**	.663**	.363**	.374**	.325**
32	Forearm-fingertip length	.556**	.827**	.313**	.243**	.247**
33	Shoulder-elbow length	.454**	.769**	.168**	.151**	.181**
34	Elbow-wrist length	.541**	.616**	.326**	.321**	.334**
35	Buttock-popliteal length (seat depth)	.442**	.596**	.259**	.233**	.348**
36	Buttock-knee length	.620**	.764**	.361**	.340**	.454**
37	Neck circumference	.813**	.455**	.690**	.709**	.589**
38	Chest circumference	.816**	.118**	1	.890**	.829**
39	Waist circumference	.809**	.093**	.890**	1	.814**
40	Wrist circumference	.715**	.306**	.643**	.667**	.623**
41	Thigh circumference	.698**	.139**	.660**	.617**	.815**
42	Calf circumference	.704**	.146**	.661**	.615**	.821**

**Correlation is significant at the 0.01 level (2-tailed)

comparatively significant linear correlations between stature and length related items, with the correlation coefficients being basically between 0.5 and 0.7.

- There're comparatively closer correlations between chest circumference/waist circumference/hip circumference and weight/circumference/thickness/width related measurements. What's more, the correlations between chest circumference, waist circumference and hip circumference are also relatively closer. The correlation coefficients are all above 0.8.
- There're comparatively weaker correlations between head/face measurements and the five independent variables, with the correlation coefficients all being below 0.5.
- Among the hand and foot related measurements, only hand length, palm length and foot length have closer correlations with stature (Their correlation coefficients are above 0.7) (Table 3).

Table 3. List of correlation coefficient (r) between the body dimensions (continued)

NO.	List of measurements	Weight	stature	Chest circumference	Waist circumference	Hip circumference
43	Hand length	.554**	.799**	.383**	.009	.119**
44	Palm length perpendicular	.569**	.805**	.399**	.013*	.124**
45	Hand breadth at metacarpals	.594**	.657**	.475**	.063**	.146**
46	Index finger length	.445**	.629**	.307**	.042**	.163**
47	Index finger breadth, proximal	.557**	.611**	.460**	.064**	.108**
48	Index finger breadth, distal	.534**	.527**	.451**	.114**	.154**
49	Foot length	.558**	.792**	.244**	.228**	.250**
50	Foot breadth	.427**	.383**	.275**	.260**	.275**
51	Head length	.309**	.290**	.222**	.225**	.180**
52	Head breadth	.348**	.431**	.171**	.110**	.213**
53	Face length	.235**	.257**	.157**	.150**	.116**
54	Head circumference	.375**	.314**	.250**	.218**	.247**
55	Sagittal arc	.205**	.321**	.066**	.056**	.078**
56	Bitragion arc	.218**	.288**	.099**	.068**	.149**

**Correlation is significant at the 0.01 level (2-tailed)

3.2 Linear Regression Analysis

As we can see from the 3.1 correlation analysis result, there're linear correlations in the sense of statistics between the basic anthropometric measurements and weight, stature, chest circumference, waist circumference and hip circumference. Usually, when the linear correlation coefficient $|r|$ is above 0.8, it is held that the two variables have a close linear correlation. Now, we shall launch the linear regression analysis on the trunk measurements and stature whose correlation coefficients are above 0.8. Please refer to Table 4 for the regression equations.

Table 4. Linear correlations (regression equation) between basic body dimensions and Stature (H_1)

		Chart is the mm units
1	Eye height	$0.953 H_1 - 50.3$
2	Shoulder height	$0.819 H_1 - 24.5$
3	Elbow height	$0.620 H_1 - 2.3$
4	Lilac spine height	$0.536 H_1 - 2.6$
5	Crotch height	$0.447 H_1 - 47.1$
6	Fist height	$0.432 H_1 - 7.9$
7	Tibial height	$0.306 H_1 - 83.1$
8	Sitting height	$0.454 H_1 - 142.7$
9	Eye height, sitting	$0.428 H_1 - 65.8$
10	Cervical height, sitting	$0.352 H_1 - 60.7$
11	Knee height	$0.308 H_1 - 25.3$
12	Forearm-fingertip length	$0.259 H_1 + 6$

3.3   Test of the Regression Equation

After checking the above regression equations by way of mathematical statistics, we've come to the conclusion that the regression equations and all variables' regression coefficients have passed the test of significance, and that the regression equations can accurately reflect the correlations between all measurements. Therefore, we can utilize the linear relations between all measurements to optimize the basic anthropometric measurements in the actual anthropometric work from now on. We can collect some major anthropometric measurements and utilize the regression equations to predict the anthropometric measurements that have closer correlations with the major measurements but are hard to collect.

4   Conclusion and Outlook

Based on the existing latest anthropometric data of the Chinese adults, we have conducted the correlation analysis between the basic measurements stipulated in GB/T 5703 and the five main anthropometric items, and set up the effective linear regression equations, which can serve as technical references for the optimization of the anthropometric measurements. This research result can be directly applied in the update work of the anthropometric data, which can lower the difficulty of anthropometric measurement work further.

In order to improve the practicability of the Chinese people's anthropometric data in industrial designs, we should continue to carry out researches on the correlations between all the human body dimensions, as well as between the industrial designs related body dimension and the basic body dimensions.

Acknowledgment. This work is supported by the National Key Technology R&D Program (2014BAK01B02 and 2014BAK01B05) and China National Institute of Standardization through the "special funds for the basic R&D undertakings by welfare research institutions" (282014Y-3353 and 522013Y-3055).

References

1. Wei, L.: Research of ergonomics application-the analysis and processing of human dimensions' data & its application research. Dong Hua University Master's degree dissertation, 2006
2. Pan, Z.G., Wang, L.M., Guo, Y.M.: Application of anthropometry to industrial design. Mach. Build. Autom. (2003)
3. Liu, B.-S., Guo, X.-C., Ma, X.: Practical characteristics of anthropometry for Chinese male pilots. Chin. J. Ergon. (2002)
4. GB 10000-88, Human dimensions of Chinese adults (1988)
5. GB/T 5703-1999, Basic human body measurements for technological design (1999)
6. Chen Wen-fei, Pan Qing. Establishment of grey models of body shapes. J. China Text. Univ. (2000)

The Experimental Research of the Thumb's Comfortable Control Area

Hui-min Hu[1], Junmin Du[2(✉)], Chaoyi Zhao[1], Fan Yang[3], and Ling-hua Ran[1]

[1] Ergonomics Laboratory, China National Institute of Standardization,
Beijing, China
{huhm, zhaochy, ranlh}@cnis.gov.cn
[2] School of Transportation Science and Engineering/
Airworthiness Technologies Research Center, Beihang University,
37 Xueyuan Road, Haidian District, Beijing 100191, China
dujm@buaa.edu.cn
[3] School of Biological Science and Medical Engineering,
Beihang University, Beijing, China
yangf@cnis.gov.cn

Abstract. Thumb control area is a significant concern for manipulating handheld controllers. In order to obtain the thumb's comfortable control area of Chinese people, experimental measurements were designed and carried out. The measuring parameters included right thumb size, comfortable control area and comfortable control angle range. The data showed that with the increase of control angle (from 0° to 90°), the thumb's comfortable control far-end limit and the near-end limit presented a monotonic increasing tendency. The thumb's comfortable control far-end limit equaled to the thumb length when control angle was about 60°. Combined with the Chinese people hand size database, typical percentiles of thumb sizes were calculated. The results can provide references for handheld controller interface design, especially those for single-handed operations.

Keywords: Thumb control area · Handheld controller · Interface design · Experimental measurement

1 Introduction

Handheld controllers, such as TV and air conditioner remote controls and mobile phones, have become a part of people's life. When using a handheld controller, most users prefer to use one hand to hold the device and control it with the thumb of the same hand. Some handheld controllers are designed poorly, which make it difficult to

This research was supported by the National Key Technology R&D Program under project: control devices ergonomics design technology and standards research (project number 2014BAK01B02). This research was also supported by Presidential Foundation of China National Institute of Standardization (project number 522013Y-3081).

© Springer International Publishing Switzerland 2015
V.G. Duffy (Ed.): DHM 2015, Part II, LNCS 9185, pp. 44–52, 2015.
DOI: 10.1007/978-3-319-21070-4_5

reach the control key with the thumb while holding it with the same hand. In such a case, the user has to adjust the holding position or use the other hand to assist operation, which makes it inconvenient to use. In order to improve operation performance, the important and frequently used buttons should be located in the area where the thumb can reach easily and control comfortably. This is also helpful for carrying out control activities smoothly with only one hand.

Previous researches showed that the controller interface size, button layout, button size, control form (physical button or touch screen), handiness and hand size have a significant impact on operation performance and user experience. For small handheld devices, such as mobile phone, most users prefer touch screen and attempt to manipulate it with the thumb of the same hand (Pekka P., et al. 2006, Min K.C., et al. 2010). Research on single-handed thumb interaction with a mobile phone showed that the location of the icons on the touch screen had significant effect on operation performance (Yong S.P., et al. 2010). For the user, interface of a mobile phone with single-handed usage, the most comfortable icons were located on the middle, followed by the upper side and the lower side; the bottom most part contributed to the worst performance. Slightly larger interface had more disadvantages for single-handed manipulation because of more zones that the thumb found difficult to touch (Yunfei X., et al. 2006, Amy K.K., et al. 2006). Whether operating hand was the preferred hand or not also had significant effect on single-handed thumb manipulation (Keith B.P., et al. 2008). When the phone was a medium size, users with three types of hand sizes (small, medium and large) have no significant difference in operation speed and accuracy. But medium hand size users got the best experience from the flexibility of finger activities, the total satisfaction of operation and the compatibility between phone size and hand size (Hongting L., et al. 2014). It could be concluded from these studies that the location of touch point on the interface had an effect on the thumb operation performance and user experience. Thumb touching position on the interface is an important issue influencing operation. The manipulation would be more comfortable and more convenient if the touching points were located within the thumb's comfortable control area.

However, there is no data to represent where the thumb's comfortable control area is based on the hand size of Chinese people. This made the designers wonder where exactly would be the comfortable location for arranging the buttons/icons, and how large should the interface size be. Based on the concerns above, the experimental measurements, addressing on the Chinese adult thumb's comfortable control area were designed and carried out. By collecting and analyzing the data, the thumb's comfortable control area for Chinese users on single-handed devices was represented. The results can provide helpful references for handheld controller interface design.

2 Method

2.1 Participants

28 participants were recruited for this experiment through online, email, and poster advertisements. Participants were eligible if they were right handed, without a history

of any disease of the right hand and were between 25 and 45 years old. All participants were Chinese residents and lived in Beijing, China. They were 14 females and 14 males, half of them were between 25–35 years old, and half of them were between 36 and 45 years old. Their basic features are shown in Table 1. There was a significant difference in the right thumb length between females and males ($p < 0.01$). Participants were paid for their participation.

Table 1. Participants' basic features

Gender	Participants	Age	Height (cm)	Weight (kg)	Right thumb Length (mm)
Female	14	32.6 ± 5.8	162.4 ± 3.3	57.4 ± 4.8	55.5 ± 3.6
Male	14	32.2 ± 5.4	171.9 ± 4.8	70.3 ± 5.6	59.7 ± 3.9
Total	28	32.4 ± 5.6	167.2 ± 6.3	63.8 ± 8.3	57.6 ± 4.3

2.2 Design

A hand scanner was used to obtain hand dimensions. The participants were required to put their palm down on the scanner screen with fingers spread and straight. The data of hand and thumb would be obtained directly from the scan picture. Thumb length refers to the distance of the transverse line between the thumb base and the tip, as shown in Fig. 1.

A thumb movement range measuring plate was designed for recording the area of thumb tip touching, as shown in Fig. 2. From the base point, the vertical upward was

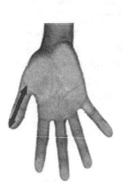

Fig. 1. Hand scanner for thumb

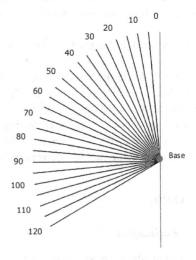

Fig. 2. Thumb movement range measuring plate

set as 0°. With the counter clockwise direction, lines were drawn evenly with 5° intervals until 120°. A nail pole was placed perpendicular to the surface of plate at the base position. Although the plate showed lines in 120° range, the actual measurement was only between 0° and 90°, because this was the thumb joint range of motion.

The measuring scene is shown in Fig. 3. The goal was to obtain the comfortable reaching area for the thumb. This was surrounded by the minimum comfortable angle, the maximum comfortable angle, the near-end comfortable line and the far-end comfortable line. When measuring, participants remained sitting, arms naturally placed on the desktop, wrist kept in neutral position, right hand held the measuring plate, part of the hand between the thumb and the index finger was close tightly to the nail pole, and the left hand assisted the fixed measuring plate. Except the thumb, all other parts of the hand, as well as the arm were still. That is, during the experiment, only the right thumb could move. If any movement occurred in the measuring process, the measurement would be taken again. A lead was pasted just below the tip of the right thumb to record the reaching area of thumb.

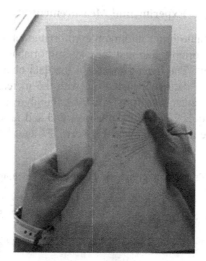

Fig. 3. Thumb control area measurement

Participants were asked to make reaching actions with their right thumbs on the measuring plate surface. The actions included reaching:

- The reachable limit line, which was composed by the maximum distance that participants could reach with effort;
- The minimum comfortable angle line, which was composed by the minimum angle that participants could reach naturally and comfortably by thumb adduction;
- The maximum comfortable angle line, which was composed by the maximum angle that participants could reach naturally and comfortably by thumb abduction;
- The near-end comfortable line, which was composed by the minimum distance that participants could reach naturally and comfortably by thumb flexion;
- The far-end comfortable line, which was composed by the maximum distance that participants could reach naturally and comfortably by thumb extension.

2.3   Procedure

Prior to measuring, the experimenter guided the participant through the following: informed consent, filling personal information, scanning right hand on hand scanner, calibrating the measuring plate holding posture for the individual participant, giving participants an overview of the experiment, teaching the participant how to perform the task, and acclimatizing the participant to keeping the arm and hand still except the right thumb. First, the right thumb reachable limit line was measured. Then the comfortable reach area was measured. Participants were told to do this task in a natural and comfortable way with their right thumb. After these setup activities, participants practiced a bit and then marked their experimental data on the measuring plate. A brand new measuring plate was provided for each participant.

3   Results

3.1   Data Obtained from Experimental Measurement

Data for the thumb reachable limit, minimum comfortable angle, maximum comfortable angle, near-end comfortable line and far-end comfortable line were collected by experimental measurement. The overall means of the data obtained at various angles are shown in Table 2. The data kept increasing with the increasing angles. It can be seen that with the increase in angles (from 0° to 90°), thumb reachable limit presented a monotonic increasing tendency, as well as the near-end and far-end comfortable reach distance. The comfortable angle range was between 35° and 75°.

Table 2. Thumb's reachable limit and comfortable reaching area (mean)

Angle(°)	0	5	10	15	20	25	30	35	40	45	50	55	60	65	70	75	80	85	90
Reachable limit	50	50	50	50	51	51	52	52	53	54	55	56	57	58	59	60	61	61	62
Near-end distance	37	37	37	37	37	37	38	38	39	40	41	41	42	43	44	45	46	47	48
Far-end distance	49	49	49	50	50	51	52	52	53	54	56	57	58	59	61	61	62	63	64
Comfortable angle								√	√	√	√	√	√	√	√	√			

3.2   The Ratio Between the Thumb's Comfortable Limit and the Thumb Length

The proximal ratio and distal ratio were used to represent the relationship between the thumb's comfortable limit and the thumb length, i.e., proximal ratio equaled to the thumb's comfortable near-end limit divided by the thumb length and distal ratio equaled to thumb's comfortable far-end limit divided by the thumb length. The proximal ratio and distal ratio could be calculated since the thumb's comfortable near-end value and far-end value had been obtained by experimental measurement, as well as the thumb's length. The results are shown in Table 3 and Fig. 4.

Table 3. Proximal ratio and distal ratio of the thumb's comfortable reaching

Angle (°)	0	5	10	15	20	25	30	35	40	45	50	55	60	65	70	75	80	85	90
Proximal ratio (female)	.64	.64	.64	.64	.64	.65	.65	.66	.67	.68	.70	.71	.73	.74	.75	.78	.64	.64	.64
Distal ratio (female)	.87	.87	.87	.88	.89	.89	.90	.91	.93	.94	.96	.97	.99	1.00	1.01	1.03	.87	.87	.87
Proximal ratio (male)	.64	.64	.64	.64	.65	.65	.66	.67	.68	.70	.71	.73	.75	.77	.78	.79	.64	.64	.64
Distal ratio (male)	.89	.89	.89	.90	.90	.91	.92	.94	.95	.97	.99	1.01	1.03	1.05	1.08	1.09	.89	.89	.89

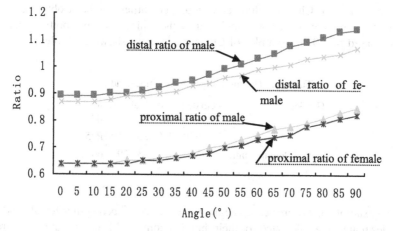

Fig. 4. Proximal ratio and distal ratio of the thumb's comfortable reaching

There was no significant difference in the proximal ratio between females and males ($p > 0.5$). There was also no significant difference in the distal ratio between females and males ($p > 0.1$). It can be seen that with the increase of control angle (from 0° to 90°), the proximal ratio and the distal ratio presented a monotonic increasing tendency. When control angle was about 60° (for female, it was 65°; for male, it was 55°), the distal ratio was approximately 1. When the control angle was less than 60°, the distal ratio was less than 1. When the control angle was larger than 60°, the distal ratio was larger than 1. It showed that when control angle was about 60°, the thumb's comfortable far-end distance equaled to the thumb length. When the control angle was less than 60°, the far-end distance was less than the thumb length. It was contrary to the situation when the control angle was more than 60°. This was perhaps mainly caused due to the following reasons:

- The hand anatomical structure. When the control angle was larger than 60°, besides the thumb, part of the metacarpal that connected the thumb to the hand was also involved during the action. Therefore, the thumb's comfortable reaching distance was increased due to the contribution of the metacarpal.
- The contact area of thumb pulp. When the control angle was small, flexion was needed to make the thumb pulp have larger contact with the plate surface. Otherwise, the contact was handled mostly by the thumb side, which was less

comfortable than when handled by thumb pulp. As the control angle kept increasing, the thumb pulp was more and more parallel with the plate surface, which made the thumb reach farther.

- Personal habits. It was maybe the personal habit of the participants to reach with thumb flexion when control angle was small and with thumb extension when control angle was large.

3.3 Calculate Chinese Adult Thumb's Comfortable Control Area

The thumb length of Chinese adults at various percentiles has been obtained by our previous measurement, which was included in the Chinese people body dimensions database, based on 20,000 samples of Chinese adults, as shown in Table 4.

Table 4. The thumb length of Chinese adults

Gender	Female (18 to 65 years old)			Male (18 to 65 years old)		
	P5	P50	P95	P5	P50	P95
Thumb length (mm)	48	54	61	53	59	66

As an example of extreme case, the thumb length of 5th percentiles female and 95th percentiles male were calculated for their thumb's comfortable control area. According to the proximal and distal ratio in Table 3 and Fig. 4, the near-end and far-end comfortable line could be calculated. This is shown in Table 5.

Table 5. Thumb's comfortable reaching area of 5th percentiles female and 95th percentiles male

Angle(°)		0	5	10	15	20	25	30	35	40	45	50	55	60	65	70	75	80	85	90
P5 Female	Near-end	31	31	31	31	31	31	31	32	32	33	34	34	35	36	36	37	38	39	39
	Far-end	42	42	42	42	43	43	43	44	45	45	46	47	48	48	48	49	50	50	51
P95 Male	Near-end	42	42	42	42	43	43	44	44	45	46	47	48	50	51	51	52	53	55	56
	Far-end	59	59	59	59	59	60	61	62	63	64	65	67	68	69	71	72	73	75	75

It can be seen that the thumb's comfortable control area was different for different populations. The thumb's comfortable far-end line of 5th percentiles female mostly coincided with the thumb's comfortable near-end line of 95th percentiles male. This meant that the comfortable control area of 5th percentiles female and 95th percentiles male was totally different. If a button/icon was located in the area that the 95th percentiles male find comfortable and convenient to manipulate, the 5th percentiles female would find it uncomfortable and difficult to reach. Of course, the comparison between 5th percentiles female and 95th percentiles male was an extreme situation. A common (overlapping) comfortable control area would definitely occur if the controller design was based on 50th percentiles females and males.

The thumb's comfortable control area of 95th percentiles male is shown in Fig. 5. For the handheld controller, if the buttons were located in the comfortable control area, 95th percentiles male could manipulate comfortably and conveniently with single-hand. An application of the thumb's comfortable control area study was the remote controller design, as shown in Fig. 6.

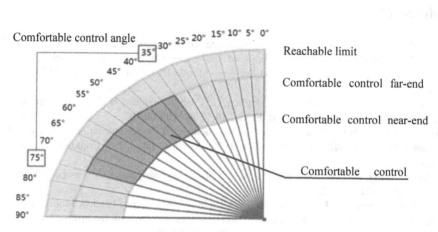

Fig. 5. Thumb's comfortable control area of 95th percentile male

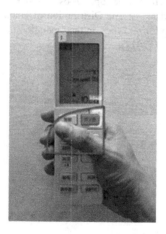

Fig. 6. Remote controller: an application of the thumb's comfortable control area

The data in this study was suitable for a Chinese adult. Diverse races and ethnic groups usually have different anthropometric features. So the proportion of each body part may vary, including the ratio of limbs and hands. Therefore, the thumb's comfortable control area for other races and ethnic groups should be measured all over again.

For a handheld controller, the operating performance and satisfaction is affected significantly by the location of the buttons/icons, especially for the single-hand manipulation. Putting the frequently used components within the thumb's comfortable control area would result in better performance, more convenience and better experience for the user. The results could provide helpful reference for handheld controller interface design, especially those for single-handed operations.

References

Pekka, P., Amy, K.K., Benjamin, B.B.: Target size study for one-handed thumb use on small touch screen devices. In: Proceedings of the ACM Conference on Human-Computer Interaction with Mobile Devices and Services, Mobile HCI 2006, pp. 12–15. ACM Press, New York (2006)

Min, K.C., Dongjin, K., Seokhee, N., Donghun, L.: Usability evaluation of numeric entry tasks on keypad type and age. Int. J. Ind. Ergon. **40**(1), 97–105 (2010)

Yong, S.P., Sung, H.H.: Touch key design for one-handed thumb interaction with a mobile phone: effects of touch key size and touch key location. Int. J. Ind. Ergon. **40**(1), 68–76 (2010)

Yunfei, X., Gang, L.: Ergonomic research on cell-phone keyboard placement design. J. Packag. Eng. **27**(2), 171–174 (2006)

Amy, K.K., Benjamin, B.B., Jose, L.C-V.: Understanding Single-handed Mobile Device Interaction. Handbook of Research on User Interface Design and Evaluation for Mobile Technology. Technical report 2006-02, pp. 86–101 (2006)

Keith, B.P., Juan, P.H.: Evaluating one handed thumb tapping on mobile touchscreen devices. In: Proceedings of Graphics Interface 2008, pp. 57–64. ACM Press, Toronto (2008)

Hongting, L., Yuanna, G., Weidan, X.: The Distribution of Hand Sizes of University Students and the Effects of Users' Hand Size Types on the Operation on Touch Screen Mobile Phone. Science paper Online, pp. 1–9 (2014)

Study on the Body Shape of Middle-Aged and Old Women for Garment Design

Xiaoping Hu[✉] and Yan Zhao

School of Design, Guangzhou Higher Education Mega Centre,
South China University of Technology, Panyu District,
Guangzhou 510006, People's Republic of China
huxp@scut.edu.cn

Abstract. The purpose of this paper is to study and determine the body shape parameters of middle-aged and old women for garment design to satisfy their needs of garment fitness. The body shape of middle-aged and old women who have been more than 50 years of age in North China, were measured by garment specialty students. The measure covered height, shoulder width, bust, waist and hip circumference. The body shape data was collected from 108 different middle-aged and old women fem. And SPSS was used for statistical analysis to reveal the change of body shape about middle-age and old women then find out the issue of size designation and the body shape of middle-age and old women. Under this premise, the difference between chest circumference and abdominal circumference as the research focus. Not only can the study provide data for the costume design of middle-aged and old women, but also provide reference data for tessellate garment size.

Keywords: Middle-aged and old · Female · Physical characteristic · Garment size

1 Introduction

The plastic of cartilage decrease, muscle atrophy, the ability of balance and posture control reduce for middle-aged and old women as the regression of human body function which led to the evident change of body shape. There are garment size standards for men, women and children, but there is no specific standard for middle-aged women, which leds to the clothing in the current market can't fit the elderly people's body characteristic properly. So it's necessary to study the body shape of middle-aged and old women for garment design. Due to the acquired factors, such as physical growth, living habits and routine work, every part of the body about the most middle-aged and old men and women have changed, which would form special body figure like potbelly, hunchback and so on. This kind of the change is particularly apparent in the body of the middle-aged and old women and it has a certain universality. Because the great changes in the outer body, more and more middle-aged and old women put forward higher requirements for the appropriateness of their clothes. And costume need adapted to the human body, and researching for different periods, different regions and different age of human body is the basic subjects of clothing

© Springer International Publishing Switzerland 2015
V.G. Duffy (Ed.): DHM 2015, Part II, LNCS 9185, pp. 53–61, 2015.
DOI: 10.1007/978-3-319-21070-4_6

structure design. Based on this issue, the research of the body of the middle-aged and old women and garment size is imperative.

2 The Issue of Garment Size in China

2.1 The Measuring Data Is Quite Old

In the late 1980s, the China has carried out anthropometric on a large scale and get the basic data of the sizes of humanity. Based on the data, the standard GB/T1335—1991 of garment size was set out. Later on, there were appeared the edition about 1997 and the edition about 2008, which is used by now. However, the two editions were just slightly adjusted based on the edition about 1991, and they were not make changes about the basic data of the sizes of humanity. With the improvement of living conditions, the condition of body type about Chinese people has changed compared with 20 years ago. So the data of current standard of garment size is too old, which is lack of reference value to guide the apparel companies produced clothing for that consumer demands.

2.2 The Classification of Garment Size Is Too Simple

The classification of the standard of garment size is detailed in many developed countries. For example, in Japan, the standard of garment size divide the body type of adult into 7 kinds which included Y, YA, A, AB, B, BE, E. They are represents the degree of fatness of people. Also the standard of garment size in Japan divides different age stages, for example, they divided the body type of female into 3 kinds which included the young girl type, the young woman type and the woman type. The classification is very detail. However, in China, the current of the standard of garment size about female only have 4 kinds of body type. And the standard of garment size is not divide age grades, which is not considered the body type characteristic of people's age grades. What's more, the standard of garment size is also not divide area. So it leads many consumers, especially the middle-aged and old women can't find suitable clothing in the market.

3 The Methods of the Classification About Body Type in the Domestic and Overseas

The partition of people's body type is the key to set out the standard of garment size. Many countries have different methods and index to divide the body type of the standard of garment size in the world. Overall, there are several kinds. Firstly, the partition based on the discrepancy of girth, mainly based on the discrepancy of chest circumference and waistline, the discrepancy of chest circumference and hipline and the discrepancy of waistline and hipline as the partitioning index. Secondly, the partition based on height, weight, age and chest circumference. Thirdly, the partition based on the index of the body, such as the index of stoop, the ratio of body and chest circumference and the ratio of chest circumference and waistline. Fourthly, the partition based on the index of the type of chest, waist and hip. The last, the partition based on clustering method, which is divided by selecting the classification of body type.

In China, the classification of body type is based on the partition of discrepancy of girth, mainly based on the discrepancy of chest circumference and waistline. However, with the change of the body characteristics of the middle-aged and old women, the discrepancy of chest circumference and waistline which as the basis to divide body type can't represent all kinds of body type characteristics. So, in this paper, we measured date of the body of middle-aged and old women who is more than 50 years old and come from the same area.

4 The Data of Anthropometry

4.1 The Analysis of Data Percentage

Statistics and classified the date of somatometry, we know that the distribution percentage of chest circumference, waistline and hipline. From the Figs. 1, 2 and 3, we can know that the chest circumference of middle-aged and old women mainly distribute in the range of 98–101 cm. And the waistline of middle-aged and old women mainly distribute in the range of 75–98 cm, and the percentage is 73 %. The hipline of middle-aged and old women mainly distribute in the range of 90–113 cm, and the percentage is 80.3 %. Compared with the waistline and hipline of the national adult, those middle-aged and old women's waistline and hipline is clearly larger. That is prove that most middle-aged and old women due to put on fat, their fat accumulated at waist and abdomen, which is led the waistline and hipline clearly larger. The figures as follow and the abscissa axis stands for percentage, the depth axis stands for girth.

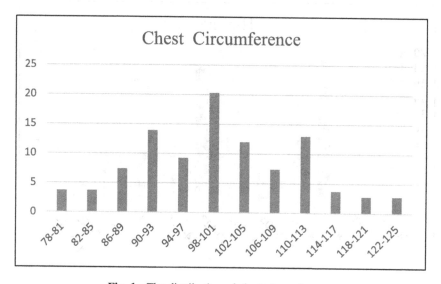

Fig. 1. The distribution of chest circumference

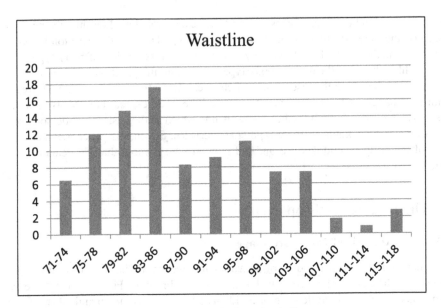

Fig. 2. The distribution of waistline

4.2   Experimental Subject

All data collection used the random sampling method. The target group is more than 50 years old middle-aged and old women who come from North China. The middle-aged and old women are covered manual workers, mental workers and people who in the leisure.

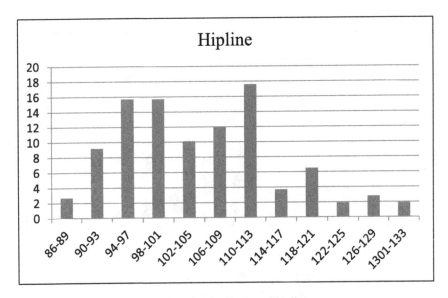

Fig. 3. The distribution of hipline

4.3   Measurement Methods and Measurement Tools

The measurement method is completed by traditional contact measurement. In order to ensure the measuring technique unified specification and the data be accurate, the whole process to assign a person to operate. All the measured women wearing thin lingerie. And they keep natural upright, visual ahead and arms natural prolapse. Finally, the people who make measurement using a tape measure to manual measurement.

4.4   The Measurement Parts and Methods

In order to combine purposes of research and requirements, in this paper, we based on the clothing making for the changes of people's body type and the system of apparel mass customization for the database require of people's body type choosing 10 kinds of representative measuring project which include height, chest circumference, waist circumference, hip circumference, neck circumference, abdomen circumference, arm circumference, the long of neck to waist, arm length and shoulder breadth. Those measuring project can not only covers the main control parts of the entire body, but also can satisfy all kinds of related analysis of the body type.

5   Body Type Characteristic Analysis

5.1   The Body Type of Current Situation of Middle-Aged and Old Women

Knowing by watch and observe survey, compared with body type between middle-aged and old women and the youth, we will find that with the increase of age, the changes of women's back type become obvious. Their posture gesture becomes anteflexion which from the muscle of hindneck to the middle back form the hunchback gradually and from side neck point the length of front decreased and the length of behind increased. At the same time, the situation of trunk obesity is more common. And the most obviously characteristic is the increase of chest circumference, waistline and hip circumference, also the abdomen bulged, the chest drooped and the nipple points down. What's more, the spine curvature increased with the growth of the age, from the normal body turn to curved back body, and finally turn to crookback.

5.2   The Analysis of Data Dispersion

The standard deviation reflects the trend of dispersion. The larger standard deviation, the larger degree of dispersion. On the contrary, the standard deviation is small, the degree of dispersion is concentrated. From the Table 1, the biggest standard deviation have 4 items as follows: the chest circumference is 10.37459 cm, the waistline is 11.12287 cm, the hipline is 10.67983 cm and the abdomen circumference is 10.38509 cm. Those are further evidence that the phenomenon of observation of the middle-aged and old women, who have the big changes in chest circumference, waistline, hipline and abdomen circumference.

Table 1. Basis statistics of measuring project

Project (centimeter)	Mean	Standard deviation
Height	160.0833	4.606233
Chest circumference	100.233	10.37459
Waistline	89.21019	11.12287
Hipline	105.4833	10.67983
Neck circumference	39.678	2.083051
Abdomen circumference	102.581	10.38509
Arm circumference	32.175	3.724027
Neck to waist	43.248	2.372914
Arm length	54.59043	2.017009
Shoulder breadth	41.5667	3.169802

5.3 The Analysis of K-Mean Cluster

In order to make the classification of body type can clearly reflect the study about the overall characteristics of body type, there need to combine several investigate of index. In this paper, we used the K-means Cluster which is belong the part of SPSS to realize. From the analysis of the above data dispersion, the mainly changes of the body type of middle-aged and old women are chest circumference, waistline and hipline and then the height. So choosing the five projects as the analysis of K-Mean Cluster index, and make sure the object can divided into 5 kinds after by testing of sample system cluster. The results of clustering statistics are shown in Table 2.

Compared with the sample which is clustered and the standard data of the same age women in China, in order to make the comparison result more clearly in Table 2, using the numerical value of reference standard to deal with the original data of sample in standardized and then making the fold point figure to compare. The results are shown in Fig. 4.

According to the compared with the reference standard, the all kinds of samples can based on their each characteristic divided into as follow:

Table 2. The number of samples of all kinds of body type and the mean of fraction index after K-mean Cluster (unit: centimeter).

	Cluster				
	1	2	3	4	5
Height	159.8000	160.8333	158.6250	163.5000	162.3333
Chest circumference	99.2	108.0	88.4	120.6	111.6
Waistline	86.6200	96.9967	77.4125	110.9875	109.3333
Hipline	103.8314	113.1967	94.3594	129.9625	101.0000
Number of samples	35	30	32	8	3

(1) The body type of normal, which is the third kind in the Fig. 4. This kind of middle-aged and women who's height and the girth of other part in the body accessed the standard values.

(2) The body type of slight chubby, which is the first kind in the Fig. 4. This kind of middle-aged and women who's girth values are more high than standard values.

(3) The body type of middle fat, which is the second kind in the Fig. 4. This kind of middle-aged and women who's girth values are more high than standard values and the girth values of the body type of slight chubby.

(4) The body type of obesity, which is the fourth kind in the Fig. 4. This kind of middle-aged and women who's girth values are more high than other values all above body type.

(5) The special body type, which is the fifth kind in the Fig. 4. This kind of middle-aged and women who's chest circumference and waistline are more high than others values, but the hipline is lower than others.

So, from the all kinds conditions and graphic above, we can know that compared with the reference research object, the figure reflects the body type characteristics of the research object.

5.4   The Determine of Body Type

In the standard of garment size in china, the body type is divided by the body's difference value of chest circumference and waistline. The standard of garment size about women in the People's Republic of China, which is the latest standard of

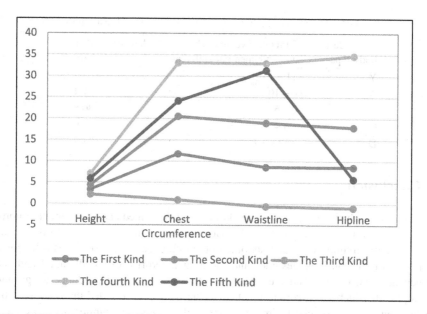

Fig. 4. The comparison of all kinds samples and the major indexes of reference standard

women's garment size stipulated that the body type is divided into Y, A, B, C. And the Y stands for slim, the A stands for standard, the B stands for a little fat and the C stands for obesity. The specific classified as follow (Table 3):

Table 3. The range of body type classification code

Body type classification code	Y	A	B	C
Difference value of chest circumference and waistline	19–24	14–18	9–13	4–8

From the all above table and figure of research data, we know that most the middle-aged and old women in the north of China are the a little fat or obesity, and their body type like a pear. In the process of statistical, some people's difference value of chest circumference and waistline is minus. So according to the difference value of chest circumference and waistline to determine the body type of middle-aged and old women is not reasonable. With the changes of body characteristic of middle-aged and old women, their abdomen is more and more bulge, so we need to adjust based on the body characteristic of middle-aged and old women and it is necessary to increase the key part size which has large difference, such as abdomen circumference. In this paper, we based on the difference value of chest circumference and abdomen circumference to divide the body type of middle-aged and old women in north China. According to the statistics, the mainly change range of difference value of chest circumference and abdomen circumference is (−12, 15), the rangeability of range difference is 27. So we classified the body type into 5 kinds, and make the range difference of each kind is 5. Then, also make Y respective thin body, A respective a little thin body, B respective normal body, C respective a little fat body and D respective obesity (Table 4).

Table 4. The ratio of body type divide suggestion and distribution

The code of body type	Difference value of chest circumference and abdomen circumference	Ratio (%)
Y	11 ~ 15	2.7
A	6 ~ 10	7.4
B	0 ~ 5	30.5
C	−6 ~ −1	37.9
D	−12 ~ −7	21.2

6 Conclusion

Based on the analysis of the body type about the middle-aged and old women in north China, we set out the new standard of divided garment size which is used difference value of chest circumference and abdomen circumference. This research is offer some reference for the clothing designer and clothing enterprise of middle-aged and old women in north China. And the research is benefit for related products design and development, which has a certain practical value. However, divided the body type by the difference value of chest circumference and abdomen circumference may have some deficiency, some special data also need pay attention and some related research need to further deepen and expand.

Acknowledgment. The project supported by The Central Colleges and Universities Basic Scientific Research Foundation NO: x2sj/D214277w and Teaching Research and reform of Higher Education in Guangdong Province NO: x2sj/Y1143330.

References

1. Qian, L.L., Wang, H.F., Hu, C.J.: The research of the classification about 50–75 years old of middle-aged and old women in Jiangsu and Zhejiang area based on the three dimensional measurement. J. Shandong Text. Technol. **2**, 40–44 (2014)
2. Liu, Y.M., Dai, H.: The research of body type of middle-aged and old women in Chengdu area. J. Text. Res. J. **31**, 110–115 (2010)
3. Zhang, W.B., Chen, H.Y.: The Statistical Analysis of Practical Data and the Application of SPSS12.0. Beijing University of Posts and Telecommunications Press, Beijing (2006)
4. Liu, R.P., Liu, W.H.: The Principle and Technique of Clothing Structure Design. The Textile Industry Press, Beijing (1993)
5. Li, Y., Wang, H.J.: The research of garment size about middle-aged and old women's body type characteristic in North of Shanxi. J. Zhongyuan Inst. Technol. **19**, 43–48 (2008)
6. Zhang, J.X.: Human Ergonomics of Costume Design. China Light Industry Press, Beijng (2010)
7. Bai, L.H., Zhang, W.B.: The research of choosing the basis part that using mathematical theory in the standard of garment size. J. Tianjin Univ. Technol. **2**, 33–35 (2006)

Estimating Ergonomic Comfort During the Process of Mechanism Design by Interaction with a Haptic Feedback-System

Evaluation of Simulated and Kinesthetically Displayed Mechanisms Using the Haptic Feedback System RePlaLink

Thomas Kölling[(✉)], Michael Krees, Mathias Hüsing, and Burkhard Corves

Department of Mechanism Theory and Dynamics of Machines (IGM),
RWTH Aachen University, Aachen, Germany
{koelling,krees,huesing,corves}@igm.rwth-aachen.de

Abstract. The use of a Haptic Feedback-System (HFS) in the mechanism design process is very promising. The RePlaLink HFS developed at the IGM - RWTH Aachen University is presented exemplarily. It is a hybrid solution combining a parallel kinematic structure with a small serial actuator in the tool-center. Therefore it is quiet powerful and still agile. Several scenarios of implementation of hand-activated motion are shown. Moreover the way of estimating the operator's ergonomic comfort and particularly, the advantage of human posture scoring techniques are discussed in detail. Finally, it is illustrated how this HFS can be used as a process driven tool for the superior design process. The simulation capabilities and the haptic real-time display in combination with special knowledge databases concerning the mechanism design and testing are a powerful enhancement for novel as well as senior design engineers. The common work flow can basically be changed, newly arranged and improved.

Keywords: Mechanism design · Ergonomics/human factor · Haptic feedback · Virtual prototyping · Simultaneous engineering

1 Introduction and Motivation

1.1 Design Process of Manually Operated Mechanisms and Usage of Haptic Feedback

When people interact with a technical product via a mechanical interface most often it is done by manually operated mechanisms. They are used to guide certain points along a given path as well as for power or signal transmission. The user impression of a product is defined primarily through the interface and the experience of the usage.

© Springer International Publishing Switzerland 2015
V.G. Duffy (Ed.): DHM 2015, Part II, LNCS 9185, pp. 62–73, 2015.
DOI: 10.1007/978-3-319-21070-4_7

Besides the technical characteristics of a product, which are sometimes difficult to interpret according to the effect on ergonomics, the personal impression of the interaction is another possibility to compare or evaluate certain products or versions of a product. Crucial for market success of such a product is therefore the perceived ergonomic comfort. The haptic impression is important to differentiate oneself from competitors, especially regarding motion devices. Since this may ultimately affect the purchase decision, huge efforts are made to create a positive haptic perception and to fulfill all ergonomic requirements. For this purpose hand-operated mechanisms often have comfort functions additionally to the basic functionality.

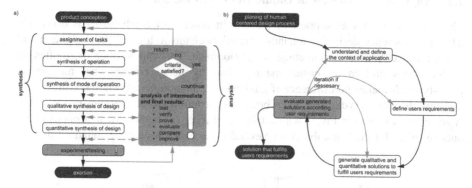

Fig. 1. Process of mechanism design in (a) conventional [1] and (b) human centered procedure [2]

In order to meet the requirements for a human-machine interface and to achieve the goals of human factor design, DIN EN ISO 9241 puts the user in the center of the design activities. Hence the comprehensive understanding of the user and the application scenarios, as well as the inclusion of users throughout the development process is fundamental. The conventional design process according to VDI 2221 [3] can be adapted to the specific requirements of the mechanism design according to [4]. What both procedures have in common is a highly iterative passing through the individual phases, in which the process can be structured. A recurring task is to evaluate the achieved results, not least at the end of a phase and to plan the following work stages accordingly. This can be perfectly enhanced by the user centered approach and the estimation assistance according to DIN EN ISO 9241, compare Fig. 1.

Evaluation of the qualitative synthesis of design in early stages and out of the users perspective is instantly supported or in some cases even enabled by haptic and visual display of virtual prototypes. Moreover it is possible to gain a deeper understanding of the context of usage when using a so called Haptic Feedback-System (HFS). Thereby the requirements can be better understood and specified more exactly.

Since it is generally not easy to evaluate ergonomic aspects, knowledge from multiple fields should be used. Also, in this case, it is hard for users to come to a clear-cut evaluation [5]. To obtain qualitatively high-grade results in a user acceptance study a trial strategy that includes several aspects is needed, see Sects. 3 and 4.

Conventionally, mechanical prototypes are used for the haptic representation of hand-driven mechanisms. The demands of a user-centered design process can only be implemented in a worthwhile manner, when financial- and time-requirements of a mechanical prototype can be lowered significantly. Haptic Feedback-Systems can achieve this by simulating a digital prototype of a mechanism and letting the user experience it immediately. Ideally, a system compromises a haptic display of sufficient scale and performance as well as providing tools for the usage of the designer.

1.2   Application Scenarios of Haptic Devices in Design Process

The usage of a HFS as support of the design process of mechanisms is especially advantageous when designing a hand-operated mechanism. It gives the designer a tool to get feedback on the current stage of development. This can be done more often, in earlier stages and in an easier manner than by using conventional mechanical proto-types. It makes no difference if guidance or function-generating mechanisms are in focus. In the everyday life, everybody uses a multitude of mechanisms by hand. A selection is shown in Fig. 2 with a tailgate of a car (a), a window that opens to the outside (b) and a kitchen cabinet (c) Several other examples can be found easily.

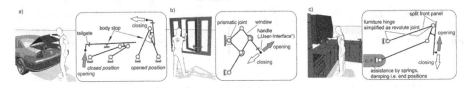

Fig. 2. Selection of different manually operated mechanisms

All of these examples have in common, that a macroscopic space is needed to operate them. It is striking, that most of the manually actuated mechanisms are planar or can be reduced to a planar mechanism. Hence, a HFS should be designed to cover these application scenarios, see Sect. 2.2. Such a system is capable to reproduce very different hand-operated mechanisms, depending on the simulation model. This can mean the simulation of a finalized product, as well as the simplified functional models in the early development phases. In this way, different paths of movement can be tested by varying the kinematic parameters. Or force potentials in the human workspace can be studied independently of the structure that is being developed.

Furthermore, a great advantage of the HFS is the immediate comparison of different variants of a development with little effort. These variants can arise from different mechanism structures, as shown in Fig. 3(a)–(e) or by a changing in the model parameters of the same structure, which leads mostly to slightly different behavior.

As already described, hand-operated mechanisms often include comfort functions. These can range from passive force assistance by springs to active electrical assistance, from dampers for the end positions to supporting openers. Depending on the requirements and to obtain a lifelike user experience, a HFS must provide a simulation of friction, inertia, elasticity and end stops. The main goal is to achieve an appropriate

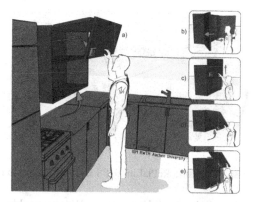

Fig. 3. Comparisson of different structural versions of kitchen cabinets

output, so that, for example, the forces required for manually operating the device are comfortable.

2   RePlaLink – Haptic Feedback-System

2.1   State of the Art of Haptic Feedback Devices

Considering the market review of haptic feedback devices one can determine different device-classes like desktop-devices, teleoperations or hand mounted. They comprise devices of similar workspace and feedback force. Additionally one may take into account further specifications like rigidity, resolution, accuracy or number of degrees of freedom. Devices covering the range of motion and the force potential needed do display a simulation of the above described manually operated mechanisms are hard to find. Hence a customized design of a haptic feedback device is needed [1].

2.2   Characteristics of the RePlaLink-HFS

The Haptic Feedback-System called RePlaLink (Reconfigurable Planar Linkage) is constructed at the IGM and meets the requirements for a haptic simulation system for hand-operated mechanisms, especially the requirements respective to rigidity, workspace and feedback force. Generally, a universally usable HFS should just be able to surpass the sensory capabilities of a human (when simulating an everyday mechanism) as well as to generate the occurring forces and velocities of the simulated application. Haptic perception can be classified in two categories; the sense of touch, tactile sensors in human skin and the sense of position, the kinesthetic sensors in muscles and tendons. While the tactile sensors are very sensitive and can resolve frequencies up to 1000 Hz and have a spatial resolution of up to 0.5 mm, the sense of position is only able to resolve frequencies of 20–30 Hz and angles between 0.8° and 2.5° depending on the joint. A parameter for the evaluation of the perception of force is the just noticeable difference. Depending on the study and the posture it is between three and seven percent. A stiffness of at least

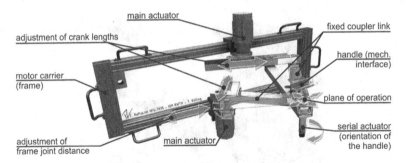

Fig. 4. Setup of the RePlaLink HFS and local adjustability

24.5 N/mm onward is classified as a solid by a human. We are capable of movements up to 20–30 Hz at velocities around 1 m/s and forces of 100 N [6–9].

Besides further requirements, the size of the workspace of the HFS plays a crucial role. The output mechanism of the RePlaLink is a partially parallel six-bar-linkage. It includes a fully parallel five-bar linkage with links of round about half a meter, actuated by two servo motors, as shown in Fig. 4. One frame joint and the cranks can be reconfigured. This ensures that the system can be adapted to the needs of the task at hand. For common applications, sufficient workspace is ensured, as well as enough engine power. The parallel planar structure provides a high rigidity, especially perpendicular to the working plane and small masses to accelerate. This leads to an improved dynamical behavior.

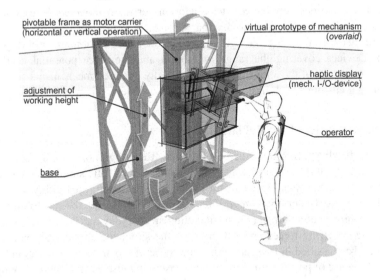

Fig. 5. RePlaLink HFS being used to explore a simulated cabinet (overlaid) and global adjustability.

Indeed, most applications only use a planar mechanism. But it can be positioned in very different heights relative to the user and vertical or horizontal orientation. That is why adaptability is also required here. Therefore the motor carrier frame of the RePlaLink is mounted on rails in such a way, that the height can be adjusted and it can be pivoted by 90°. Thus, an operation in a horizontal- and vertical-mode in every desired height is possible. See Fig. 5 for a depiction the RePlaLink with an overlaid simulation model.

2.3 Control and Data Processing

Four quadrants can be made out during the operation of a HFS as shown in Fig. 6. The operator interacts primarily kinesthetically with the haptic display, which functions as the input-output-unit of the HFS. The tactile sense is served by the usage of a realistic handle piece. Depending on the control strategy, either the force applied by the user or the position of the handle is measured and used as an input for a dynamical multi body simulation. The user interaction necessitates a real time calculation, since not all the states of the system can be calculated in advance. Subsequently, the reaction of the simulation model is transformed via inverse kinematics or dynamics respectively, in such a way that the signal provided matches the configuration of the output unit. Based on this signal the output unit is controlled. This completes the circle and the user obtains a haptic feedback.

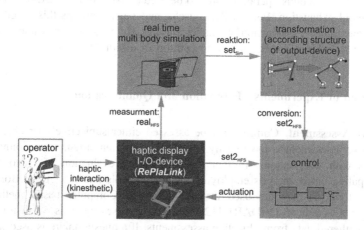

Fig. 6. Four basic quadrants of HFS operation (visualization and configuration excluded)

3 Design of Experiments Using a HFS to Estimate Ergonomic Comfort

3.1 Designer and Customer Tests

The classic design process of mechanisms focuses on stability and reliability of the function of the mechanism itself. The accommodation of human operators of mechanisms is usually accomplished by applying principles of ergonomics or human factor design. These principles widen the focus of design to include accessible and safe working spaces and the quantitative calculation and evaluation of static operation forces as well as the design of user interface hardware. The aim of this widened focus is to ensure the capability of the operator to reliable perform the tasks required and the safety of the operator as well as minimizing the risks of musculoskeletal disorders.

Dimensioning According to Human Factors. Parameters not generally considered by this approach to design are dynamic loads of interfaces of hand-operated mechanisms and the possibility of operational forces concerning their direction. Several standards, e.g. DIN 33411 [10], provide the designer with maximum operating forces or maximum operating torques, often in relation to relative height and reach of the point of application. These maximum forces are usually determined for different directions of the force and angles of the arm or arms. One drawback of those tables is their generation through the use of young test persons in good physical health, omitting the possibility of older operators, as well as the short term and static nature of the forces. In this way dynamic forces are not adequately considered. Also missing is a definition for calculating comfortable operating forces, in magnitude as well as in direction.

Quantifying Comfort and Discomfort. The German Bundesanstalt für Arbeitsschutz und Arbeitsmedizin (Federal Institute for Occupational Safety and Health) [11] states the maximum continuous operating force to be used as 10 % of the maximum possible force to avoid exhaustion. For smaller muscles and muscle groups this is reduced to 5 %–7 % due to faster exhaustion of smaller muscles. But these too are values provided for medical safety, not directly linked to comfort or discomfort.

3.2   Design of Experiments - Estimation and Quantification

Subjective Assessment. Comfort can be assessed either subjectively or objectively. A subjective assessment is most easily obtained through employing questionnaires or interviews with test persons. Further possibilities are evaluation of video footage or participative video analysis employing evaluation tools like the CR-10 Borg scale or similar tools as they are used in the Video and Computer based method for Ergonomic Assessment (VIDAR) [12]. Subjective assessment is vital for cross-checking gathered data from objective assessments. If a questionnaire is used it has to be specifically tailored to the task to be evaluated to complement objective assessment of the task.

Objective Assessment. A more objective way of assessment of comfort or discomfort is provided by methods to evaluate workload or posture. Table 1 list a representative selection of such methods covering several different types based on an evaluation and comparison of several methods by Takala [13]. These methods can be differentiated by several factors. Foremost is the purpose of the method. Most of the methods are used to assess possible health risks, especially musculo-skeletal disorders, of lifting tasks, postures or movements. Another possible aim of a method is the assessment of the comfort or more often the discomfort of these lifting tasks, postures or movements. Another way to differentiate between these

Table 1. Representative selection of methods of workload assessment and posture evaluation

Method	Aim	Dim.	Posture	Move.	Forces	Duration	Evaluation	Comments
HAL TLV	MSD	Move.	-	D, F	M	Workcycle	Discrete	Only distal upper limbs
HSE	MSD	Check	M D F	-	M D F	Workcycle	Discrete	Only upper limbs
LUBA	com	Angles	M	-	-	Posture	Discrete	Only upper body
MMGA	com	Angles	M D	M D	-	Single task	Continuous	Based on LUBA
NIOSH-LE	MSD	Weight	M	-	M D F	Single task	Continuous	Only lifting tasks
OWAS	MSD	Post.	M F	-	M F	Workcycle	Discrete	Widely used
QEC	MSD	Check	M D F	-	M D F	Workday	Discrete	Widely used
REBA	MSD	Angles	M	M	M	Posture	Discrete	Rapid to use
RULA	MSD	Angles	M F	-	M F	Posture	Discrete	Rapid to use
VIDAR	MSD	Post.	M F	M F	M F	Workcycle	Discrete	Uses discomfort score

Method: *name of method*, Aim: *aim of method*, Dim.: *dimensions of target exposures*, Posture: *observation of body posture*, Move.: *observation of movements*, Forces: *observation of external forces*, Duration: *duration of observation*, Evaluation: *resulting score*,
Abbreviations: MSD: *musculoskeletal disorders*, com: *comfort*, move.: *movement*, check:*checklist*, weight: *handled weight*, post.: *body posture*, angles: *joint angles*, M: *magnitude*, D: *duration*, F: *frequency*

methods are the observed target exposures. Some of the most widespread methods like the Quick Exposure Check (QEC) [12] or the Health & Safety Executive Upper limb Risk Filter and Risk Assessment (HSE) [12] utilize simple checklists to assess the existence and severity of health risks. These methods are designed for rapid assessment of possible risks, ease of use and to help in making decisions regarding improvements.

Most methods designed to evaluate lifting tasks require additional input to calculate the strain of lifting on the body. Some of the most common, like the National Institute for Occupational Safety and Health Lifting Equation (NIOSH-LE) [12], calculate a risk factor or a recommended lifting weight out of the horizontal and vertical location in relation to the body, the travel distance, angle of asymmetry, the coupling of the grip, task frequency and the weight.

A few methods use the evaluation of movements, like the American Conference of Governmental Industrial Hygienists Threshold Limit Value for Hand Activity Level (HAL TLV) [12], which was designed to evaluate the risk of repetitive hand movement.

Other methods evaluate comfort on the basis of body posture. For the observation and recording of postures two main methods are utilized. One is a comparison with predefined postures or partial postures which have been assessed by medical or ergonomic professionals during the design of the method. A good representative of this kind of method is the Ovako Workload Assessment System (OWAS) [12], a method originally developed to assess the workload of workers in a steel mill.

A second method of recording body postures is the estimation or measuring of joint angles. Two of the user friendliest methods are the Rapid Upper Limb Assessment (RULA) [12] and Rapid Entire Body Assessment (REBA) [12]. Both of these methods are used to observe the joint angles and determine separate risk factors for each joint. Both methods utilize a division of the range of joint movement into two to four segments, associated with their own risk score. These risk factors are then grouped and used to determine a grand score describing the need for improvement of the task. The main difference is that while REBA observes the entire body, RULA only observes the upper body.

Another use of observing the joint angles in a body posture or during movement is the assessment of perceived discomfort. Out of the selection in Table 1, two methods share this aim, the postural loading on the Upper Body Assessment (LUBA) [14] and the Method for Movement and Gesture Assessment (MMGA) [15]. LUBA has been designed for the assessment of body postures using a division of the range of joint movement into four to seven segments similar to RULA. Each of these segments is associated with an increasing discomfort score when deviating further from the neutral position. These scores are added for each section of the upper body; arm, neck and back. This allows for an evaluation of the observed posture regarding the total discomfort and the grading of the perceived comfort, by means of correlation of the LUBA score and maximum holding times of postures. MMGA is based on LUBA and expands the scope of observation. With this method it is possible to assess complete movements of the whole body, not only body postures of the upper body. This is achieved through the measuring of additional joint angles in the lower body and the observation and recording during a movement, usually through motion capturing. Additionally the segments of the joint angles have been converted to splines, enabling the assessment of small angles and changes of the angles. The individual discomfort scores of joints are weighted by the distal bodyweight supported by this joint.

Evaluation of Movement Tasks. The evaluation of the comfort of movement tasks using hand-guided mechanisms requires a certain set of minimal requirements. These are a measurement of all joint angles in the arm, because the arm usually experiences the most movement and changes of joint angles while operating a hand-guided mechanism. Second would be a precise measuring of joint angles to register small changes. Third is the possibility to assess the posture and its change during movement. These requirements are not all met by either LUBA or MMGA, since MMGA discards several joint angles in the arm. The observation of small changes of joint angles is met by MMGA, while the segmentation of joint angles of the LUBA method is not fine enough to register these changes. Preliminary studies showed that during operation of white goods there were usually no changes in the LUBA score. If the joints reached positions that were assessed uncomfortable by LUBA, the score spiked due to the often rather large difference in the discrete discomfort scores in neighboring segments, limiting the use of this method. The third requirement, the observation of movements was met by MMGA, while LUBA is designed to assess a single body posture.

Customized Method of Evaluation. Due to these requirements outlined above a new method of evaluation was devised. The method is based partly on the LUBA method and partly on the MMGA. The joint angles observed are based on LUBA (depicted in Fig. 7), covering the upper body. The angles are the flexion and extension of the wrist, elbow, shoulder, neck and back, the radial and ulnar deviation and the supination and pronation of the wrist, the medial and lateral rotation of the upper arm, the abduction and adduction of the shoulder and the rotation and lateral bending of the neck and back.

To complement the objective data a questionnaire has been devised to collect subjective data. This helps to gather impressions and perceived comfort of the operator.

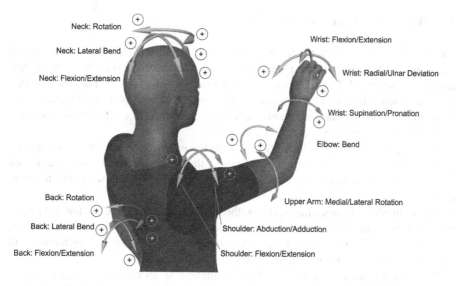

Fig. 7. Observed angles of human movement, more important ones on the right

This questionnaire is tailored to specific movement tasks using a hand-operated mechanism. Typical questions for the operation of a lift-up flap door on a kitchen cupboard are the possibility to reach the working space of the door, the comfort of reaching specified points of the movement, especially the end. Another important point is the subjective assessment of the magnitude of the operating forces, their uniformity and direction. Directly related to this is the accessibility of the handle and its size. At the same time different modules of the mechanism can be assessed, e.g. dampers, springs, locking mechanisms and supports.

These angles can be measured either by motion capturing, an accurate depth camera (i.e. time of light) or photo and video analysis, depending on available equipment and pace of movement. A photo analysis can be used for mainly static postures, while movements should be registered and measured with the video camera or the other methods. Photo and video analysis should be conducted from at least two different angles at the same time to capture the complete spatial movement and allow the calculation of all joint angles. Another method of registering the joint angles are goniometers attached to each joint. These measuring instruments allow for constant measuring of joint angles but optical measuring has been shown to be less intrusive, allowing for more natural movements and is reasonably accurate.

These angles of the joints enable a calculation of discomfort scores, based on the modification of the LUBA steps into splines similar to MMGA, for every angle. Following this, the same sums are calculated as in LUBA. In addition the development and changes of the discomfort score during the movement are shown, as are maximum deviations. This allows for a more exact evaluation and comparison of movement tasks.

4 HFS as Process Oriented Tools

The HFS is more than just the hardware device. It includes simulation, modelling and visualization. Additionally, the planning, execution and evaluation of the experimental testing are facilitated. The HFS can support the design process as a whole and together with the extension of a suitable software-system it functions as a development environment for hand-operated mechanisms. The advantages of the HFS from a process- and economical-perspective are discussed in [16].

The software system of the HFS can guide the engineer through the development process and can prompt a recurrent evaluation of the design parameters and a validation of the results. Additionally, the data storage can be used in finding solutions to design challenges.

As outlined in the preceding sections, there are a multitude of factors that have to be taken into account when performing a user acceptance study. For the most part these are recurring tasks, since user acceptance studies on hand-operated mechanisms all share similar aspects. Hence, support by software makes sense.

User acceptance testing can aid the development in all phases. The feasibility of a project in principle can be tested in explorative studies. Isolated functions or improvements can be validated during every phase of development and alternative solutions can be compared. In the end, the validated results can be compared with the requirements. [17].

References

1. Kölling, T., Paris, J., Hüsing, M., Corves, B.: Enhancement of mechanism design process by interaction with haptic feedback-systems. In: Petuya, V., Pinto, C., Lovasz, E.-C. (eds.) Second Conference MeTrApp 2013. Mechanisms and Machine Science, vol. 17, pp. 293–300. Springer, Heidelberg (2014)
2. Deutsches Institut für Normung: DIN EN ISO 9241-210 Ergonomie der Mensch-System-Interaktion, Teil 210: Prozess zur Gestaltung gebrauchstauglicher interaktiver Systeme. Beuth Verlag, Berlin (2011)
3. Verein Deutscher Ingenieure: VDI 2221 – Methodik zum Entwickeln und Konstruieren technischer Systeme und Produkte. VDI, Düsseldorf (1993)
4. Niemeyer, J.: Methodische Entwicklung von Prinziplösungen bei der Auslegung ungleichmäßig übersetzender Getriebe unter Verwendung eines praxisorientierten interaktiven Wissensspeichers. Dissertation, IGM der RWTH Aachen (2002)
5. Goodman, E., Kuniavsky, M., Moed, A.: Observing the User Experience. Elsevier, Waltham (2012)
6. Schmidt, R.F., Thews, G. (eds.): Physiologie des Menschen, pp. 216–221. Springer, Heidelberg (1997)
7. Kern, T.A. (ed.): Entwicklung haptischer Geräte, pp. 97–104. Springer-Verlag, Berlin, Heidelberg (2009)
8. Hale, K., Stanney, M.: Deriving haptic design guidelines from human physiological, psychophysical and neurological foundations. In: IEEE Computer Science (2004)
9. Tan, H., Srinivasan, M., Ebermann, B., Cheng, B.: Human factors for the design of force-reflecting haptic interfaces. In: DSC, vol. 55-1; ASME Book No. G0909A (1994)

10. Deutsche Institut für Normung.: DIN 33411-1 Körperkräfte des Menschen, Teil 1: Begriffe, Zusammenhänge, Bestimmungsgrößen. Beuth Verlag GmbH, Berlin (1982)
11. Steinberg, U., Liebers, F., Klußman, A.: Manuelle Arbeit ohne Schaden – Grundsätze und Gefährdungsbeurteilung. Bundesanstalt für Arbeitsschutz und Arbeitsmedizin, Dortmund (2014)
12. Finnish Institute of Occupational Health. http://www.ttl.fi/en/ergonomics/methods/ workload_exposure_methods/table_and_methods/Pages/default.aspx
13. Takala, E.-P., Pehkonen, I., Forsman, M., et al.: Systematic evaluationof observational methods assessing biomechanical exposures at work. Scand. J. Work Environ. Health 36(1), 3–24 (2010)
14. Kee, D., Karwowski, W.: LUBA: an assessment technique for postural loading on the upper body based on joint motion discomfort and maximum holding time. Appl. Ergon. 32, 357–366 (2001)
15. Andreoni, G., Mazzola, M., Ciani, O., Zambetti, M., Romero, M., Costa, F., Preatoni, E.: Method for movement and gesture assessment (MMGA) in ergonomics. In: Duffy, V.G. (ed.) ICDHM 2009. LNCS, vol. 5620, pp. 591–598. Springer, Heidelberg (2009)
16. Kölling, T., Paris, J., Hüsing, M., Corves, B.: Optimierung des Entwicklungsprozesses von handbetätigten Bewegungseinheiten durch Simulation digitaler Prototypen in einem universellen haptischen Feedbacksystem. In 10. Kolloquium Getriebetechnik. Technische Universität Ilmenau, Ilmenau (2013)
17. Kölling, T., Paris, J., Hüsing, M., Corves, B.: Einsatz haptischer Feedbacksysteme im Entwicklungsprozess von Mechanismen. In: Bewegungstechnik 2014: 17. VDI Getriebetagung, pp. 203–214. VDI-Berichte 2237, Düsseldorf (2014)

The Role of Virtual Ergonomic Simulation to Develop Innovative Human Centered Products

Daniele Regazzoni[1(✉)], Caterina Rizzi[1], and Giorgio Colombo[2]

[1] Department of Management, Information and Production Engineering,
University of Bergamo, Dalmine, BG, Italy
{daniele.regazzoni,caterina.rizzi}@unibg.it
[2] Department of Mechanical Engineering, Polytechnic of Milan, Milan, Italy
giorgio.colombo@polimi.it

Abstract. The paper concerns the use of integrated methodologies and tools to perform innovative human centered development of products. Digital simulation of ergonomics by means of DHM is shown together with advanced tools for design, taking into account Knowledge-based systems, Design Automation and design of highly customized goods. Two different applications of the proposed approach are described, the first refers to an industrial product, the second to the medical domain. Both applications, even if belonging to completely different fields benefit from putting the human at the center of the developing paradigm from the very first step of product development. Some results and discussion highlight benefits and limitation of the approach and of the adopted tools.

Keywords: Digital human modeling · Ergonomics · Human centered design · Design Automation · Knowledge-based systems · Lower limb prosthesis

1   Introduction

Digital Human Modeling (DHM) enables designers to face several design issues, such as comfort and posture prediction [1] for envisaged groups of users, task evaluation and safety, visibility of products [2] (machinery, equipment, vehicles, etc.), reaching and grasping of devices (buttons, shelves, goods, etc.) [3], and multi-person interaction to analyze if and how multiple users can cooperate among them and with the product. DHM can be used for product ergonomics [4], crash testing, product virtual testing, workplace design, and maintenance allowing a fast redesign and reducing the need and realization of costly physical prototypes, especially for those applications dealing with hazardous or inaccessible environments.

The aim of this work is to present a method and different ways in which DHM can be used to improve product development process, obtaining either flexible design tools or highly customized products. The paper, after a presentation of the method shows two applications in different domain to clarify the potentiality of DHM integrated with other design methods and tools.

© Springer International Publishing Switzerland 2015
V.G. Duffy (Ed.): DHM 2015, Part II, LNCS 9185, pp. 74–83, 2015.
DOI: 10.1007/978-3-319-21070-4_8

2   Methodology

The potential of digital humans at a methodology level can be exploited to define a new design framework for managing new product development processes and product innovation (Fig. 1).

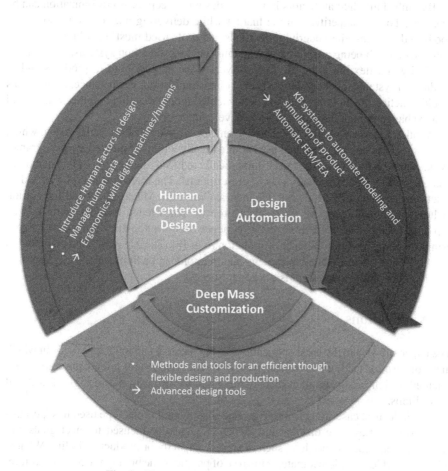

Fig. 1. Human centered methodology framework

Actually, the capability to handle human factors in a design activity constitutes a deep change crossing many existing methods and tools.

Human centered design can be the starting point for the conceptual design phase. Technicians can start dealing with human data from the very first step of product development to embed customer's personal requirements at the beginning of the pipe rather than at the end. This is the base also for a broad Computer Aided Ergonomic approach [5] to design the environment in which operators will carry out their tasks, no matter which is the application sector (e.g., industry, medical, transportation) who is the operator (taking into account also his/her skills, characteristics and culture) and what is the task to be performed. Tools available on the market, such as Siemens Jack [6] or Dassault System Delmia [7], are perfectly suited for most of the ergonomics issues and allow users to addresses practically any task of an industry-oriented scenario. By the way, there are still some open challenges for a better characterization of human models in terms physical details and of their behavior.

By embedding human factors in product design, a deep mass customization can be achieved. To be competitive on the market while delivering one to one personalized goods and services, the underlying methods and tools used must meet high efficiency standards though being adaptable, and so must be the production systems. Modularity, scalability and flexibility are the main drivers to be applied both to products and to production systems to gather a higher level of customization. For instance, design tools would benefit from an improved function-oriented modularization together with a fluid data exchange though the entire product development process.

Another key issue strictly connected to enhanced customization is the way in which design tools can be integrated and used automatically within a knowledge-based framework. Actually, time and costs can be dramatically reduced by changing design paradigm according to Design Automation (DA) prescriptions. The main features of a good DA practices are Advanced Modeling, Parametric/Constraint Management and Integration of Iterative Steps/Interactive Analysis. Moreover, Knowledge Based systems can be exploited to embed senior technicians' experience into an automatic design environment using, for instance, Finite Element simulation tools [8]. The capability of a company to quickly define the most suitable strategy and to implement a light and effective product development process paradigm is the key to success.

3   Applications

The paper shows two different applications in the medical and industrial fields in which many of the cited methods have been integrated. The applications refer to the ergonomic-oriented design of supermarket display units and to the custom-fit design of artificial lower limbs.

The industrial case study is a refrigerated display unit of the type used in supermarkets and groceries. The display unit design is generally focused to meet goals and constraints centered on product, such as storage capacity or product visibility. What is missing, or at least underestimate, is the role of people in the buying process. Therefore, in a human centered approach, the display unit will have to meet as much as possible the requirements of a variegated population of users characterized by different anthropometric measures. Moreover, besides customers picking up goods during opening time, also maintenance technicians and workers filling out the shelf with fresh products must be considered. For each category of people interacting with the display unit, some ergonomic aspects are more relevant than others: i.e., visibility and reachability of goods for customers, reachability of some display components for technicians and, the most important, posture and stress for operators who repeat the same task for hours and may suffer from musculoskeletal disorders. An integrated method based on parametric modeling and DHM simulation of human-machine interaction provides the designers with a tool that updates ergonomic evaluation indexes at each modification of the display unit design.

The medical case study refers to the design and test of lower limb prosthesis required by a person who had a leg amputated. The artificial leg is composed by standard parts (e.g., knee, foot, connectors) and by the socket that is a highly customized part. In this case, the patient is already the main reference for any design step, but the weakest link in the design process is the lack of digitalization of the available tools. Actually, in most of orthopedic labs the realization of sockets is still accomplished in a manual way. What is proposed according to the novel approach is to switch to a complete virtual approach and automated design, while taking into account that the final users will be an orthopedic technician who is not supposed to have a deep expertise in IC technologies. Input data are generated at the beginning of prosthesis development by acquiring patient's geometry with a MRI scanner. After that, the design module has the goal to (i) create the virtual socket relying on patient's anatomy and (ii) define a consistent assembly of standard components chosen accordingly to patient's history. The test module has the goal to forecast the prosthesis behavior when used by the patient and different kind of numerical simulation (FE analysis and gait simulation with DHM) are performed almost automatically to check comfort and performance of the final product. All the knowledge related to routine steps of both design and test have been embedded into the system and the human intervention is required only to control the procedure and evaluate partial and final outputs.

The two different applications are better described and discussed in the followings.

3.1 Industrial Application

This application refers to a vertical display unit and to its ergonomic evaluation method based on a full virtual approach. We propose a method based on DHM commercial tool and a CAD software in order to evaluate in details accessibility and visibility of products, generating results that are both numerical and graphical for an easy comprehension and usability.

Human modeling tools are used to simulate the person physically interacting with the product and the environment. This allows a quantitative assessment of accessibility and visibility of products, as requested in this specific application, but, for instance, posture analysis and tasks evaluation can be carried out with the same approach.

The application exploits the potential of a parametric approach for both modelling of the product people is going to interact with, and the digital human models. Depending on the case of use, the parameters to be considered can be different: the product may be designed so that any potential geometric variant is achieved only modifying a few independent variables; human models can be varied as well, for instance, depending on gender, age, height and build. In this case, we adopted two software solutions by Siemens: Solid Edge ST4 for the CAD side and Jack as DMH solution.

When dealing with a display unit it is very important to have a flexible approach. On one side, the supermarket is visited by every kind of people and the larger portion of population is satisfied by the buying experience, the better it is. On the other side, the display unit can be easily configured by repositioning shelves at different heights or using shelves with a different depth. These variations impact on the way people will be able to see and to reach product they want to buy, and thus the efficiency of the overall process.

Even if designers know very well generic issues, or can easily forecast some of them, (e.g., the highest shelf is the less reachable) it is not easy at all to gather a quantitative index measuring the comprehensive change of performance of the product/human system whenever one or more parameters are changed. The following examples show how this can be done and how a graphical representation of results can improve usability of results during product development.

The example reported in Fig. 2 addresses the visibility of a vertical, open (without doors), display unit. Colors are used to highlight the hidden zones for respectively a man whose height correspond to the 95th percentile, and a woman corresponding to the 25th percentile of the European population. By changing avatars' height, distance from the display unit and shelves vertical position it is possible to quickly gather a new configuration and the related visibility results.

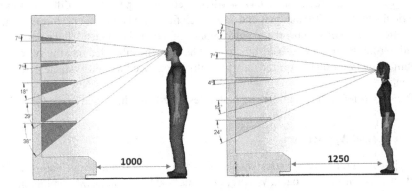

Fig. 2. Open display unit visibility test for different human models (Color figure online)

When dealing with reachability the test campaign can be much more complex respect to visibility because it imply a study on the posture assumed while measuring the maximum reachable distance. Moreover, different postures can lead to different results in terms of both distance reached and comfort [9].

Another notable example of exploiting parametric models to gather ergonomic results consist in assessing the reachability of the horizontal surface of a shelf in a display unit with doors. Actually, for any point on a 50 × 50 mm grid in which each shelf has been divided, the avatar assumes a different position and it may interfere with the display. Figure 3 shows the results of a reachability analysis in which collision (red cells) or proximity (yellow cells) are detected among different parts of the display unit and of the avatar. Mapping the results using colors directly on the 3D model of the product allows technicians to easily and quickly interpret simulation outcomes. The results can be obtained for each shelf and varying the digital human model to cover the desired target of population.

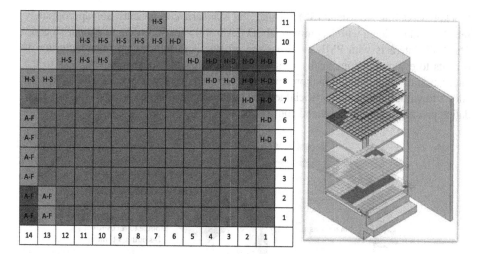

Fig. 3. Closed display unit reachability test and collision detection. The cells colors mean: Gray: not reachable; Red: collision; Yellow: proximity; Green: good reachability. Letters inside the yellow and red cells refer to the colliding parts: H: head; A: arm; F: frame; S: shelf; D: door (Color figure online).

3.2 Medical Application

This example of methods and tools integration refers to the design and simulations of lower limb prosthesis, with particular attention to the most customized component i.e., the interface between the patient's residual limb and the artificial leg, namely, the socket.

In this context, the main goal has been to implement an automatic design and simulation procedure. The rationale beside this goal is, uncommonly, not just to save time in performing the computer-based design process, but to let it be feasible. Orthopedic technicians and prosthetists, actually, have not got the competences required to handle CAD systems and simulation tools required to virtualize the process of making a socket. Thus, the need for a system that highly support the technicians to generate the geometry of the socket and automatically runs FE analysis to validate it, is crucial.

In order to obtain a proper design platform the point of view is shifted from the tools available to the final user of the socket, or, better, to its 3D digital avatar. A huge research effort allowed to gather an environment in which a non-technical user is able, exploiting his/her medical expertise, to obtain the design of the socket, the results of the simulation of socket-residuum interaction, and the chance to apply the entire prosthesis to a digital avatar to analyze the gait.

The design platform integrates tools to acquire patient's data, CAD tools to model prosthesis components, a finite element analysis (FEA) package to study the socket-residual limb interaction, and a digital human modeling (DHM) system to perform gait analysis. It consists of two main environments (Fig. 4): (i) the prosthesis modeling laboratory (PML) and (ii) the virtual testing laboratory (VTL). The PML allows the prosthetist to design the whole prosthesis, for both transtibial and transfemoral amputees. The 3D socket model is created onto the residual limb digital model using a dedicated CAD tool

(Socket Modeling Assistant (SMA)) and the standard components are appropriately selected and modeled with a commercial 3D CAD software according to patient's needs. The VTL interacts with PML to assess the prosthesis design before manufacturing. It permits to evaluate automatically or semi-automatically the socket shape thanks to the integration of numerical simulations tools. Furthermore, by the use of a DHM system, it allows to virtually set up the artificial leg and simulate patient's posture and walking, validating prosthesis functionality and configuration.

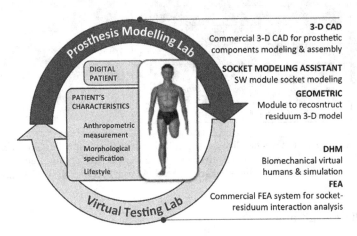

Fig. 4. Prosthesis design platform

Within the VTL, the numerical simulation has been implemented embedding a FEA solver. Among the various FE solvers commonly used in this field, we adopted Abaqus package and use it through the Abaqus Scripting Interface for executing a series of "jobs" without user's intervention.

Once the prosthetist has created the 3D socket model, the system acquires the input for the analysis, produces the files required to generate the FE model and calls the module to execute the analysis. The FE model is automatically created; Abaqus solves the analysis, and generates the file output containing the pressure values. These are imported in SMA and visualized with a color map. SMA evaluates pressure distribution and highlights the areas that should be modified. Figure 5 shows an example of the geometric modelling of the socket (Fig. 5a) and the pressure map identifying the load zones to be evaluated (Fig. 5b). Thus, technicians are only requested to evaluate the level of intensity of the modifications to be applied to the geometric model before running the few simulation requested until the result is satisfying. Such a process, in the manual procedure, implied the production of at least one check socket and some trials with the patient, while in this new way the patient is involved only when the design of the socket is much more likely to be correct.

Moreover, having the digital models of all the components of the prosthesis allows introducing new manufacturing technologies, as the Fused Deposition Modelling 3D printing we are testing to create a fast and reliable product while preserving full customization for each patient.

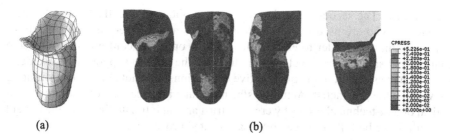

(a)   (b)

Fig. 5. Socket model (a), Socket/residuum pressure map obtained by FE analysis (b)

Another important aspect of the change of paradigm in leg prosthesis design is related to the use of DHM for the prosthetized patient. Human modelling tools, actually, could be used to analyze the virtual gait of the patient's avatar wearing his/her virtual leg before it is manufactured. Figure 6 shows an image of the model of the patient in which the left leg has been replaced by the prosthesis.

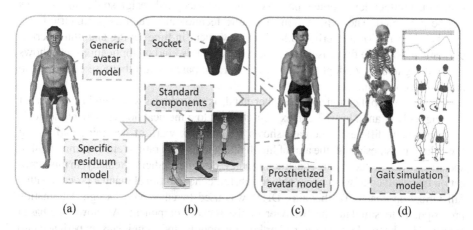

(a)   (b)   (c)   (d)

Fig. 6. Model of the patient having the residuum of the limb reconstructed by RMI Dicom images (a), assembled with the custom socket and standard components (b) to create the complete model (c) to be used for gait analysis (d).

The analysis of the gait of the patient can be performed either on the virtual avatar or on a patient already having and using a lower limb prosthesis. In this last case, the Motion Capture (MoCap) techniques can be used to gather gait data. Optical markerless low cost sensors have been tested for this aim and results can be found in [10].

Since a patient walking with a prosthesis may encounter a set of well-known and classified abnormalities respect to a standardized correct gait, we defined a module to support expert personnel in identifying these abnormalities so that the prosthesis can be tuned at its best. To this aim two sources of knowledge have been used. First, we formalized the knowledge of the Atlas of Limb Prosthetics [11] and embed it in the module to automatically assess key parameters of the gait, compare those values with a set of reference values and highlight eventual deviations for each specific case. The second set of knowledge was obtained directly from orthopedic technicians who are used to correct design issues and to fine-tune the regulations of the prosthesis in order to empirically find the optimum configuration to ensure comfort and safety. The developed module has the goal to support and ease decisions by means of automatic quantitative evaluations, it is not aimed at substituting the work of the prosthetist. Actually, s/he must take into account also other psychological or non-technical issues by creating trust and an intimate link with the patient that will never be fully replaced by an automated procedure.

4   Discussion and Conclusions

The results gathered with this work are still at a methodological level and the case study have the goal to clarify potentiality of the integrated approach but they do not represent a validation. By the way, it is undeniable that shifting the focus on human models each time a person interact with a machine brings notable benefits. Ergonomics can be brought inside the product development process from the conceptual design so that main issues can be prevented. The exploitation of mature technologies such as parametric CAD together with DHM may bring to huge improvement in time saving and, thus, permit deeper analysis. The first case presented deals with this kind of applications and shows a way designers may adopt to shorten the test campaign that, otherwise could be too much time consuming.

The second application, on the other hand, is not addresses at refining the use of existing tools in an industrial context, but it refers to a medical domain where the goals are completely different. The case shows the complex work of designing and testing lower limb prosthesis with the aim of highlighting tools integration (either commercial or specifically developed) while constructing a new design paradigm. Actually, in this application the result consists in being able to substitute the traditional manual process with a full virtual approach. To this aim, DHM was used together with Design Automation prescriptions to simulate the behavior of the socket component. A knowledge-based approach has been adopted to embed orthopedic notions and technicians' experience into a system able to detect gait abnormalities and suggesting how to fix them. Using digital data instead of physical copy of patient's body segments allows storing human data and creating a database, for instance, of residual limb geometries and gait motion characteristics, so that they can be reused or set as a reference. The digital representation opens the way also to flexible manufacturing technologies, such as 3D printing, that can cut costs while preserving the required level of customization.

Several other potential integrations among the methods shown in Fig. 1 are feasible and may vary depending on the specific aim and domain. Even if some barriers exist (data exchange, personnel training, and psychological resistance) and are slowing down this process, in the future many other works will exploit the centrality of DHM and ergonomics to improve product development process.

References

1. Marler, T., Bataineh, M., Abdel-Malek, K.: Artificial neural network-based pre-diction of human posture. In: Duffy, V.G. (ed.) DHM/HCII PART II. LNCS, vol. 8026, pp. 305–313. Springer, Heidelberg (2013)
2. Colombo, G., De Vecchi, G., Regazzoni, D., Rizzi, C.: Motion capture and virtual humans to enhance ergonomic design and validation of refrigerated display units. In: Proceedings of the ASME IDETC-CIE, pp. 1–9. ASME (2012)
3. Lau, H.Y.K., Wang, L.: Digital human modeling for physiological factors evaluation in work system design. In: Duffy, V.G. (ed.) DHM/HCII PART II. LNCS, vol. 8026, pp. 134–142. Springer, Heidelberg (2013)
4. Liem, A.: Digital human models in work system design and simulation. In: Proceeding of the Digital Human Modeling for Design and Engineering Symposium, Rochester, MI, USA (2004)
5. Ortengren, R., Sundin, A.: Handbook of Human Factors and Ergonomics. Wiley, New York (2006)
6. Siemens, J.: http://www.plm.automation.siemens.com. Accessed 6 Mar 2015
7. Delmia. www.3ds.com/products-services/delmia. Accessed 6 Mar 2015
8. Colombo, G., Facoetti, G., Regazzoni, D., Rizzi, C.: A full virtual approach to design and test lower limb prosthesis. Virtual Phys. Prototyp. 8(2), 97–111 (2013)
9. Colombo, G., Regazzoni, D., Rizzi, C.: Ergonomic design through virtual Humans. Comput.-Aided Des. Appl. 10(5), 745–755 (2013)
10. Regazzoni, D., de Vecchi, G., Rizzi, C.: RGB cams vs. RGB-D sensors: low cost motion capture technologies performances and limitations. J. Manuf. Syst. 33, 719–728 (2014)
11. Atlas of Limb Prosthetics. http://www.oandplibrary.org/alp. Accessed 6 Mar 2015

Anthropometric Casualty Estimation Methodologies

Daniel Rice[✉] and Medhat Korna

Technology Solutions Experts Inc., Natick, MA, USA
{daniel.rice,medhat.korna}@tseboston.com

Abstract. The design of Personal Protective Equipment (PPE) for force protection is critical to soldier survivability and effectiveness for a range of combat operations. This ongoing research project will support US Army technology priorities for force protection through the research and development of new approaches for analyzing fit and form of PPE, specifically body armor systems, to better account for a range of individual body shape differences and enhance protection. By leveraging high-resolution digital 3D scans and building on existing models, this project will provide improved analysis capabilities to scientists engaged in the design of current and future PPE systems. This paper describes the ongoing research and development process for the creation of a methodology to study PPE fit and form and describes potential technological solutions and integration into existing systems.

Keywords: Anthropometry · Body armor · Personal protective equipment · Casualty estimation · Force protection

1 Background

Anthropometric casualty assessment consists of methodologies and algorithms that: (1) use of accurate three-dimensional (3D) models of soldiers and PPE; (2) determine interaction of munitions with PPE, taking into account fit and form; and (3) determine casualties from munitions effects. The design of PPE for force protection is critical for soldier survivability and effectiveness for a range of combat operations. The Army Science and Technology (S&T) strategic direction includes the Soldier and Small Unit (SU) Force Protection, Technology Enabled Capability Demonstration (TECD), which identifies the critical need for new technologies to increase protective gear performance by reducing PPE weight and volume, providing protection from weapon threats and ultimately reducing the number and severity of soldier injuries and casualties (Association of United States Army 2011). Protective equipment is subject to many design considerations; the most fundamental are "form" and "fit." Form is the PPE design elements that are derived by functional choices, such as which areas of the body must be protected for anticipated combat operations. In determining the optimal form, tradeoffs must be made – for example, between level of protection and limits on weight. Fit is how well a specific individual is protected by the form and how the individual's freedom of motion is impeded by the form. To achieve the designed level of protection, proper fit is essential. Optimal fit maximizes protection

© Springer International Publishing Switzerland 2015
V.G. Duffy (Ed.): DHM 2015, Part II, LNCS 9185, pp. 84–91, 2015.
DOI: 10.1007/978-3-319-21070-4_9

while minimizing encumbrance. Less-than-optimal fit can result in inadequate protection or obstruct the soldier's ability to perform operational tasks.

Lt. Col. Jon Rickey, product manager for soldier protective equipment at Program Executive Office (PEO) Soldier, stated in a 2011 interview with *National Defense* magazine that having accurate anthropometric sizes of soldiers to ensure proper fit is the crucial first step in designing future body armor (Beidel 2011). The Army has invested significant time and resources into collecting accurate 3D data of active-duty soldiers. Through the most recent activity, the U.S. Army Anthropometric Survey II (ANSUR II), the Army has collected over 12,000 3D scans as of May 2012. Anthropometrists collect this data using laser scanning to produce high-resolution 3D models of each soldier. This technology also can capture high-resolution scans of PPE body armor such as vests or helmets in specified sizes.

With new Army sizing charts under development as part of ANSUR II, the Army needs advanced analysis tools to evaluate the impact of current and future PPE sizing decisions. For example, the Interceptor Body Armor (IBA) Improved Outer Tactical Vest (IOTV) comes in 11 sizes, with modular configurations for lower back, groin, and deltoid protective pieces based on the soldier's mission. The Advanced Combat Helmet (ACH) comes in five sizes and adds a protective pad between the bottom of the helmet shell and the top of the IBA collar. PPE designers need sophisticated analysis tools to improve form and fit metrics to improve soldier protection.

Live-fire testing of all permutations of PPE sizes, configurations, and individual body types is impractical, but computer Modeling and Simulation (M&S) provides a valid, safe way to study armor effectiveness in preventing or reducing injury from combat hazards such as fragmenting explosives. To analyze PPE fit for a soldier population, it is insufficient to place a static equipment model over a static human model. Soldiers in the battlefield frequently are in motion, and changes in posture may cause the area of PPE coverage to change. The soldier's position and posture at the moment of an attack ultimately determines if the armor is in the right place to stop an incoming bullet or fragment. To account for variations in PPE coverage that may result from less-than-optimal fit, the equipment model must predict variations in fit due to shifts in posture when applied to digital soldiers.

Fit and PPE effectiveness are influenced greatly by the dynamics of the combat situation. Anthropometric casualty assessment should provide a capability to examine fit in operational scenarios in which soldier agents are engaged in a combat mission. For example, the Infantry Warrior Simulation (IWARS) is a force-on-force constructive combat simulation, because it is the current state-of-the-art for evaluating equipment performance in operational scenarios. Developing anthropometric casualty estimation in a simulation like IWARS will have clear benefits for the evaluation and procurement of future equipment systems.

Furthermore, linking ANSUR II anthropometric data, improved digital models of humans and equipment, and state-of-the-art computer simulations will provide scientists and engineers engaged in the design and analysis of current and future PPE with powerful new tools to assess the protective capabilities of alternative armor configurations. Testing variations in PPE size and configuration in simulation against a representative soldier population enables scientists to use the simulation results to identify potential gaps in armor coverage caused by inadequate fit.

2 The Need for Anthropometric Casualty Estimation

We conducted comparative analysis of existing tools to identify the current state of the art, enabling technologies, and potential transition partners. We examined the Integrated Casualty Estimation Methodology (ICEM) (Simulation Technologies, Inc. 2003) platform and its use of the ORCA (Neades et al. 1998) casualty estimation model. Based on this research, we determined that the body models being used by ICEM had no capability to account for individual body variations. Additionally, we consulted with potential transition partners to determine needs and capability gaps in current analysis tools. The Army identified a need to be able to perform analysis with a constructive simulation that will enable analysts to substitute their own models for certain components, including alternative casualty assessment models and munitions flyout models.

3 Analysis Process to Study PPE Fit and Form

We developed an analysis process consisting of three primary analytical components: (1) input; (2) DHM/DEM configuration; and (3) output and analysis components. This analysis process is illustrated in (Fig. 1).

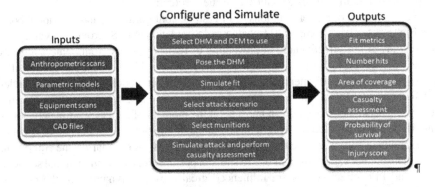

Fig. 1. The ACES analysis process

The development of the analysis process led to the construction of a system concept that combines different methodologies. The ACES concept combines multiple models and methodologies into a single system where each component model or methodology fulfills a particular requirement of anthropometric casualty assessment. We defined the initial ACES concept to consist of the following six component models:

1. DHM – 3D model of the human form.
2. DEM – 3D model of equipment/PPE.
3. Penetrating Projectile Model – Represents impacts by penetrating projectiles (e.g., fragments, bullets, pellets).
4. Ballistics Material Model – Calculates the critical velocity required to penetrate the material and the residual velocity of the projectile.

5. Translation to Casualty Assessment – Translates from the DHM to casualty body model.
6. Casualty Assessment Methodologies – Quantifies harm caused by penetrating projectiles.

By connecting these low-level models and software components into a single package, the ACES concept will be a comprehensive tool for analysts. A depiction of the components of the ACES concept can be seen in Fig. 2.

¶

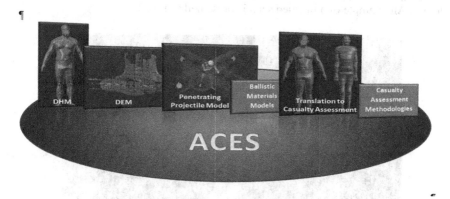

Fig. 2. Components of the ACES concept

4   Analysis Methodologies to Access Fit, Form, Wound Severity, and Level of Protection for Anthropometric DHM and DEM

In order to support the analysis process, we researched and developed methodologies and algorithms to perform the following tasks:

1. Clean the mesh, fill gaps, and reconstruct missing areas of scan data to ensure water-tightness.
2. Rig and weight[1] the DEM to model the characteristics of sizing components used to fit the DEM to the DHM.
3. Rig and weight the DHM to support posing the DHM into operational postures (e.g., prone, kneeling, standing).
4. Detect intersection of projectile with DEM, determine material type at point of impact, and use material type to calculate critical and residual velocity.
5. Determine intersection and entry angle of projectile with DHM and associate with Sperrazza-Kokinakis (SK) casualty estimation body region (Kokinakis and Sperrazza 1965).

---

[1] Rigging and weighting is the process of binding an articulated control structure (the rig) to the 3D mesh so that adjustments to the control structure translate into deformation (bending and flexing) of the mesh.

We researched and developed methodologies for converting full-body laser scan data to create DHMs. We investigated the conversion workflow by converting several scans from the Civilian American and European Surface Anthropometry Resource (CAESAR®) data set. (CAESAR® data currently is being used because it is commercially available). The methodologies created in this R&D will be applicable to ANSUR II data. We focused the research on investigating existing methodologies for converting digital human laser scans to DHM suitable for anthropometric casualty assessment, identifying technology and research gaps, and analyzing competing methods and technologies. An example of a finished scan is presented in Fig. 3.

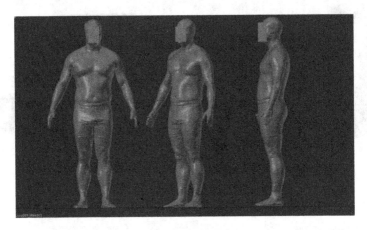

Fig. 3. Cleaned, Decimated Scan: shows the scan in its final state prior to rigging. The scan is free of all geometrical errors, decimated, and watertight.

We used digital artists to investigate a mix of available automated and manual tools used for converting scans to DHM and documented the process steps requiring special tools and/or manual conversion. We identified the following process steps as requiring digital artist manual intervention: (1) find and remove non-manifold edges; (2) find and remove artifacts; and (3) find and remove intersections and overlapping faces. We identified the methodology for preparing DHM scan data as consisting of three critical process steps: mesh decimation, mesh simplification, and mesh sealing. Again, we used digital artist to perform these process steps using three sets of anthropometric data selected from data that had been collected from previous projects.

The initial merged scan data produced an extremely dense, non-uniform mesh containing approximately 300,000 to 600,000 polygonal faces. This data was unnecessarily large for both visualization and simulation purposes, so the digital artists loaded the mesh into Meshlab (MeshLab 2012) to begin the optimization process. We selected MeshLab because it offered several of the required mesh processing algorithms. TSE digital artists first decimated the scan using the quadric edge collapse decimation tool to a target size of 20,000 polygonal faces, creating a less dense and therefore more workable mesh. The quadric edge collapse decimation tool works by specifying the target amount of polygonal faces for the final mesh, allowing options to preserve surface area and form after decimation. This allowed the final mesh to have fewer polygonal faces while still accurately representing the original form. Figure 4 includes an image of the original scan and the processed DHM, which is indicative of how the original form was preserved.

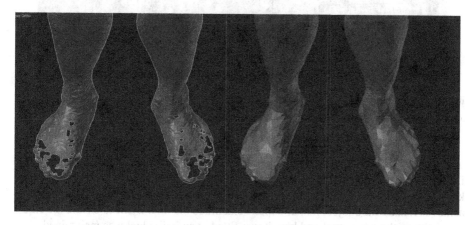

Fig. 4. A comparison between the feet of the original scanned file and the scan in its final state. On the left, the scan is of an overly dense resolution and full of holes and intersections. On the right, the intersections are cleaned up, and all of the holes in the mesh are filled.

The scans were re-topologized using the surface reconstruction algorithms with Meshlab and resurfacing to create a uniform mesh. By the end of this step, the mesh holes and irregularities were corrected so the resulting form was as close as possible to the original scanned form. A before-and-after example of this process is shown in Fig. 4. We also researched methodologies for rigging and weighting DHM and evaluated the capabilities of Commercial Off-The-Shelf (COTS) software solutions such as the 3ds Max software application, which contains prebuilt rigs that could be used on scan data.

The rigged and weighted DHMs could be posed into different postures. We posed the three DHMs in operational postures and positioned the scans into a set of operational poses, including armed standing, kneeling, and prone postures (illustrated in Fig. 5). Digital artists made continuous alterations to the positions of the clavicle, pelvic, spine, and limb controls until realistic poses were achieved and used orthographic and perspective views to increase the efficiency of the process.

The DEM is a 3D representation of the equipment form used to determine if a piece of equipment can fit a given DHM. It determines where and how well the DHM is protected and if a projectile traveling along a certain vector will strike the equipment. The DEM must meet the following requirements:

- Simulate adjustments realistically to achieve a better fit, such as pulling or loosening straps.
- Support testing for geometric intersection by a ray and report the location of all intersections.
- Be watertight.

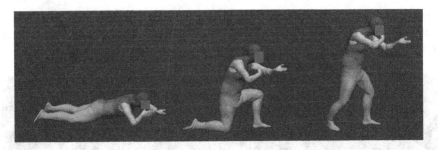

Fig. 5. A rigged DHM in an armed prone posture (left), armed kneeling posture (middle), and armed standing posture (right).

TSE digital artists created a digital model of the IOTV and ACH as a use case to understand the process of PPE rigging and enabling flexible elements for fitting to the DHM. These were modeled using photographic references and the artist's firsthand knowledge and were rigged to enable flexible elements to bend realistically in order to achieve realistic fit. Subject matter experts examined the final DEM to ensure the characteristics of the equipment and how it was fitted to an individual was maintained.

We researched physics-based methods for simulating clothing dynamics for modeling equipment fit and investigated existing technologies, including the cloth solver in Blender (Blender 2012), a 3D modeling program, and the soft body physics capability provided by the Bullet Physics engine. Our analysis of these technologies indicates that while they provide realistic draping behavior over a human model, they assume a uniform, non-elastic material type. Because PPE typically is a combination of flexible, rigid, and adjustable components, the usual assumptions of clothing models are inadequate. We concluded that a more sophisticated simulation approach should be identified or created for use as a tool to investigate clothing dynamics and model fit. We investigated and evaluated options for modeling clothing dynamics and determined the level of work required to implement a clothing dynamics model was extensive. Alternatively, we developed a methodology using standard rigging and weighting of DEM in such a way that it could be fitted realistically. Three DHM poses, fitted with the IOTV, are shown in Fig. 6.

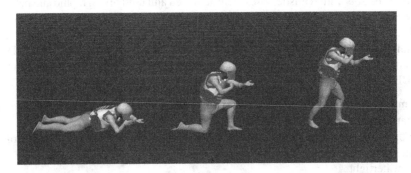

Fig. 6. A DHM equipped with PPE in each posture – the end result of the fitting process

5   Conclusions and Future Work

This paper describes the ongoing research and development of approaches for analyzing fit and form of PPE, specifically body armor systems, to better account for a range of individual body shape differences and enhance protection. Future work on the project will include the investigation of commercial applications and extending capabilities to reach a broader community of users such as law enforcement, firefighting, and other hazardous occupations.

Acknowledgements.   This work is funded in part by the U.S. Army Natick Soldier Research, Development, and Engineering Center (NSRDEC) and the Small Business Innovation Research (SBIR) program under contract W911QY-12-P-0650.

References

Association of United States Army: Army Science & Technology, Army Science and Technology Strategic Direction, 12 October 2011

Beidel, E.: Army Looks Ahead to Next Generation of Body Armor and Helmets, February 2011. National Defense: NDIA's Business and Technology Magazine. http://www.national defensemagazine.org/archive/2011/February/Pages/NextGenerationOfBodyArmorAndHelmets. aspx

Blender, December 2012. Blender: http://www.blender.org/

Kokinakis, W., Sperrazza, J.: Criteria for Incapacitating Soldiers With Fragments and Flechettes. BRL Report No. 1267. Aberdeen Proving Ground, U.S. Army Ballistic Research Laboratories, MD (1965)

MeshLab, August 2012. Sourceforge Web Site: http://meshlab.sourceforge.net/

Neades, D., Klopcic, T., Davis, E.: New Methodology for the Assessment of Battlefield Insults and Injuries On the Performance of Army, Navy, and Air Force Military Tasks. RTO MP-20. RTO HFM Specialists' Meeting on "Models for Aircrew Safety Assessment: Users, Limitations and Requirements", Ohio, October 1998

Simulation Technologies, Inc.: ICEM Analyst Manual. Integrated Casualty Estimation Methodology (ICEM) Analyst Manual, December 2003

Experimental Study on Grip Ergonomics
of Manual Handling

Ai-ping Yang[1], Guang Cheng[1], Wen-yu Fu[1], Hui-min Hu[2(✉)],
Xin Zhang[2], and Chau-Kuang Chen[3]

[1] Department of Industrial Engineering, Beijing Union University, Beijing, China
[2] Ergonomics Laboratory, China National Institute of Standardization, Beijing, China
huhm@cnis.gov.cn
[3] Department of Institutional Research, Meharry Medical College, Nashville, TN, USA

Abstract. Improper design for the grip structure will lead to inefficient operation or work injuries. The study purpose was to simulate the shape, size, and position of a gripping structure by using a 30 kg rectangular box as a heavy object, to enhance the health and comfort for an operator. Ergonomic evaluation experiments for grip structural factors were performed by samples testing and virtual simulation methods for operational tasks. Research methods and results in this study have some reference meanings and guidance for the man-machine adaptation design regarding the shape, size, and location of manual handling gripping structure of products, supplies and equipment.

Keywords: Grip ergonomics · Samples testing · Virtual simulation · Manual handling · Man-Machine adaptation

1 Introduction

Both the shape and position of the gripping structure for heavier objects directly affect the efficiency of manual handling operations. Prolonged and frequent use of improper shape and position of the gripping structure will lead to work-related acute or chronic injuries to the operator, especially when manually handling heavy loads. Tooley [1] considered participatory ergonomics activities, with the appropriate ergonomics infrastructure, should reduce work-related musculoskeletal disorders. Alzuheri, Atiya [2] proposed a framework that allows for the consideration of multiple ergonomics measures to assess ergonomics stresses resulting from work postures in manual assembly work. In order to study the manual operator comfort, some scholars performed human motion modeling and analysis related to arm and finger movements. Chaffin [3] developed a set of human motion prediction models to resolve the dynamics of the motions of people reaching and moving which were measured by a motion capture system. Bae [4] established a model describing human finger motion for simulation of reach and grasp for selected objects and tasks. Dickerson [5] defined the quantitative relationship between external dynamic shoulder joint torques and calibrated perceived muscular effort levels for load delivery tasks. Jung [6] implemented a two-handed reach prediction

© Springer International Publishing Switzerland 2015
V.G. Duffy (Ed.): DHM 2015, Part II, LNCS 9185, pp. 92–99, 2015.
DOI: 10.1007/978-3-319-21070-4_10

model that the human upper body was modeled as a seven-link system with thirteen degrees of freedom, being regarded as a redundant open kinematic chain with two end-effectors.

In order to facilitate the operational efficiency and reduce the operator fatigue, many ergonomics experts performed the man-machine interface adaptation regarding products or equipment by using experimental study or virtual simulation analysis. Mallam [7] optimized the design and the layout of ship engine control room utilizing human factors and ergonomics knowledge. Määttä [8] evaluated the impact of Virtual Environments on safety analysis and participatory ergonomics. Ekandem [9] assessed the ergonomics of BCI (brain computer interface) devices for research and experimentation. Otten [10] provided thumb reach envelopes to help guide the placement of controls on handheld devices and useful methods to gather and analyze thumb reach data. Freeman [11] determined optimal pedal positioning for automobiles using Jack modeling software. Carey [12] identified ergonomics hazards using the Jack software system at the very early design stages of new vehicle programs. Freeman [11] determined simulations of pedal positioning, using Jack modeling software for 1st percentile female to 99th percentile male, the optimal fore/aft positioning of the accelerator pedal for joint comfort, and the resulting consequences on strength and comfort for the using of brake pedal. Lu [13] introduced a new method which combined grasping plan with posture prediction to realize grasping strategy for ergonomics simulation. Clift [14] discussed the appraisal of the fit between operating theatre tables and the surgical staff who have to use them.

Focusing on the grip structure and location of a product or device to facilitate manual handling operation, the ergonomics theory was applied through samples testing via the human motion capture system VICON and ergonomics analysis platform JACK. In this study, a 30 kg rectangular box was used to simulate a heavy object, in which six pairs of slots on both sides of the box were treated as the installation locations of the gripper structures. These structures with fixed opening width, seven depths, and five tilt angles were designed, and the gripping structure samples were manufactured. Two types of experimental studies were conducted for this study by performing the following key steps. First, two samples of the same size were inserted into the slots on both sides of the box. Secondly, the study subjects lifted the box and evaluated their operating comfort levels regarding the slot depth and the tilt angle of the gripping structures, respectively. Thirdly, actions were repeated using different sized samples with the corresponding test data being recorded. Finally, repeated actions using the same box with different slot positions lead to the operating position data which allowed subjects to feel more comfortable while being recorded. By analyzing the experimental data, reasonable geometry shape parameters, position, and size, range of the gripping structure were obtained.

2 Methods

In this study, virtual simulation and sample testing were applied, as shown in Fig. 1.

The sample testing method was a specific process. First, corresponding series of hand groove samples with different size were developed by analyzing the factors of structural dimensions that affect the efficiency of the use of hand-clasping in actual use. After considering the characteristics of the user groups, subjects were recruited to perform the operational task with analog samples. Finally, the results of the experimental study were analyze, and geometry values of gripping hand groove structure that subjects felt operation convenient and comfortable were obtained.

Virtual simulation was completed by analyzing manual operation of the man-machine system, the factors of shape, size, and position of gripping groove affecting the efficiency of manual operation and comfort were extracted. Subjects performed specific operating actions similar to the actual work scene. The experimental action data were recorded via the human motion capture system VICON. The size and location of the manual device for the comfort of operation were obtained through a comprehensive analysis of human joint activity satisfaction and muscle tension force via the ergonomics analysis platform JACK.

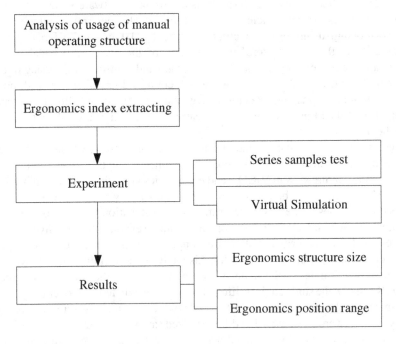

Fig. 1. Technical route of this study

2.1 Experimental Study of the Shape for the Gripping Structure

Twenty-four male participants ranging from ages 21 to 40 years old without physical defects or diseases, or healthy, contributed to this experiment. The test procedure contained many steps. First, the main factors affecting the operation efficiency and comfort levels of the manual handling of heavy objects were analyzed which included opening width, depth and tilt angle of the gripping structure of the box. Secondly, the opening width of grasping slot was generally greater than 25 mm according to the middle finger thickness of the 95th percentile male and experimental data, Thirdly, samples of the buckle groove of different depths were designed based on the finger length of the 95th percentile male (See Fig. 1). The specific depth values were 25 mm, 35 mm, 45 mm, 55 mm, 65 mm, 75 mm, and 85 mm, respectively. Fourthly, five samples were manufactured according to the actual common tilt angles of gripping structures (See Fig. 2) with the increased value of the tilt angle being 15°. The specific values of the tilt angles were 15°, 30°, 45°, 60°, and 75°, respectively as shown in Fig. 2. Finally, twenty young men with similar careers were recruited as study subjects whose feedback was recorded. The size range of the grip structure in ergonomic design was achieved by analyzing the experimental data (Fig. 3).

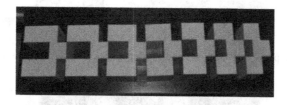

Fig. 2. Simulation samples of groove depth of grasping structure

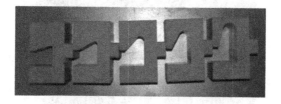

Fig. 3. Simulation samples of groove inclination angle of grasping structure

2.2 Experimental Study of the Position for the Gripping Structure

Twenty-four male participants ranging from ages 21 to 40 years old without physical defects or diseases participated in this experiment.

An experimental cube sample with a mass of 30 kg was designed and built, representing a heavy object of 775 mm length, 540 mm width, and 240 mm height as shown in Fig. 4. The experimental positions of the gripping slot were located on both sides of the cube sample. There were seven heights measured from the top face of the cube sample to the center of the gripping slot incremented by 30 mm. Specific values of the heights were 30 mm, 60 mm, 90 mm, 120 mm, 150 mm, and 180 mm, respectively. After inserting buckle samples into the slots on both sides of the cube sample, the comfort assessment for the height test related to manual lifting was performed. Then, a randomly selected study subject and an assistant lifted the cube sample using the grip structure and walked five steps forward. The action of the two operators carrying the cube sample was recorded by the human motions capture system VICON. The experimental scene was shown in Fig. 5. Finally, the motion capture data was imported into the JACK ergonomics simulation platform and the change in waist forces of the movement for the subjects was analyzed. By analyzing the experimental data, the appropriate height location range of the ergonomic design for the gripping structure was attained.

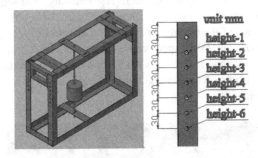

Fig. 4. Prototype for heavy objects and experimental location set of grasping structure

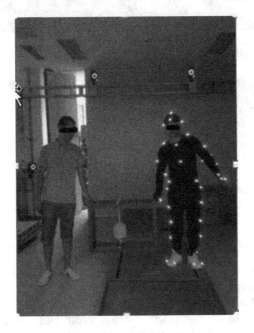

Fig. 5. Experimental scene

3   Results

3.1   Ergonomic Structure Size of Grip Groove

(1) Gripping groove depth. Of the twenty-four healthy male subjects participating in this experiment, twenty subjects selected 55 mm as the optimal groove depth, three subjects thought 45 mm groove depth was comfortable and one subject preferred 65 mm. Eighteen of these healthy male subjects thought that a groove depth of 25 mm was an acceptable minimum limit. However, the results showed that 55 mm was the optimum grove depth and 25 mm was the worst. The proportion of subjects who selected groove depth was shown in Fig. 6.

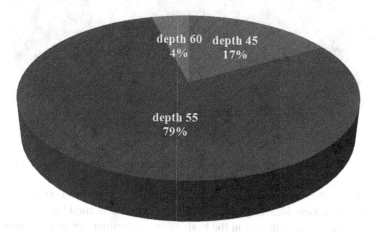

Fig. 6. Representation of subjects and their preferred groove depth

By analyzing the correlation between the above test results and the dimensions of the human hands, groove depth was described as: the middle finger distal phalanx Length + 0.5 * middle of the second knuckle lengths of the 95th percentile male population, as shown in Fig. 7. Therefore, the recommended groove depth was at most 45 mm. The minimum groove depth should not have been less than 30 mm.

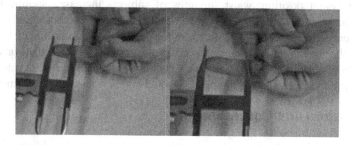

Fig. 7. The length of the middle finger distal and proximal knuckle to fingertip length

(2) Inclination angle of gripping groove. Based on the twenty-four healthy male subjects who participated in this experiment, 2 % preferred a groove angle of 60° and 56 °% preferred an angle of 45°. A 30° inclination angle was the acceptable minimum value. Most of the subjects considered 15° too low because they were easily slipped from the user's hands. Figure 8 showed results of the proportion of subjects who selected the optimal groove inclination angle.

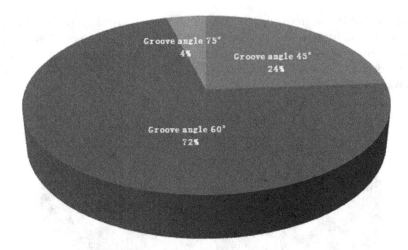

Fig. 8. Proportion of subjects that selected the preferred groove inclination angle

According to the experimental test results, ergonomic evaluation criteria of groove inclination angles were identified as the bend angles of the second knuckle relative to the first knuckle of four fingers. On the basis of the experiment results, the ergonomic recommended range of gripping groove angle was greater than 45°.

3.2   Position Height of Grasping Groove

There were eighteen sets available out of twenty-four healthy male subjects who participated in this experiment. Test data showed that when subjects lifted the test bench with their right hands in different height positions as shown in Fig. 4, their waist strengths gradually increased with the decrease of the position of the gripping groove. At the fourth experiment height position, waist strengths of subjects increased significantly. By analyzing the objective and subjective data of all subjects, 59 % considered the fourth position as easy to operate, while 91 % considered the fifth position as difficult to operate. Therefore, the recommended height for gripping grooves was less than or equal to 150 mm (about position 4). The acceptable height limit of the gripping slot was position 5. The maximum height of the gripping slot should not have been greater than 180 mm.

4   Discussions and Conclusion

By conducting these experimental studies, the appropriate groove depth, angle, and position of the gripping structure could be determined. The empirical results were summarized. First, the recommended groove depth was between 30 mm and 45 mm. Second, the ergonomic recommended range of gripping groove angle was greater than 45°. Third, the acceptable height of the gripping slot was position 5. However, the maximum height of the gripping slot was 180 mm.

The research methods and results had some implication and guidance for the adaptation of the shape and location for gripping structures. Therefore, they could be used to prevent acute or chronic injuries to the operator in the work environment. Follow-up experiments should consider how to reasonably determine the step size of sample geometry sizes based on experience with actual usage, which would lead to an increase in the accuracy of the experimental results.

Acknowledgment. This research was supported by the National Key Technology R&D Program (2014BAK01B02,2014BAK01B04 and 2014BAK01B05), 2015 Beijing Municipal Education Commission Research Project (Title: Comfort model research of human upper limb movement), and China National Institute of Standardization through the "special funds for the basic R&D undertakings by welfare research institutions" (282014Y-3353 and 522013Y-3055).

References

1. Tooley, S., Holtman, K.: The effects of ergonomics, lean manufacturing, and reductions in workforce on musculoskeletal health. In: Proceedings of the 7th Annual Applied Ergonomics Conference 2004 (2004)
2. Atiya, A., Luong, L., Xing, K.: Ergonomics design measures in manual assembly work. In: 2010 2nd International Conference on Engineering System Management and Applications (2010)
3. Chaffin, D.B.: On simulating human reach motions for ergonomics analyses. Hum. Factors Ergon. Manuf. Serv. Ind. **12**(3), 235–247 (2002). Summer
4. Bae, S., Armstrong, T.J.: A finger motion model for reach and grasp. Int. J. Ind. Ergon. **41**(1), 79–89 (2011)
5. Dickerson, C.R., Martin, B.J., Chaffin, D.B.: The relationship between shoulder torques and the perception of muscular effort in loaded reaches. Ergonomics **49**(11), 1036–1051 (2006)
6. Jung, E.S., Shin, Y.: Two-handed human reach prediction models for ergonomic evaluation. Hum. Factors Ergon. Manuf. **20**(3), 192–201 (2010)
7. Mallam, S.C., Lundh, M.: Ship engine control room design analysis of current human factors & ergonomics regulations & future directions. Proc. Hum. Factors Ergon. Soc. Annu. Meet. **57**, 1521–1525 (2013)
8. Määttä, T.J.: Virtual environments in machinery safety analysis and participatory ergonomics. Hum. Factors Ergon. Manuf. Serv. Ind. **17**(5), 435–443 (2007)
9. Ekandem, J.I., Davis, T.A., Alvarez, I., James, M.T., Gilbert, J.E.: Evaluating the ergonomics of BCI devices for research and experimentation. Ergonomics **55**(5), 592–598 (2012)
10. Otten, E.W., Karn, K.S., Parsons, K.S.: Defining thumb reach envelopes for handheld devices. Hum. Factors **55**(1), 48–60 (2013)
11. Freeman, R., Haslegrave, C.M.: The determination of optimal pedal positioning for automobiles using Jack, In: SAE Technical Papers, Digital Human Modeling for Design and Engineering Symposium (2004)
12. Carey, E.J.: Application of ergonomics in vehicle assembly-Early design to on-site analysis. Contemp. Ergon. **2007**, 139–144 (2007)
13. Lu, Z., Yan, L., He, H.: Research on hand grasping strategy for ergonomics simulation. In: Proceedings of the World Congress on Intelligent Control and Automation (WCICA), Proceedings of the 7th World Congress on Intelligent Control and Automation, WCICA 2008, pp 5721–5727 (2008)
14. Laurence, C., Maxine, C., Elton, E.: Evaluating the fit of operating theatre tables-Using basic ergonomics to help improve procurement of medical technology. In: Proceedings of the Human Factors and Ergonomics Society, Proceedings of the Human Factors and Ergonomics Society 55th Annual Meeting, HFES, pp 710–714 (2011)

Moment Analysis of Virtual Human Joint Based on JACK

Qianxiang Zhou[1], Qingsong Yin[1], Zhongqi Liu[1(✉)],
Fang Xie[2], and Shihua Zhou[3]

[1] Key Laboratory for Biomechanics and Mechanobiology of the Ministry of
Education, School of Biological Science and Medical Engineering,
Beihang University, Beijing 100191, China
liuzhongqi@buaa.edu.cn
[2] General Technology Department, China North Vehicle Research Institute,
Beijing 100072, China
[3] Astronaut Center of China, Beijing 100094, China

Abstract. The purpose of this study is to explore the torque size of the joints of
the ankle, knee, and hip under the static posture of car driving when an external
force is exerted to the low limb joint. Twenty five anthropometric parameters of
ten participants were sampled. The personalized digital model of ten participants
was set up with sampled anthropometric data in the senior digital modeling of
JACK. By simulating the driving posture and using the static strength prediction
module of JACK, external force was imposed on front foot to calculate moment
of low limb joint when the degree of ankle joint and knee joint was changed. The
results indicated that the moment of knee joint and ankle joint produced by
external force gradually decrease with the increase of ankle joint angle and the
rate of decrease was faster and faster. The moment of hip joint gradually
decreased with the increase of ankle joint angle and the decrease amplitude was
uniform and linear trend. The moment of ankle joint monotonously increase with
the increase of knee joint angle and the increase rate was slower and slower. The
moment of knee joint first decreased and then increased with the increase of knee
joint angle and the moment of knee was minimum when the angle of knee joint is
110°. The moment of hip joint gradually increased and made a linear increase
with the increase of knee joint angle. The results calculated by JACK were
compared to the data measured by Primus RS system and their results were
consistent. Conclusions can be made from the result: the drivers can properly
increase their ankle joint angle or decrease their knee joint angle, so as to reduce
the low limb joints torque produced by external force imposed on foot because of
braking; it is suggested that 108° to 113°of knee joint angle is the best.

Keywords: Human digital model · Lower limb joint moment · Driving
posture · Computer simulation

1 Introduction

Human body joints are important load-bearing parts of the force and moment under
different working posture and movement. It is of great significance to study the stress
state and the change trend of related limb joints under the particular position in order to

© Springer International Publishing Switzerland 2015
V.G. Duffy (Ed.): DHM 2015, Part II, LNCS 9185, pp. 100–109, 2015.
DOI: 10.1007/978-3-319-21070-4_11

plan working posture reasonably, prevent joint damage, improve working comfort, and guide the design of artificial joints and so on. But it is difficult to measure the stress state of the joint parts directly because of the osculating coupling between limb joints musculoskeletal and other tissues. JACK which is currently acknowledged as the software of modeling and simulation of human body and ergonomic evaluation has a function of the strength prediction. People can easily calculate the force and torque in the digital body joint by with JACK [1]. Digital human model based on JACK software has been widely used in scientific research and optimized engineering design of many fields [2–5].

At present, with the rapid development of modern society, automobile driving gets wide attention. Understanding for driving force of the lower limb joints, especially in a particular driving position and joints angle will have great guiding significance for the analysis of driving fatigue and design of the comfortable driving position, etc.

Domestic and international Scholars have carried out extensive research work about the comfortableness of driving posture and appropriate joint angle. Rebiffe et al., established human biomechanics model to simulate the automobile driver's posture and position [6]. They calculated out of the comfortable joint angle theoretically. Ma et al. combining the characteristics of Chinese human body, quantitatively proposed the mean value and range of joint angle about comfortable driving posture, compared and analyzed the differences of comfortable driving angle between the body of Chinese and foreign body through a large number of vehicles driving tests [7]. Zhao et al. established a three-dimensional biomechanical model that can be used to calculate the force and torque of each limb joint which is based on the driving position of tank drivers [8]. However, in the context of present literature survey, the researches related to the main joint torque of lower limbs under the driving position are not enough. This requires further study to validate and supplement the result of the present research.

In this paper, by modeling individualized digital human based on JACK and using its static strength prediction module researchers got the moment of the ankle, knee and hip joints from the right lower limb of human body under static posture in the car driving. And they hope to get the change rule and trend of joint torque with the change of the angle and external force of the lower limb joints. The results will provide reference for the design of automotive cockpit and man-machine interface.

2   Modeling of Digital Human

Module of JACK that can accurately establish the digital human model contains 25 static measurements items. Ten participants who are fit and healthy adult males and the age is form 20 to 25 (mean 23) were selected in this study. Twenty five static anthropometric parameters of human body were measured. The results were shown in Table 1.

Because the database of human body size of JACK does not match the participants and there are internal functions to restrict coupling among some body size data of advanced digital human modeling modules in JACK, the body size data measured above cannot be completely input to JACK. When creating a personalized virtual human,7 parameters need to be set—the height, the distance between hip and knee, the

Table 1. The results of 25 static anthropometric parameters (cm)

Parameters	Results	Parameters	Results
Stature	174.5 ± 6.6	Hand length	17.6 ± 1.1
Abdominal depth	19.8 ± 2.0	Head width	15.7 ± 0.6
External ankle height	7.1 ± 0.7	Head height	24.2 ± 1.2
Shoulder height	144.3 ± 6.0	Head length	18.9 ± 0.4
Upper extremity length	75.8 ± 3.7	Hip breadth	33.2 ± 1.7
Shoulder peak width	32.7 ± 1.8	Papillary distance	7.7 ± 0.4
Maximum shoulder breadth	44.6 ± 2.4	Shoulder-elbow length	3.6 ± 1.5
Hip-knee length	55.8 ± 1.9	Shoulder height sitting	63.9 ± 2.8
Elbow height sitting	27.7 ± 1.9	Eye height sitting	84.4 ± 2.2
Forearm-fingertip length	45.1 ± 2.6	Sitting height	95.1 ± 2.7
Foot breadth	9.3 ± 0.6	Knee height sitting	52.4 ± 2.3
Foot length	25.1 ± 1.3	Thigh depth sitting	14.2 ± 0.7
Hand width	8.1 ± 0.4		

knee height in sitting, the height of lateral malleolus, the foot length, the foot width and the thighs thick in sitting. The rest of the body size was calculated by the functions of JACK. In the digital modeling senior module of JACK, the personalized digital human model corresponded to 10 participants were established, as shown in Fig. 1.

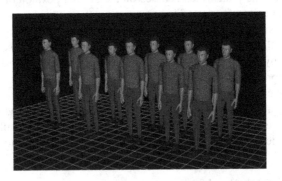

Fig. 1. Ten digital human models

Based on the results of Ma [7] the angel range of ankle, knee and hip joint of the right lower limb with driving position in this study was determined as, the ankle 90° ~ 110°, the knee 100° ~ 140°, the hip joint 95° ~ 115°. An external force is applied to the front end of the foot to simulate force of the foot when braking. Moreover the force is set in the plane of the right lower limb. The driving position of digital human in JACK was shown in Fig. 2.

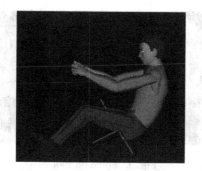

Fig. 2. Driving posture of digital human

3   The Influence on the Joint Torque by Changing Joint Angle

The method of controlling variables was used in this study which means to observe the changes of each joint torque by fixing the joint angle of two joints and changing the joint angle of the third joints. It included two cases as follows.

1. Fixed the hip joint angle to 100°and the knee joint angle to 120°. The ankle joint angles were changed form 90° to 110° which are set in step of 5°, that is 90°, 95°, 100°, 105°, 110°. Meanwhile, at each position, the force F was sequentially set to 10 N, 20 N and 30 N. Joint torque of ankle, knee and hip joint were recorded respectively.
2. Fixed the hip joint angle to 100°and the ankle joint angle to 100°. The knee joint angles were changed form 100° to 140° which are set in step of 10°, that is 100°, 110°, 120°, 130°, 140°. Meanwhile, at each position, the force F was sequentially set to 10 N, 20 N and 30 N. Joint torque of ankle, knee and hip joint were recorded respectively.

3.1   The Joint Torques Change of the Right Lower Limb with Ankle Joint Angle

In the module of JACK of advanced digital human modeling, the personalized digital human that correspond to the 10 participants was set up with anthropometric data of this study. Each digital human was adjusted for driving position. Using static strength prediction module and external force was applied at the location of the forefoot of the digital human. External force was located in the plane of the right lower limb, the direction of which has a 45° angle with horizontal direction of the earth coordinate system pointing in the direction of digital human (Fig. 3). Each joint under specific static force was calculated.

The digital human was adjusted for driving posture. The hip joint angle was adjusted to 100°, and the knee angle to 120°. The ankle joint angle was changed gradually in steps of 5° between the 90° to 110° which is sequentially set to 90°, 95°, 100°, 105°, 110°. Meanwhile, at each position, the force F was sequentially set to 10 N, 20 N and 30 N, and joint torque of ankle, knee and hip joint was recorded respectively.

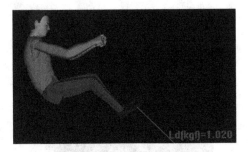

Fig. 3. Force on foot

Table 2. Joint torque of ankle, knee and hip with 10 N of external force (N·m)

Ankle joint angle	Ankle joint torque	Knee joint torque	Hip joint torque
90°	1.404 ± 0.211	1.050 ± 0.168	4.194 ± 0.671
95°	1.326 ± 0.199	0.972 ± 0.146	4.116 ± 0.645
100°	1.237 ± 0.186	0.884 ± 0.124	4.028 ± 0.604
105°	1.140 ± 0.182	0.787 ± 0.129	3.930 ± 0.589
110°	1.033 ± 0.144	0.681 ± 0.114	3.823 ± 0.573

Table 3. Joint torque of ankle, knee and hip with 20 N of external force (N·m)

Ankle joint angle	Ankle joint torque	Knee joint torque	Hip joint torque
90°	2.808 ± 0.422	2.101 ± 0.336	8.388 ± 1.342
95°	2.651 ± 0.398	1.945 ± 0.292	8.232 ± 1.290
100°	2.475 ± 0.372	1.769 ± 0.248	8.055 ± 1.208
105°	2.280 ± 0.364	1.574 ± 0.258	7.860 ± 1.178
110°	2.067 ± 0.288	1.361 ± 0.228	7.647 ± 1.146

The analysis was made with static strength prediction module of JACK when external force is 10 N, 20 N, 30 N. The mean and standard deviation for each joint torques of the right lower limb were shown in Tables 2, 3 and 4. It could be seen from the results of the table that the torque on the ankle generated by the external force show a declined trend and the rate of torque reduction becomes higher when the angle of the ankle joint increase gradually. This was because when the angle of the ankle joint is larger, the increase of angle of the ankle joint make the force arm in the center of the ankle joint determined by external force reduce in larger amplitude. Thus the reduce rate of the torque was bigger. The change trend of the torque generated by external force at the knee joints is the same at the ankle. The joint torque at the hip joint decreased gradually along with the increase of the angle of the ankle joint, and reduced uniformly in a linear decrease trend basically.

Table 4. Joint torque of ankle, knee and hip with 30 N of external force (N·m)

Ankle joint angle	Ankle joint torque	Knee joint torque	Hip joint torque
90°	4.212 ± 0.633	3.151 ± 0.504	12.582 ± 2.013
95°	3.977 ± 0.597	2.917 ± 0.438	12.347 ± 1.935
100°	3.712 ± 0.558	2.653 ± 0.372	12.083 ± 1.812
105°	3.419 ± 0.546	2.360 ± 0.387	11.790 ± 1.767
110°	3.100 ± 0.432	2.042 ± 0.342	11.471 ± 1.719

Table 5. Joint torque of ankle, knee and hip with 10 N of external force (N·m)

Knee joint angle	Ankle joint torque	Knee joint torque	Hip joint torque
100°	0.798 ± 0.119	0.818 ± 0.123	2.327 ± 0.326
110°	1.033 ± 0.155	0.054 ± 0.008	3.178 ± 0.411
120°	1.237 ± 0.185	0.884 ± 0.131	4.028 ± 0.564
130°	1.404 ± 0.210	1.707 ± 0.256	4.851 ± 0.679
140°	1.528 ± 0.230	2.478 ± 0.371	5.621 ± 0.784

3.2 The Joint Torques Change of the Right Lower Limb with Knee Joint Angle

The digital human was adjusted for driving posture. The angle of hip joint and the ankle joint was fixed to 100°. The knee joint angle changed from 100° to 140° in steps of 10° which was 100°, 110°, 120°, 130°, 140°. Meanwhile, at each angle position, the force F was sequentially set to 10 N, 20 N and 30 N. The mean and standard deviation for each joint torques of the right lower limb were shown in Tables 5, 6 and 7.

The results of tables showed that the ankle joint torque increased monotonously with the increase of the knee joint angle and the increase rate became slower and slower. It was obvious that the change of the knee joint angle has a big effect on the ankle joint torque within the scope of a comfortable driving position when the knee joint angle is small, And when the knee joint angle increased gradually, the effect on the additional torque generated by the external force on the ankle reduces with the knee joint angle change. However, in general, the increase of the knee joint angle caused the increase of the ankle joint torque.

With the gradual increase of knee joint angle, there was a variability characteristic that the knee joint torque increase after the first reduce. When the knee joint angle was 110°, the additional torque generated by the external force on the knee joint reached to the minimum. Since then, the knee joint torque increased along with the increase of joint angle. This was because when the knee joint angle is 110°, the knee joint center fall in the near of the action line of the external force, and the force arm to the center of the knee joint generated by the external force reached to the minimum, so reduced the balance of torque at the knee joints at the same external force. In the process of the knee joint angle gradual increase after reaching 110°, the distance between the center of the knee joint and the action line of the external force which is called the force arm increased gradually, so the torque took the trend of gradual increase.

Table 6. Joint torque of ankle, knee and hip with 20 N of external force (N·m)

Knee joint angle	Ankle joint torque	Knee joint torque	Hip joint torque
100°	1.596 ± 0.238	1.637 ± 0.246	4.655 ± 0.652
110°	2.067 ± 0.310	0.109 ± 0.016	6.356 ± 0.822
120°	2.475 ± 0.370	1.769 ± 0.262	8.055 ± 1.128
130°	2.808 ± 0.420	3.413 ± 0.512	9.701 ± 1.358
140°	3.055 ± 0.460	4.955 ± 0.742	1.243 ± 1.568

Table 7. Joint torque of ankle, knee and hip with30 N of external force (N·m)

Knee joint angle	Ankle joint torque	Knee joint torque	Hip joint torque
100°	2.394 ± 0.357	2.455 ± 0.369	6.983 ± 0.978
110°	3.100 ± 0.465	0.163 ± 0.024	9.534 ± 1.233
120°	3.712 ± 0.555	2.653 ± 0.393	12.083 ± 1.692
130°	4.212 ± 0.630	5.120 ± 0.768	14.552 ± 2.037
140°	4.583 ± 0.690	7.433 ± 1.113	16.864 ± 2.352

Along with gradual increase of the knee angle, the hip joint torque increased monotonically. Moreover, with the gradual increase of the knee joint angle, the torque of the external force in the hip joint increased steadily in an approximate linear growth trend.

4   Test and Analysis

In order to compare to the results of JACK, the data of static stress on the foot front-end of right lower limbs was collected from previous10 participants on Primus RS function simulation system with simulating driving posture. Because it was difficult to measure the torque of the knee and hip with the measurement system, only the data of the ankle was collected in this study.

In the test, the participants sat on the chair with his upper torso and waist fixed and the right lower limb was in a driving posture, while the right thigh, the right shank and the right foot in the same vertical plane, and feet were placed on the training tool. In order to simulate the force of the front end of foot, a force transducer was fixed in the front end of the test tool 701. The front of participants' feet put on a sensor and exerted the force of 30 N. After the readings of force sensor were stabilized, click "start" button on the Primus RS interface. The system measured the torque transferred from the practice center of Primus RS which is approximately regarded as the torque of the ankle of the participants. In the test, the participants maintained the angle of the hip joint to 100°and the knee joint to 120°. Moreover they adjusted the angle of the ankle joint to 90°, 95°, 100°, 105°, 110° in turn. Test scenario was shown in Fig. 4. Table 8 was the experimental data.

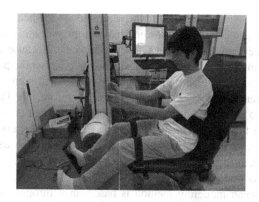

Fig. 4. Test scenarios

Table 8. Joint torque measured by Primus RS system (N·m)

Joint angel	90°	95°	100°	105°	110°
Joint torque	8.3 ± 0.4	7.7 ± 0.5	6.8 ± 0.3	5.6 ± 0.3	4.2 ± 0.5

It could be seen from Table 8 that with the gradual increase of the angle of the ankle joint, the torque of the ankle joint decreased in a faster and faster reducing rate. The change trend of the data was consistent with the results of JACK. Therefore, during driving drivers could increase properly the angle of the ankle joint to reduce the moment generated by the external force imposed on the foot at each joints of the lower limb when braking. But in the process of test, by asking participants' comfort degree, it was found that the participants feel uncomfortable in different degree when the ankle's angle was close to the upper limit of threshold, So, although the torque on the lower limb joint is smaller with the greater of ankle's angle, it make drivers feel uncomfortable. Because when the joint's angle was larger, the difficulty of muscular contraction force increased so that it is more difficult for participants to maintain position. Therefore, as to the angle of the ankle under the driving position, it was not the bigger the better. The ankle angles should be increased moderately. At the same time, by reducing the knee joint angle, the torque can be reduced generated by the force which is imposed from the brake pedal to the foot on the ankle and hip of the lower limb. But the torque of the knee joint came to minimum at the 108°of the knee joint's angle. In addition when the knee joint angle was a little bit small or large, the drivers will feel uncomfortable because their position was constrained by cabin space. Thus it was advisable that the knee joint angle is between108° and 113°.

There were significant differences between the data in Table 8 and in JACK ($p < 0.05$). When the participants were measured with Primus RS system, the front foot of the subjects is forced. Although the stress could be controlled by the force transducer, it was difficult to accurately control the direction of the force, thus the error that cannot be ignored was produced. The measurement results of Primus RS system was not the real moment of the ankle. However, when the center of the ankle joint of the participants was aimed at the center of the equipment tool head axis, the moment conduct by external pedal tools into the internal equipment was considered approximately as the moment of the ankle of the participants. Because the foot had the characteristic of human tissue biomechanics, muscle contraction produced complex stress environment to the tissue around the ankle, so the measurements of Primus RS contained part influence factors of biomechanics. Therefore, the Primus RS system measurement method could obtain the experimental results that are relatively close to the actual stress, but the measurement location was limited. The ankle moment could only be measured approximately. It was difficult to obtain the torque of the knee and hip, and the adjustment of the subjects' posture and the external environment settings would produce errors that cannot be ignored.

JACK digital human modeling method is based on anthropometric parameters to establish a digital human model. The balance torques of the joints was obtained by internal biomechanical calculation functions of static prediction module of JACK. The main error sources of this method are that the size of JACK digital human model doesn't exactly match with the size of the real people. Because the JACK prediction module of the static strength calculation is based on the size of the digital human, the joint torque of the personalized digital human calculated by JACK is not exactly the ankle joint torque. However JACK has the powerful function in modeling and simulation of digital human, it can easily adjust the digital human position and set its stress environment, conveniently obtain the stress of the joints.

5   Conclusion

In this study, based on JACK and simulation of car driving, personalized digital human models were set up, the stress of the right lower limb joints was analyzed, and data obtained from JACK and Primus RS system was compared. Through calculation and analysis, this research can draw the following conclusion:

(1) Within the scope of the comfortable driving posture, when the knee joint angle and the hip angle are fixed, the moment of the ankle, the knee joint and the hip joint will gradually decrease with the increase of the ankle joint angle. Therefore, the moment of lower limb joints that imposed on the foot in the brakes by external force can be reduced by properly increase the ankle joint angle when drivers are driving. (2) Within the scope of the comfortable driving posture, when the ankle joint angle and the hip angle are fixed, the moment of the ankle joint and the hip joint will gradually increase with the increase of the hip joint angle. Therefore, in consideration of the driving space of the car and the factors of stress on lower limbs, in driving it is advisable that the driver's knee joint angle should keep from 108° to 113°. (3) Digital human modeling method by JACK which can conveniently obtain the stress of the joints, is a reliable and efficient method.

Acknowledgement. This work is supported by the Technology Foundation of National Science (A0920132003), the Natural Science Foundation of China (31170895) and the opening foundation of the Science and Technology on Human Factors Engineering Laboratory, Chinese Astronaut Research and Training Center (HF2013-K-06).

References

1. Niu, J.W., Zhang, L.: The Basis of Human Factors Engineering and Instance of Beijing. Electronic Industry Press, Beijing (2012). (in Chinese)
2. Kessler, G.D.: Virtual environment models. In: Stanney, K.M. (ed.) Handbook of Virtual Environments Technology, pp. 255–276. Lawrence Erlbaum Associates, Mahwah (2002)
3. Kallmann, M., Thalmann, D.: Modeling objects for interaction tasks. In: Arnaldi, B., Hegron, G. (eds.) Process Euro graphics Workshop on Animation and Simulation, pp. 73–86. Springer, Wien (1998)
4. Tan, Z.W., Xue, H.J., Sun, R.E.: Research on visibility for cockpit of civil aircraft based on JACK. Aeronaut. Comput. Tech. 40(5), 79–81 (2010). (in Chinese)
5. Liu, S.M., Wang, X.P., Chen, D.K., Wang, S.X.: Cockpit simulation and ergonomics analysis based on JACK. Comput. Mod. 8, 106–110 (2013). (in Chinese)
6. Rebiffe, R.: The driving seat: its adaption to functional and anthropometric requirements. In: Proceedings of a Symposium on SittingPosture, pp. 132–147 (1969)
7. Ma, J., Fan, Z.S., Ruan, Y.: The test of comfortable driving posture and the fuzzy evaluation of the comfort. Ind. Eng. Manage. 13(4), 121–125 (2008)
8. Zhao, Y.L., Liu, W.P., Jiang, K.L.: A three-dimensional biomechanical human model of tank driver for ergonomics. Veh. Power Technol. 4, 51–54 (2008). (in Chinese)

Motion Modeling and Tracking

Parameter Estimation from Motion Tracking Data

Csaba Antonya[1(✉)], Silviu Butnariu[1], and Horia Beles[2]

[1] Department of Automotive and Transport Engineering, Transilvania University of Brasov,
Braşov, Romania
{antonya,butnariu}@unitbv.ro
[2] Faculty of Engineering and Technology Management, University of Oradea, Oradea, Romania
horia.beles@gmail.com

Abstract. User tracking for gesture recognition, object manipulation and finger-based interaction within an immersive virtual environment represents challenging problems. The motion capture system is providing the data for the user's motion recognition, but the uncertainty remains in obtaining the exact motion of the user due to the deformations, especially when the markers are attached to the clothes or to the skin. This paper address the question how can this uncertainty be solved, how can be obtained the geometrical parameters of the users based on tracking data. The tracking data obtained from markers cannot be independent and had to satisfy the physical constraint between the different body parts, represented by the joints of the human skeleton. The Bayesian filtering technique provides an efficient way to obtain the distributional estimate of the unknown parameters. The obtained algorithm is well-suited to identifying parameters of articulated models in the presence of noisy data.

Keywords: Parameter estimation · Uncertainty · Tracking

1 Introduction

Gesture recognition, object manipulation and finger-based interaction within an immersive virtual environment represent challenging problems. In the interactive virtual reality application the computer generated environment is responsible to provide visual, force (pressure) or vibro-tactile haptic feedback to the user [1].

Tracking of the user can be made by one or more of the commercially available mechanical, magnetic, optical, acoustic and inertial tracking systems [2]. The body, arm, head, hand and the fingers can be tracked by using reflective markers, magnetic markers, gloves with bending sensors, image processing techniques or a combination of all these. The motion capture system is providing the input data for the user's motion recognition. Even if the motion capture system is calibrated and the tracking data is recorded with high frequency, the uncertainty remains in obtaining the exact motion of the user due to the deformations, especially when the markers are attached to the clothes or to the skin.

Physical parameters estimation of mechanical systems is the subject of several researches. The estimation process can be based on statistical methods, optimization functions or machine learning algorithms. Renaud et al. [3] presented an approach to

© Springer International Publishing Switzerland 2015
V.G. Duffy (Ed.): DHM 2015, Part II, LNCS 9185, pp. 113–121, 2015.
DOI: 10.1007/978-3-319-21070-4_12

minimize the error between the measured variables and their corresponding values in the forward and inverse kinematic model obtaining kinematic parameters, describing the geometry, and the dynamic physical parameters, describing the effects of masses, inertias and friction. The identification process can be based on manipulation data and a decision-theoretic formulation [4], pushing or pulling object to discover and learn how to manipulate the environment's degrees of freedom [5] or kinematics [6] and the kinematic cues can be used for person identification and how can the observers learn to identify walkers [7].

Probabilistic uncertainty quantification in mechanical simulations with rigid and elastic elements has been used to propagate uncertainty from model inputs to outputs. The sources of the uncertainty could be the inaccuracy of available data, approximations in the mathematical model or discretization error. To compute the propagation of uncertainty in numerical simulations mainly stochastic models are employed, but also sampling method with Monte Carlo simulations, polynomial chaos methodology, stochastic collocation or other probabilistic models [8, 9]. Knowing the parameters of the user is important during interaction with virtual words, because the interaction process and virtual objects are expected to obey the laws of physics with respect to the simulated environment.

Bayesian filtering techniques provides a powerful statistical tool for solving problems in the presence of uncertainty and can be used to obtain a distributional estimate of the unknown parameters. The Bayesian statistics defines how new information can be used and combined with prior belief and objectives to make optimal decisions [10]. The advantage of the Bayesian method is that is not defining the probability as a frequency of occurrence [11], but as a reasonable degree of belief. The Bayesian probability theory returns the best estimate of a parameter from the data and prior information.

This paper address the question how the uncertainty be solved, how can be obtained the exact parameters of an articulated model based on tracking data and without assuming that the probability density function of the searched parameters are known in advance. An accurate parametric model is important in virtual reality applications, especially for force rendering in haptic feedback and to produce realistic interactions with virtual words [12–15].

2   The Articulated Model

The articulated model of the user can be constructed with interconnected rigid element, but subject to deformations. The connection between the rigid elements (corresponding to the bones) corresponds to mechanical joints, with different degree of freedom. The virtual model of the articulated system can be constructed based on the following assumptions:

- each of the rigid componenets can be seen as an individual element of the simulation,
- the joints are ideal joints, and for the planar case all axis of rotation are parallel,
- in case the markers on the elements belong in the same plane during the simulation, the model can be seen as two-dimensional.
- the markers' positions on the elements are not fixed during the simulation, due to the deformations the measured data obtained from the tracking devices are corrupted by

noise; in the simulations this will be replicated by a Gaussian probability density function.

For each mechanical joint the constraints equation can be formulated [16], the number of them is depending on the degree of freedom of the joint [17]. The sum of the number of constraint equation and the degree of freedom of the joint is equal to the associated space dimension, 3 in the planar case and 6 in spatial case. These holonomic constraint equations represent the relationship between the coordinates of the points (markers) and geometrical characteristics (length, angles). Other constraint equations can be formulated to describe the constant distant between two points belonging to the same rigid element.

Different types of parameters are included in the constraint equations: motion tracking data, parameters of the model and coordinates of the point of interest [18]. The motion tracking data are the coordinates of markers obtained from the measurements. The constant parameters of the model are the geometrical characteristics of the rigid elements and position of markers on the rigid elements. The coordinates of the point of interest (like the coordinates of the joints) are variables and their values will modify during the simulation. To estimate the number of parameters of the virtual model which can be computed, first the constraints equations have to be formulated.

The maximum number of equation which can be solved in each frame of the simulation is equal to the number of independent data obtained from the measurements (tracking data). The number of independent data is according to the type of marker and number of markers on each rigid body:

- In case of one marker attached to a rigid element and the marker is returning the space position (x, y and z), then the number of independent coordinates is three;
- In case of one marker attached to a rigid element and the marker is tracking the position in plane (retro-reflective marker or position obtained by image processing), then the number of independent coordinates is two;
- If two markers are attached to a rigid element, then the number of independent coordinates are five in the spatial case, and three in the planar case;
- If three markers are attached to a rigid element, then the number of independent coordinates is six in the spatial case (in the planar case no new information can be retrieved from the third marker).

The value of the desired parameters can be obtained using noise rejection by filtering and will be presented in the next section). The following two case studies are demonstrating the proposed method.

2.1 Case A

In Fig. 1 are presented three elements (1, 2, 3) linked with revolute joint M and N (corresponding to three linked body parts as leg, arm, hand or fingers). The 2D (plane) movements of the elements are tracked with optical marker (A, B and C) on each. The total number of independent data available for the reconstruction of the virtual model is 6 (the x and y coordinates of the markers).

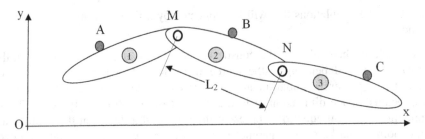

Fig. 1. The articulated model of the tracked elements, Case A

This model has two revolute joints between the rigid parts 1–2 and 2–3. The joints have one degree of freedom, so two constraint equations can be formulated. These equations correspond to the fact that the center of the revolute joints (M and N) are belonging to both of the connected elements, so the distances between these two point and the markers attached to the elements are constant during the simulation. Five constraint equations can be formulated between the coordinates of the points A (x_A, y_A), B (x_B, y_B), C (x_C, y_C), M (x_M, y_N) and N (x_N, y_N) (1):

$$\begin{cases} ((x_M - x_A)^2 + (y_M - y_A)^2)^{1/2} = d_{MA} \\ ((x_B - x_M)^2 + (y_B - y_M)^2)^{1/2} = d_{BM} \\ ((x_N - x_B)^2 + (y_N - y_B)^2)^{1/2} = d_{NB} \\ ((x_C - x_N)^2 + (y_C - y_N)^2)^{1/2} = d_{CN} \\ ((x_M - x_N)^2 + (y_M - y_N)^2)^{1/2} = L_2, \end{cases} \tag{1}$$

where d_{MA} represents the distance between the points M and A (similarly for the other points), and L_2 is the unknown length of element 2. In (1) the coordinates of M and N are not known and their values are modifying during the simulation (four unknowns), so only one of the other parameters can be computed. Presuming that the position on 1 and 3 of the marker A and C are known, and the distance between the MN line and B (known location of B on 2) is also known, then equations in (1) can be solved by iterative methods to obtain L_2 for each position of the articulated system given by the measurement of the tracking system. But the measurements are corrupted by noise, so the length of 2 has to be obtained by filtering.

2.2 Case B

In this case the movements of the same three elements are tracked by four markers (Fig. 2): three markers as in the previous case on each elements and marker D rigidly attached to element 2. The total number of independent data available for the reconstruction of the virtual model in this case is 7. To the five constraint equations of (1), two more constant distance constraints can be added:

$$\begin{cases} ((x_D - x_M)^2 + (y_D - y_M)^2)^{1/2} = d_{DM} \\ ((x_D - x_N)^2 + (y_D - y_N)^2)^{1/2} = d_{DN} \end{cases} \tag{2}$$

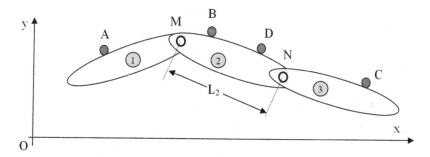

Fig. 2. The articulated model of the tracked elements, Case B

The unknown length of L_2 can be obtained also if the positions of the markers on each element are known. The nonlinear Eqs. (1) and (2) were solved using the Newton-Raphson algorithm.

3   Parameter Estimation with Bayes Filter

The inputs in the Bayes filter are measured parameters obtained from motion tracking as coordinates of the markers (CoordM) attached to the elements (A, B, C and D). Each of the marker's position is providing two parameters (assuming that the model is two dimensional). An example of tracking data is presented in Fig. 3 for Case A and Fig. 4 for Case B. The data is corrupted by noise, caused by the tracking process, replicated by a Gaussian probability density function.

In the first step the value of the searched parameter is estimated and the true will be chosen from an interval given by a minimum and a maximum of the estimation. In the case studies presented the searched parameter is L_2, and the proposed algorithm will find the true value between $L_{2\,min}$ and $L_{2\,max}$. This interval is discretized using a small step of ΔL_2, so the true value will be searched in following set of $L_{2estimation}$:

$$L_{2estimation} = \left\{L_{2min},\ L_{2min} + \Delta L_2,\ L_{2min} + 2\Delta L_2,\ldots L_{2max}\right\} \tag{3}$$

The Bayesian filter converts each measurement in the most likely hypothesis. The probability density function will be computed separately for each estimation of L_2. One by one, for each of the available tracking data the following process is repeated for every possible value of the searched parameter:

(a) for the current coordinated of the markers (CoordM) the length of L_2 is computed solving (1) for Case A and (1) and (2) for Case B;

(b) The likelihood of the measurement is computed for each estimation of L_2 (3), comparing each estimation with the current length of L_2 offerend by the measurements and assuming Gaussian distribution of the noise:

$$\Pr(L_2|L_{2estimation},\text{CoordM}) = \frac{1}{\sigma\sqrt{2\pi}}e^{-\frac{(L_2 - L_{2estimation})^2}{2\sigma^2}} \tag{4}$$

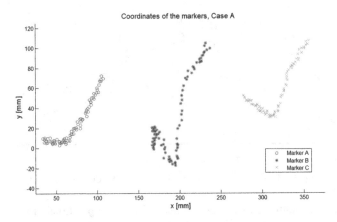

Fig. 3. The recorded coordinates of the markers, Case A

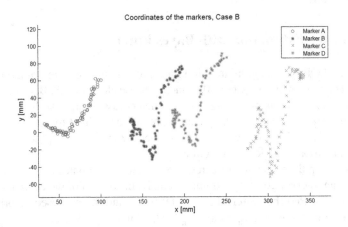

Fig. 4. The recorded coordinates of the markers, Case A

where σ is the standard deviation, as a measure of the amount of dispersion of the tracking data. High standard deviation indicates that the measured coordinates are spread out over a large range of values from the real locations.

(c) According to the Bayes rule, the likelihood and the prior can be combined to obtain the posterior probability:

$$\Pr(L_{2estimation}|L_2, \text{CoordM}) = \Pr(L_2|\text{CoordM}) \cdot \Pr(L_2|L_{2estimation}, \text{CoordM}) \qquad (5)$$

(d) The posterior probability is normalized and used as prior in the next iteration and tracking data.

These four steps are repeated for each of the available coordinates of the markers. The modification of the probability distribution after 50, 100 and 500 steps is illustrated in Fig. 5. After 200–300 steps the maximum value of the probability is already an indication of the true (Fig. 5).

The true length of L_2 will correspond to the highest value of the maximum proba-bilities from each of the investigated estimation of the set (3). Figure 6 (for Case A) and Fig. 7 (for Case B) are showing the computed length of L_2 corresponding to the maximum values of the probabilities obtained from the first 500 noisy measurements. These results correspond to a standard deviation of 15 mm for the positions of the markers in each frame of the simulation.

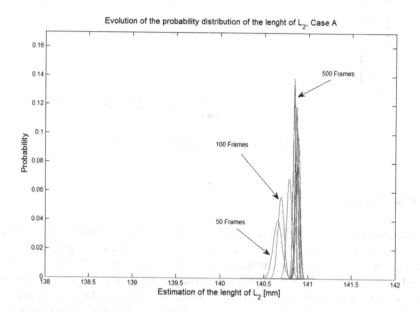

Fig. 5. The evolution of the probability distribution

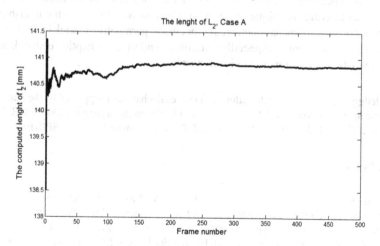

Fig. 6. The most likely length of L_2 (Case A)

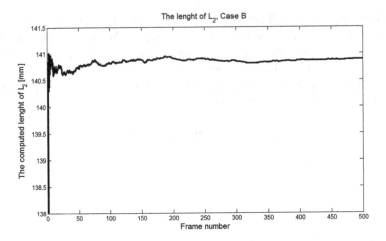

Fig. 7. The most likely length of L_2 (Case B)

4 Conclusions

The obtained algorithm is well-suited to identifying parameters (geometrical characteristics) of articulated models in the presence of noisy data. The tracking data obtained from markers attached to the articulated model has to satisfy the physical constraint offered by the mechanical joints. The constraint equations of the joints are providing the parameters of the articulated model, but it is subject to uncertainty due to noisy tracking data. The number of parameter of the virtual model which can be found during the simulation is depending on the number of constraint equation of the articulated model. The Bayesian filtering technique provides an efficient way to obtain the distributional estimate of the unknown parameters. An accurate parametric model is important in virtual reality applications, especially for force rendering in haptic feedback and to produce realistic interactions with virtual words.

Acknowledgments. The research leading to these results has been supported by the Partnership Programme in priority domains - PN-II, which runs with the financial support of MEN-UEFISCDI, Project no. 227 /2014, System for Diagnosis and Therapy of Spine Diseases (SPINE).

References

1. Iglesias, R., Prada, E., Uribe, A., Garcia-Alonso, A., Casado, S., Gutierrez, T.: Assembly simulation on collaborative haptic virtual environments. In: The 15th International Conference in Central Europe on Computer Graphics, Visualization and Computer Vision 2007 WSCG'2007 in Co-operation with EUROGRAPHICS 2007, pp. 241–248 (2007)
2. Burdea, G.C., Coiffet, P.: Virtual Reality Technology. Wiley, New York (2003)
3. Renaud, P., Vivas, A., Andreff, N., Poignet, P., Martinet, P., Pierrot, F.: Kinematic and dynamic identification of parallel mechanisms. Control Eng. Pract. **14**(9), 1099–1109 (2006)

4. Barragán, P.R., Kaelbling, L.P., Lozano-Pérez, T.: Interactive bayesian identification of kinematic mechanisms. In: IEEE International Conference on Robotics and Automation (ICRA 2014), pp. 2013–2020. IEEE (2014)

5. Otte, S., Kulick, J., Toussaint, M., Brock, O.: Entropy-based strategies for physical exploration of the environment's degrees of freedom. In: IEEE/RSJ International Conference Intelligent Robots and Systems IROS 2014, pp. 615–622. IEEE (2014)

6. Katz, D., Brock, O.: Manipulating articulated objects with interactive perception. In: IEEE International Conference on Robotics and Automation ICRA 2008, pp. 272–277. IEEE (2008)

7. Westhoff, C., Troje, N.F.: Kinematic cues for person identification from biological motion. Percept. Psychophys. **69**(2), 241–253 (2007)

8. Batou, A., Soize, C.: Rigid multibody system dynamics with uncertain rigid bodies. Multibody Sys. Dyn. **27**(3), 285–319 (2012)

9. Sandu, A., Sandu, C., Ahmadian, M.: Modeling multibody systems with uncertainties. Part I: theoretical and computational aspects. Multibody Sys. Dyn. **15**(4), 369–391 (2006)

10. Körding, K.P., Wolpert, D.M.: Bayesian decision theory in sensorimotor control. Trends Cogn. Sci. **10**(7), 319–326 (2006)

11. Bretthorst, G.L.: An introduction to parameter estimation using Bayesian probability theory. In: Fougère, P.F. (ed.) Maximum Entropy and Bayesian Methods. Fundamental Theories of Physics, pp. 53–79. Springer, The Netherland (1990)

12. Endo, Y., Kanai, S., Miyata, N., Kouchi, M., Mochimaru, M., Konno, J., Ogasawara, M., Shimokawa, M.: Optimization - based grasp posture generation method of digital hand for virtual ergonomics assessment. SAE Int. J. Passeng. Cars - Electron. Electr. Syst. **1**(1), 590–598 (2009)

13. Rusák, Z., Antonya, C., Horváth, I.: Methodology for controlling contact forces in interactive grasping simulation. Int. J. Virtual Reality **10**(2), 1–10 (2011)

14. Abhishek, S., Vance, J.M., Oliver, J.H.: Virtual reality for assembly methods prototyping: a review. Virtual Reality **15**(1), 5–20 (2011)

15. Tzafestas, C., Coiffet, P.: Computing optimal forces for generalised kinesthetic feedback on the human hand during virtual grasping and manipulation. In: IEEE International Conference on Robotics and Automation, vol. 1, pp. 118–123. IEEE (1997)

16. Haug, E.J.: Computer Aided Kinematics And Dynamics of Mechanical Systems. Allyn and Bacon, Boston (1989)

17. Talabă, D.: Mechanical models and the mobility of robots and mechanisms. Robotica **33**(01), 181–193 (2015)

18. Antonya, C., Butnariu, S., Pozna, C.: Parameter computation of the hand model in virtual grasping. In: 5th IEEE International Conference on Cognitive Infocommunications CogInfoCom 2014, pp. 173–177 (2014)

Body Tracking as a Generative Tool
for Experience Design

Monica Bordegoni, Serena Camere[✉], Giandomenico Caruso,
and Umberto Cugini

Department of Mechanics, Politecnico Di Milano, via La Masa 1,
20156 Milan, Italy
{monica.bordegoni, serena.camere, giandomenico.caruso,
umberto.cugini}@polimi.it

Abstract. Beyond ergonomic measurements, the study of human movements can help designers in exploring the rich, non-verbal communication of users' perception of products. This paper explores the ability of human gestures to express subjective experiences and therefore, to inform the design process at its early stages. We will investigate the traditional techniques used in the Experience Design domain to observe human gestures, and propose a method to couple Experience-driven design approach with Motion Capture technique. This will allow integrating qualitative user observations with quantitative and measurable data. However, the richness of information that Motion Capture can retrieve is usually inaccessible for designers. This paper presents a method to visualize human motion data so that designers can make sense of them, and use them as the starting point for concept generation.

Keywords: Motion Capture · Body Tracking · Concept design · User experience · Data visualization

1 Introduction

Human movements are a physical representation of the way people perceive a space, a product and more in general, their world. We interact with products moving around them, touching them, with bodily expressions that are totally subjective and reflect our personal experiences. The movements we perform to interact with an object define the boundaries of a space where subject and object are interrelated (i.e. the space of interaction). The notion of spatial interaction refers to a spatiality of sensation, which should be distinguished from a spatiality of position [1]. Thus, human movements are interesting for the design domain in their ability to embody the user experience, offering a rich amount of knowledge on the human-product interaction. Traditionally, the study of human postures and gestures has been carried out with a quantitative approach for ergonomic assessments, to check functional requirements and usability features of products. Product designers tend instead to prefer qualitative observations of users' movements for their greater feasibility in conditions of limited time and resources. To study human movements quantitatively, Motion Capture is considered the most accurate technique, giving a rich set of information on trajectories, position,

V.G. Duffy (Ed.): DHM 2015, Part II, LNCS 9185, pp. 122–133, 2015.
DOI: 10.1007/978-3-319-21070-4_13

orientation and speed of users' movements. It is commonly employed, coupled with Virtual Reality technologies, at the end of the design process to assess aspects such as ergonomics and usability. However, designers rarely adopt this technique. Surely, the technical skills required implementing a tracking session, the complex amount of data retrieved, and the absence of guidelines discourage designers to make use of Motion Capture technologies. Moreover, the computational form of tracking data results largely inaccessible for designers: they need a flexible and meaningful representation that can be "read" from their perspective. For instance, to effectively support the design process, motion data should be elaborated to suit 3D modelling software tools. No extensive method was found in literature addressing the visualization of human movements for concept design purposes. In this research, human movements are studied for their ability to nurture and inform subsequent design actions. The traditional methods used to observe human gestures will be explored, comparing the quantitative/qualitative approaches. Subsequently, we will reflect on the possibilities offered by Motion Capture technologies, and the limitations and barriers they present to be used in the design process. This paper introduces a method to use Motion Capture technologies with a designers' perspective, at the beginning of the design process. Finally, we will describe the application of the method on a case study in the automotive design sector.

2 The Study of Human Movements in Design

Human movements are commonly considered a matter of ergonomic studies, to assess products' usability and fitness to users. In some applications, for example workplaces, health care, design for impairments or transportation design, it involved the study of human postures to create products that do not harm users, but rather facilitate physical well being. Thus, being a matter of health and security, ergonomic studies sometimes could exploit expensive technologies as Body Tracking and Motion Capture to measure users' anthropometry in relation to the product. In these fields, in fact, a quantitative assessment is necessary to gather a specific and punctual knowledge on a broad spectrum of users, and therefore shape a product that matches users' needs. This kind of user tests is usually conducted at the end of the design process, when the design concept has already been formed, and it needs to be validated. Motion Capture technologies have been used in several studies to support these validations [2–5].

Conversely, product designers traditionally prefer to employ qualitative methods to observe users. These methods differ on knowledge claims, strategies employed and nature of data. Qualitative research uses instead a vertical approach to dig deeper in users' latent desires and needs [6]. In this way, the focus of research is not only the functional requirements of the product, but the holistic user experience [7]. Human movements are therefore approached with a different attitude and they are usually studied through video-recorded user observations. The analysis of these videos provides designers with qualitative insights that heavily rely on their subjective interpretation, and it is often conducted without a structured approach. Yet, the richness of information that comes from a qualitative observation is undoubtedly a source of inspiration for designers, to infer knowledge on the human-product interaction. Thus, the study of human movements can give important insights even in the early phases of the design process. To improve the significance of the user observations, we believe that a mixed-method approach [8] is the most effective, combining quantitative measurements and qualitative observations. The traditionally dualist perspective of quantitative vs. qualitative research faded over the last years, leaving room for the collection of numeric information (i.e. measurable data) simultaneously or sequentially to text information (i.e. interviews, etc.).

Recently, the study of human motions gained attention in the field of Interaction Design. The possibility to capture the embodied experience and use it as the starting point of the design process inspired several studies on the topic, adopting Motion Capture technologies. From an art perspective, the project Bodycloud [9] captured the movements of a dancer to generate a sculpture visualizing his graceful gestures. The work is rooted in the figurative arts, yet it provides a reference framework to understand how the visualization of movement has been tackled in the artistic domain. Another study presented a reverse engineering of human movements for architectural design [10]. The concept of the architectural space was designed as a negative shape of users' volumes of motions. The grounding work of Hansen and Morrison [11] adopts instead a semiotic approach to organise the properties and peculiarities of human motion data. The core modalities of movement (e.g. the velocity) are related to their specific characteristics (e.g. the speed) and to the corresponding best visual description (e.g. the size of mark) in a Movement Schema [11]. In this way, the richness of motion data is organised according to semiotic criteria, to be represented in a meaningful visualization. This approach can be considered the first step to make sense of human motion data and integrate them in the design process. However, literature does not offer a comprehensive method or structured guidelines to support designers facing the complexity of motion tracking. From the studies analysed, it emerges a necessity to preserve a degree of interpretation from the designer, not over-imposing meaning to the visualization of movement data. Furthermore, there is no clear agreement on which modalities of movement should be represented and, more important, how they should be characterised visually. The approach suggested by Hansen and Morrison [11] seems the most valid. Yet, we argue that designers need a representation that fits their traditional design skills, so that they can use them as reference to shape the concept design. In the next section, we present a method to capture human movements with a mixed-method approach, combining quantitative and qualitative observations of the user experience, to generate a 3D representation that can be used as the starting point of the design process. The method has been applied in a case study in the automotive design domain.

3 The Method

The method presented here couples Motion Capture techniques with traditional qualitative observation of human movements. Motion Capture technology offers a large number of benefits but also some limitations. The information retrieved through these systems must be processed in order to effectively support designers. A tracking session needs a careful setup, expensive equipment and technical skills that are unusual for designers. Moreover, the data generated with Motion Capture are usually largely inaccessible for designers due to their computational form. They are often presented as a complex aggregate of numerical data, which are difficult to interpret. This research is a first attempt to face these issues and make the use of Motion Capture techniques more accessible for designers. Figure 1 presents an overview of the method that we are now going to illustrate. The first thing designers need to understand is the focus of their study: basically, what they want to record with Motion Capture systems. To effectively define the specific focus of the experiment and to identify the 'key phenomena' to track quantitatively, we suggest relying these choices on some preliminary user observations. In our approach, we recommend a qualitative user observation in field-research modality, using video recordings, interviews, questionnaires, etc., to identify the critical issues of the user-product interaction. More generally, designers should implement a quick user observation adopting the traditional methods and tools employed for co-creation and participatory design [6], according to the specific design case. The most common and effective method to collect rich records of user experience is the "recall and describe" [12]. Participants to the study are first video-recorded while performing an action (e.g. trying a product or going through their morning routine). Soon after the task has been completed, they are asked to look at the video and comment on their subjective experience, while the interviewer asks them specific questions. The results can be then analysed to establish which are the most relevant issues to investigate in the subsequent tracking session.

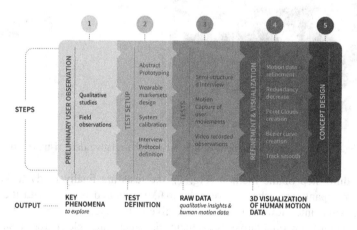

Fig. 1. Outline of the method and the output for each step

The second step of the method (Fig. 1) involves the setup for the Motion Capture testing phase. At this stage, a number of choices must be taken. First of all, designers need to consider, according to the specific design problem, which areas of the human body to track. In our method, we defined eight areas of interest (Fig. 2), which altogether outline the boundaries of human body. This step is crucial to understand the output data: the higher number of tracked areas, the greater will be the complexity of the information retrieved. Secondly, basing on this choice, wearable marker-sets must be designed to comply with several criteria. For example, marker-sets must be asymmetric and of three-dimensional shape as much as possible, to prevent occlusions and failures in tracking. In this study, we produced a set of wearables combining a rigid body that supports the markers and a flexible and adjustable strip that can fit any user. Another important issue to face at this stage is the testing environment: Motion Capture systems involve a lab setting, but users need a physical representation of the product they must interact with. This method adopts the Abstract Prototyping technique from Human Centred Design [13] to create a rough and synthetic prototype of an artefact, avoiding realistic details. Abstract Prototyping allows the creation of quick and cheap setup so that users can interact with a prototypical object. As an example, the abstract setup in Fig. 2 reconstructs half of a car's interiors, to physically limit the users space of interaction. Lastly, in this stage designers must face the Motion Capture system calibration, considering how many cameras are needed, which configurations, at what distance, etc.

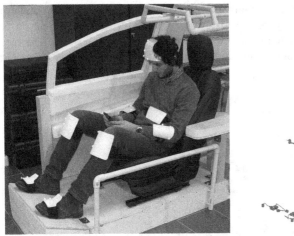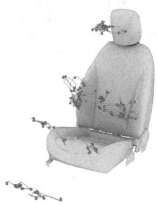

Fig. 2. The user in a moment of the test and the relative data visualization

In the third step of the method (Fig. 1), the tests are finally ready to be implemented. Participants are asked to wear the marker-sets and interact with the abstract prototype, while interviewed on their subjective experiences. Basing on the themes discovered in the first qualitative assessment, designers are able to focus on the key phenomena that are meaningful to tackle the design problem. In this method, we suggest the choice of the semi-structured interview technique [14], which enables the interviewer to follow new ideas and paths of research that might come up with users, although still basing him/herself on a pre-determined set of questions. The users' movements and interaction are tracked with the Motion Capture system and video-recorded as well. Videos are in fact relevant as a reference to refine the motion data, when, for example, some occlusions may occur.

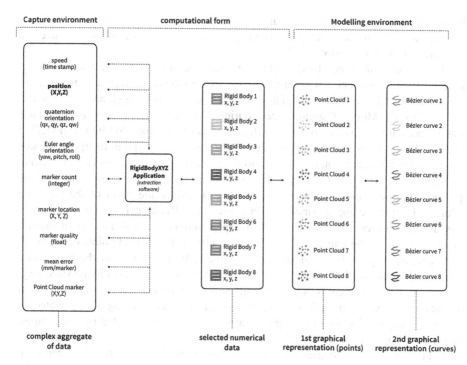

Fig. 3. Steps of data visualization necessary to achieve a 3D representation in a standard NURBS modelling software.

The fourth phase represents the core of the method (Fig. 1). In this step, we provide a method to manage the results of the tracking session and to visualize them in a 3D modelling environment. During the tracking session, a large set of raw data has been acquired. Although several measures can be taken to prevent the greatest part of possible accidents, occlusions, parts to be trimmed, misidentification of markers and other issues can occur. Once refined, data can be exported as a datasheet that gathers numerical information on the tracked movements (Fig. 3). For this reason, data are difficult to manage for designers, who need instead a 3D representation to use them as the starting point of their design process. Moreover, at this step designers might choose to extract only specific information on the users' motion. This method focuses on the visualization of the trajectories (i.e. position over time and orientation) of human movements. To identify this information in the complex datasheet, we developed a simple software application able associate it to each marker-set and generate sub-files listing the X, Y, Z position of the centroid of the marker configuration for each frame. The goal was here to generate new datasheets that could comply with standard NURBS-based modelling software. Once imported the sub-files into the 3D environment, numeric data are represented as Point Clouds, which represents the first step towards a sensible visualization of data. Yet, Point Clouds have still limited possibilities in terms of characterisation and modifications possible: for example, it is not possible to differentiate participant, tasks and the specific marker-sets associated to each area of the human body.

The creation of Point Clouds yields the construction of curves that show the trajectory of the movement. To generate curves, which effectively represent trajectories, the raw Points Clouds have to be elaborated. At first, due to the high amount of points collected by the Motion Capture system during a single trial, the sampling frequency was reduced from 100 fps to 16 fps. Then the data were imported into a modelling software and various curve-generation methods were tested. Spline interpolation was considered not effective since errors due to the precision of the Motion Capture system make the curve irregular. Consequently, the visualization and the interpretation of the generated spline is difficult. Bézier curve, instead, reduce the effect of the precision errors and the curve appear smoother. In particular, a Bézier curve with degree = 11 was used. However, the curves may still appear redundant in some part of the trajectory. To reduce the number of the redundant curves, the control points of the curve were deceased up to 10 % of the original ones. At this point, all the trajectories corresponding to users' movements and interactions can be generated in the same way. In order to visualize them in a more significantly, the assignment of a graphical representation reference to each variable is needed. This can be highly correlated to designers' subjectivity; as an example, trajectories can be represented by small pipes, each participant can be attributed a specific colour, and symbols can highlight the differentiation between themes (Fig. 4). In other cases, the distinction between each marker-sets can be more meaningful than the one on participants, and colours can be distributed according to this criterion. Anyhow, at the end of this phase, designers will achieve a structured visualization of human movements that depict the user-product interaction in a 3D modelling software. Thus, they are able to exploit these data as the starting point of the design process, to start shaping the concept design.

4   The Case Study

The method presented here was used during a case study developed in collaboration with Design Innovation, a design agency based in Milan, and the R&D department of Fiat Chrysler Automobiles Group (FCA Group). The design agency was commissioned a user-centred research to redefine the car interiors for passengers aside the driver seat. More specifically, the passenger seat is usually designed as the symmetrical counterpart of the driver seat, sometimes even lacking some features (such as the lumbar support). However, driver and passenger have highly different needs in terms of comfort, safety and freedom of movements. The automotive company asked then to generate new concepts of the passenger seat with a special focus on comfort and UX. Following our method, Design Innovation conducted a first round of user observations with 9 participants, 5 male and 4 female, video-recording them with a frontal GoPro© [15] camera and one hand-camera in the back seats. Participants were brought on a medium-length journey in a car (average 40 min), seating on the passenger side, after which they were interviewed about the level of comfort, their needs and their expectations. Through these first results, designers identified five key issues to further explore: (1) the assessment of comfort in posture; (2) the interaction with either people or objects in the back seats; (3) the placement of personal items, such as bags, coats etc.; (4) the interaction with smart devices; (5) the users' perception of the space. These problem areas were established as correlated to alterations in posture and gestures. As in the second step of the method, the test setup has been implemented by building the Abstract Prototype of half a car interior, to reconstruct the car space around the test participants and to physically limit their space of interaction. In this setup, the longitudinal left side of the car was considered to prevent the Motion Capture system from visual occlusions, which would affect the capture results.

The tests were conducted using a Motion Capture system based on 6 Flex 3 cameras by OptiTrack© [16]. The cameras were placed at a height of 220 cm, equally distant from each other. The human movements have been tracked using 8 wearable marker-sets composed of a rigid part mounted onto a flexible strip. For each marker-sets, a different configurations of retro-reflective markers was arranged, changing the number and disposition to prevent misidentification and tracking errors. The Motion Capture system was capturing the position and orientation of each marker-sets, corresponding to the selected parts of the human body. In the Motion Capture system, Rigid Bodies are defined as clusters of reflective markers in a unique configuration, which allows them to be identified and tracked in a cloud of 3D points. It is possible to track multiple Rigid Bodies at a time in full 6 degrees of freedom (position and orientation, 6DOF). The shapes of the marker-sets were chosen to maximize tracking capability. Spherical reflective markers were preferred, as they guaranteed the most stable and accurate 3D tracking. Markers were arranged in asymmetrical and unique configurations to reduce the likelihood of misidentification and swapping.

In our study we selected 9 participants (5 female, 4 male, age 25-52). They have been informed of video recording and told about the test goals and objectives. The participants claimed to be at ease with the wearable devices and the researchers could notice that after few minutes of testing, people tended to forget about cameras and markers, focusing on their own experiences. The test was split in two phases: during the former participants were asked to recall one meaningful experience as a passenger in the car. This first phase relied on the Open Interview technique. The second part of the interview was instead using a semi-structured approach, following a set of pre-determined questions to tackle the problem areas defined in the pilot study. Participants were interviewed on their subjective perceptions of the car interior and to recall and describe their personal experiences as passengers. While doing so, they were asked to show the positions they assume in the car and the movements they perform, for example, to grab their personal belongings in the back seats. During the tests, we tracked the users' movements and gestures inside the abstract set-up. The 3D capture of their movements generated a set of human motion data, from which it was possible to obtain a volumetric 3D model representing the (desired) space of interaction for passengers.

As in the fourth step of the method, the raw data needed to be processed before taking shape in the 3D modelling environment. We performed all the operations described at this stage to discard any error occurring during the tests, and we exported the datasheet including the whole aggregate of information generated in the tracking

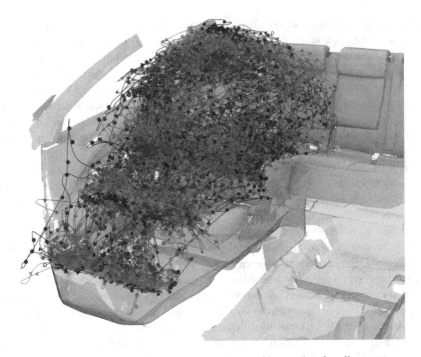

Fig. 4. Rendering of the complete volume of interaction for all users

session. Through the software application developed specifically for this method, we were then able to extract the eight sub-files listing the X, Y, Z position of every marker-set for each tracking session. At this stage, we were then able to import the sub-files in a NURBS-based modelling software and to create the associated Point Clouds. Following the last steps of the method, it was possible to achieve the visualizations in Fig. 4. The complete 3D model gathering the data of every user, some specific visualizations and the qualitative analysis of the interviews was submitted to the designers and the R&D department to start and inform the design process.

5   Results and Discussion

The amount of data obtained in the case study, coupling Motion Capture technique with qualitative observations of users, supplied information on the trajectories of the human movements and the areas where users interact the most. This will give the possibility to shape new concept of the passenger seat as a negative model, using the data as a starting point for the design process. The interview results provided other interesting insights, outlining some critical issues for every task. These suggestions reflected the users' movements in the corresponding 3D visualization (Fig. 4). Most of the results confirmed the insights collected in the first user observation, yet they provided deeper information. For instance, the tests showed the need of a greater flexibility in the movements, highlighting the participants' willingness to interact with the back seats, especially in presence of children, pets and, in general, for long journeys. They showed also to be uncomfortable in their postures, especially with their legs and arms. They claimed to perceive the need of a flexible lumbar support and more space for legs, as well as they would appreciate to have armrests. The design team was then asked for feedbacks on how they would use the complete package of results coming from the user tests. Through a questionnaire, they asserted the significant value of the method in the former stages of the design process, to inspire and inform them. The 3D nature of data was specifically found as an interesting standpoint to design the seat *"as a negative shape"*, making the *"form follow the data"*. In this way, *"the design of the style is based on solid, reliable data, merging effectiveness and style"*. Yet, they also suggested some improvements of the methods. For instance, they claimed the need for an interface to navigate through the several variables, as well as the possibility to explore other information on the users' movements (e.g. *"sudden changes"; "the time spent in a certain posture"; "the frequency of a specific gesture"*). Moreover, they would largely appreciate the integration of a mobile system for Motion Capture, and the absence (or at least flatness) of markers.

As shown here, the results of this first case are encouraging, although the method still presents some limitations. However, this study clearly showed the possibility to use Motion Capture systems as generative tools able to inform the design process and stimulate the generation of design concepts, rather than simply validating them. What is particularly interesting for designers is the chance to have a flexible 3D representation of users' movements, in a modelling environment they commonly use in their design process. This makes the data generated much more useful and appreciable for them, as designers can directly exploit them as the starting point to shape the new product. Our method, providing a step-by-step guidelines and a careful description of every action, supports designers who wish to integrate a semi-quantitative approach in their user observations. Obviously, some technical limitations are still present: as mentioned before, the system calibration, the design of the wearable marker-sets, and more in general the test setup may heavily influence the delicate phase of capturing human gestures and generate unexpected errors in the tracking session. Other difficulties lie in the intrinsic nature of Motion Capture systems: for example, to suit better the traditional approach of designers, a portable toolkit could give unexpected possibilities. Lastly, even if the method simplifies the transition from computational data to their 3D representation, a user interface that allows a greater integration between NURBS-based modelling applications and Motion Capture system could largely increase the chances of adopting this technology for user observations in the design process.

6   Conclusions

In this paper, we presented a novel method to use Motion Capture systems to inform and nurture the design process at the early stages. This method exploits the richness of information that can be gathered in a tracking session, to generate a flexible, three-dimensional representation of human movements in a modelling environment, so that designers can use it to start shaping a new product. The method describes a step-by-step guideline to implement a tracking session and couple a quantitative observation with qualitative interviews, following a mixed-method approach. In this way, human movements can be used to infer users' personal space of interaction with a product and give important insights for the design process. Adopting this method guarantees the possibility to extract the raw data of the tracking session to refine them and to generate a meaningful visualization for designers. In this paper, we presented one case study in the automotive design domain. Meanwhile, all the products involving a spatial interaction could be potentially suitable to test the method, since, in these cases, the study of human gestures acquires more value. More specifically, other case studies can be conducted easily on other transportation means, such as airplanes or trains. Other fields, as for example the design of home/office stationeries, furniture, and workstations can be also a source of interesting applications. Lastly, many sports can be an interesting field of application. As a conclusion, we argue that the issue of visualizing motion data for the design process has been sufficiently addressed by this study. Future studies can instead focus on designers' viewpoint, to understand how they can exploit this kind of data and the subsequent design actions.

Acknowledgements. The authors gratefully acknowledge the support of FCA Group and Design Innovation. We wish to sincerely thank Enrico Pisino and Giorgio Masoero (CRF), Carmelo Di Bartolo, Duccio Mauri, Filippo Lorini and Mark Salerno (Design Innovation) for their precious technical and methodological support to develop the case study. We also express our gratitude to Matteo Troiani for his contribution in processing the Motion Capture raw data.

References

1. Merleau-Ponty, M.: Phenomenology of Perception. Routledge & Kegan Paul, London (1962)
2. Bordegoni, M., Caruso, G.: Mixed reality distributed platform for collaborative design review of automotive interiors. Virtual Phys. Prototyping 7(4), 243–259 (2012)
3. Du, J., Duffy, V.G.: A methodology for assessing industrial workstations using optical motion capture integrated with digital human models. Occup. Ergon. 7(1), 11–25 (2007)
4. Chaffin, D.B.: On simulating human reach motions for ergonomics analyses. Hum. Factors Ergon. Manuf. 12(3), 235–247 (2002)
5. Mengoni, M., Peruzzini, M., Mandorli, F., Bordegoni, M., Caruso, G. Performing ergonomic analysis in virtual environments: a structured protocol to assess humans interaction. In: 28th Computers and Information in Engineering Conference, Parts A and B, vol. 3, pp. 1461–1472. ASME, New York (2008)
6. Visser, F.S., Stappers, P.J., Van der Lugt, R., Sanders, E.B.: Contextmapping: experiences from practice. CoDesign 1(2), 119–149 (2005)
7. Hassenzahl, M.: Experience Design: Technology for all the Right Reasons. Morgan & Claypool, San Francisco (2010)
8. Creswell, J.W.: Research Design: Qualitative, Quantitative, and Mixed Approaches. Sage, Thousand Oaks, CA (2003)
9. Perret, R.: Bodycloud (Unpublished work, 2010). http://raphaelperret.ch/bodycloud/. Accessed 24 Nov 2014

10. Vroman, L., Naveda, L., Leman, M., Thierry, L.: Generating tacit knowledge through motion: a vision on the matter of space. Art, Des. Commun. High. Educ. **10**(2), 255–270 (2012)
11. Hansen, L.A., Morrison, A.: Materializing movement. designing for movement-based digital interaction. Int. J. Des. **8**(1), 29–42 (2013)
12. Laurans, G.: On the Moment-to-moment measurement of emotion during person-product interaction. Unpublished Ph.D. thesis, TU Delft (2011)
13. IDEO Human Centered Design Toolkit (2008). http://www.hcdconnect.org. Accessed 24 Nov 2014
14. Denzin, N.K., Lincoln, Y.S.: The discipline and practice of qualitative research. In: Denzin, N.K., Lincoln, Y.S. (eds.) Handbook of Qualitative Research, pp. 1–28. Sage Publication, Thousand Oaks (2000)
15. GoPro Official Website (2014). http://it.gopro.com/. Accessed 24 Nov 2014
16. Motion Capture Systems (2014). http://www.naturalpoint.com/optitrack/. Accessed 30 Nov 2014

Modeling and Simulating Lifting Task
of Below-Knee Amputees

Yan Fu[✉], Shiqi Li, Qian Chen, and Wei Zhou

School of Mechanical Science and Engineering, Huazhong University of Science
and Technolgy, Wuhan 430074, Hubei Province, China
Laura_fy@mail.hust.edu.cn

Abstract. Lifting is a common activity to below-knee amputees (BKA) in
occupational and living occasions. Appropriate lifting posture is crucial to
physical safety and health to those BKAs. Often healthy parts of BKAs might be
hurt due to extra and asymmetric force exertion compensating for deficiency of
disabled body parts. To prevent further hurt, a validated biomechanical model
describing lifting is essential to analyze lifting behavior of those handicapped. In
this study, twelve BKAs were recruited to lift 45 N weights from the floor.
Subjects are asked to lift three levels of weights (0 N, 30 N, 60 N) by two
postures: squat lifting and stoop lifting. Twelve non-BKAs were recruited as
comparison group to study the variance caused by disability. Calculated forces
based on Anybody were compared with EMG signals of body parts on spine and
thigh. A framework of three-level constraints models were applied to adjust the
difference between calculated forces and EMGs and the results validate the
model.

Keywords: Below-knee · Amputees · Lifting · Modeling

1 Introduction

Among various work-related activities, lifting, awkward posture, and heavy physical
work have been indicated to have strong relationship with lumbar musculoskeletal
disorders (MSDs) [1]. Combination of lifting with lateral bending or twisting has been
identified as a frequent cause of back injury in the workplace [2, 3]. Search for an
appropriate lifting technique has thus attracted considerate attention due to high risk of
injury. Compression force limits have been recommended [4] for safer material
handling maneuvers based on the premise that excessive compression loads could
cause injury.

Role of lifting in low-back injuries is well recognized in the literature as described
before. Despite researches in low-back injuries, literatures on safer lifting methods are
still controversial. Among all methods lifting low-lying objects, squat lifting (i.e., knee
bent and back straight) and stoop lifting (i.e., knee straight and back bent) are two main
methods, and the former is considered safer than the latter, for squat lifting brings the
load closer to the body center compared to stoop lifting and reduce the extra demand on
back muscles to counterbalance additional moments. Few further researches comparing
two methods from a biomechanical view and the importance of selection between two

© Springer International Publishing Switzerland 2015
V.G. Duffy (Ed.): DHM 2015, Part II, LNCS 9185, pp. 134–143, 2015.
DOI: 10.1007/978-3-319-21070-4_14

postures are downplayed [5]. And many workers, without any occupational safety guidelines, prefer the stoop lift over squat lift. There are other conclusions that there is an increased physiological cost and more muscle fatigue are developed when squat lifting [6]. The inability to accurately determine the loads on trunk active and passive components as well as the system stability margin appears as a critical hindrance towards the development of ergonomics guidelines for the design of safer lifting tasks. Evidently, an improved assessment of risk of injury depends on a more accurate estimation of the load partitioning in human trunk.

As a special population, it is of interest to determine if it is feasible to apply a discount factor in terms of the differences in the mass selected by disabled workers in comparison to non-disabled workers for the varying task. There have been many studies conducted involving manual materials handling (specifically lifting). However, not many tools and researches involve a separation between the ordinary and special populations. Wright and Mital have done two studies involving lifting and carrying [7]. These studies were done in order to recreate the situations presented by Snook and Ciriello [8] to investigate the muscle strengths used by an older population when performing routine activities in industrial and home environments. Chen observed older (50 years and older) and younger (20–30 years old) manual materials handlers and made comparative analysis on the maximum acceptable lifting masses differed between young and older female workers, potential age-related differences in kinematic lifting strategies, grip strength, ratings of perceived exertion [9].

The goal of ergonomics is to design the job to fit the individual performing the job. This includes the worker's mental and physical capabilities, limitations and tolerances [10]. There are many different ways in order to measure the various tool and safety thresholds for workers. Some examples of tools used to evaluate occupations are rapid upper limb assessments (RULA), National Institute for Occupational Safety and Health (NIOSH), Snook and Ciriello tables, and 3D Static Strength Prediction Program (3DSSPP). It was also of interest to determine if the biomechanical model induced from observations on non-disabled people still work for handicapped. Data collected in this study are expected to increase biomechanical data activating biomechanical lifting model assisting the development of evidence-based disability-specific guidelines for safely designing manual materials handling tasks.

There are many approaches to study the biomechanical model of the spine and the force-exertion muscles. Kinematic-based approach is quite useful to compute muscle forces and spinal loads at different spinal levels in static lifting activities involving flexion of trunk and lower limbs. The study is to validate a novel kinematic-based approach applied in El Rich's research in the case that the BKAs maneuver lifting tasks with two methods: squats lifting and stoop lifting [11]. The kinematic-approach was conducted within a framework of three-level model, which integrate the two kinds of constraints: task constraints and handicapped function constraints, and thus model the specific behavior of the physical handicapped in the virtual environment. Based on 3 levels of constraints, the model predicts the optimization of strength and torque under physical and dynamic constraints of physical disability. The simulated results were compared with experiment results and validity of three-level model was validated.

2 Method

Twelve male BKAs were recruited to participate in the experiment with another group of non-BKAs with no recent back complications volunteered for the study after signing an informed consent form. The mean (± S.D.) age, body weight and mass of the BKA group were 36 ± 4 years, 169 ± 5 cm and 65 ± 9 kg, while the mean of non-BKAs were 34 ± 3 years, 172 ± 6 cm and 68 ± 5 kg. The experiment was set as Fig. 1, where the kinetic and muscle EMG signals were collected for the biomechanical analysis of two different lifting methods. A six-camera VICON system (VICON, UK) was employed to collect lifting motion of all subjects. Markers were attached to body parts (see Fig. 1). Simultaneously, four pairs of surface electrodes were positioned bilaterally over longissimus dori (∼3 cm lateral to midline at the L1), external obliques (∼10 cm to midline above umbilicus and aligned with muscle fibers), rectus abdominis (∼3 cm to midline above umbilicus) and rectus femoris. The raw EMG signals were amplified and filtered at 30 Hz.

Subjects were instructed to hold no load, 30 N and 60 N in hands with a bar hanging weights. Subjects were expected to finish stoop lifting and squat lifting with 2 s pause at each posture shown in Fig. 3. For each subject, the experiment levels are 2 × 3. There are six repetitions for each level. Thus there are altogether 36 trials for each subject. For each three trials, subjects took one minute rest. One way ANOVA for repeated measure factors were used to study how BKAs and non-BKAs behave differently during lifting tasks. Three-way analysis of variance (ANOVA) for repeated measure factors were performed to study the effect of disability, lifting techniques (stoop lifting and squat lifting) and load (0 N, 30 N and 60 N) on EMG activities of extensor muscles and abdominal muscles. Besides, one-way ANOVA for repeated measure factors were used to study the effect of disability on EMG activities of the working muscles. Interactive effects between disability, lifting methods and loads were

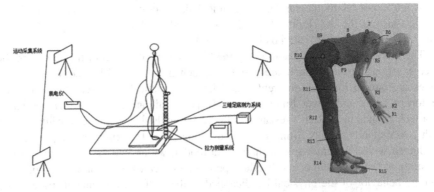

Fig. 1. Set of the experiment instrumented with 3D force plate, VICON motion capture and EMG electrode system. *Motion markers were attached to the body shown as dots on the body. Numbering both with number and letter means one pair on both sides of the body. R is on the right body part and L is for the left (unseen due to the cover from the right body part) plus number indicates the number of the right part of the body while numbering without letters*

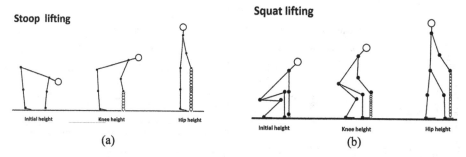

Fig. 2. Lifting postures for two lifting methods: (a) stoop lifting and (b) squat lifting. *Three stages of each lifting technique were paused for 2 s. In (a), subjects started to lift a weight with the arm and leg extended straight and marked as stage I; subjects reached stage II when the weight is at the same level with the knee; Stage III is when the subjects finish the lifting task with arm, lumbar and leg straight. In (b), during stage I, subjects started to lift a weight with the arm and lumbar extended straight and bent knees while the two feet were separated 30° from coronal plane; subjects reached stage II when the weight is at the same level with the knee; Stage III is when the subjects finish the lifting task with arm, lumbar and leg straight.*

evaluated to understand how disability, interacting with lifting methods and the loads in hands, affects muscle activities of extensor, abdominals and rectus femoris. Tukey's post hoc tests were performed to further reveal any significant trends ($p < 0.05$) (Fig. 2).

3   Results

After the experiment, the RMS of EMG was computed for each exertion by Matlab software. The percentage of maximum muscle EMG on extensors (the longissimus, iliocostalis), abdominals (external oblique, rectus abdominals) and rectus femora were compared with the normalized EMG (reflected as percentage of the maximum). The most apparent difference between BKAs and non-BKAs lies in longissimus as shown in Fig. 3. For BKAs, EMG activities in global extensor muscles (LGPT and ICPT) increased, though not significantly, in stoop lifting compared with those in squats lifting for the case with no loads in hands. EMG activity of extensor muscles significantly increased when the weight was added as 60 N and then for 30 N is not obvious. EMG muscles of rectus femoris changes most significantly in case of squat lifting with 60 N loads at hand although changes of rectus femoris is least in case of stoop lifting with no load at hand. Abdominal muscles, though relatively quiet in all tasks, demonstrated a significant change for two lifting methods and load (especially 0 N and 60 N). Disability has biggest effects on abdominal muscle activity across different lifting methods and loads. And the extensor muscles were affected least. Interactive effect between disability and lifting methods is more obvious than that between disability and loads. Tukey's tests revealed that the extensor muscle activity of BKAs increased more significantly from stoop lifting to squat lifting compared with non-BKAs. Activities of BKAs' abdominal muscles increased most significantly from stoop lifting to squats lifting compared to non-BKAs.

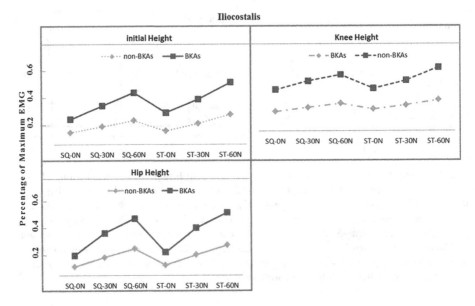

Fig. 3. Comparison of EMG of Longissimus between BKAs and non-BKAs

To determine whether the model calculating muscles forces specific for non-BKAs is still applicable to BKAs. Muscle forces of extensors, abdominal and femoral were predicted in AnyBody Modeling System™. "StandingModel" in the AMMRV1.3.1 was modified so that hand forces in "LeftArmDrivers.any" and "RightArmDrivers.any" were defined as 0 N, 30 N and 60 N (including the net weight of the bar). Body segment angles from electrogoniometers and sagittal photos were inputted to "Mannequin.any", and subsequently the inverse dynamic studies defined in "StandingModel. Main.any" were run using the infinite order polynomial optimization criterion. Similarly, "StandingModel" in the AMMRV1.3.1 was modified so that hand forces in "LeftFootDrivers.any" and "RightFootDrivers.any" were defined as the mean foot force recorded by 3D foot plate. Body segment angles from electrogoniometers and sagittal photos were inputted to "Mannequin.any", and subsequently the inverse dynamic studies defined in "StandingModel.Main.any" were run using the infinite order polynomial optimization criterion. The percentage of maximum muscle forces on the longissimus, iliocostalis, external oblique, rectus abdominals and rectus femoral were further calculated, and compared with the normalized EMG as shown in Fig. 4.

The percentage of maximum between EMG RMS and predicted muscle forces was not the same. In this study, the AnyBody Modeling System™ scaled the model linearly to fit the 50th percentile Asian population according to the subject's weight and height, so the maximum muscle force defined in the AnyBody Modeling System™ may not be the same as that of the individual subject. To solve the problem, the AnyBody Modeling System™ provides a mechanism to scale the model more accurately according to some external force measurements, individual segment length and weight.

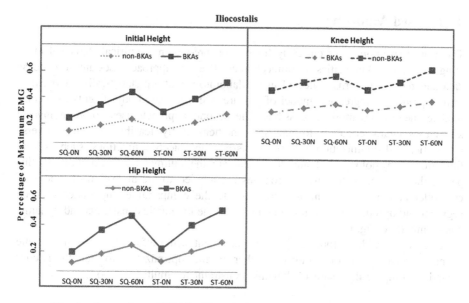

Fig. 4. Comparison of EMG of Longissimus between BKAs and non-BKAs

As expected, EMG and predicted forces of both muscles increased as hand loads increased in two lifting methods. The increasing trend of EMG was somewhat variable but the predicted muscle forces obey the similar trend. The Pearson's correlation coefficients between EMG and predicted muscle forces reached 0.7105. To improve the model predictability, further modification can be made to the model (Fig. 5).

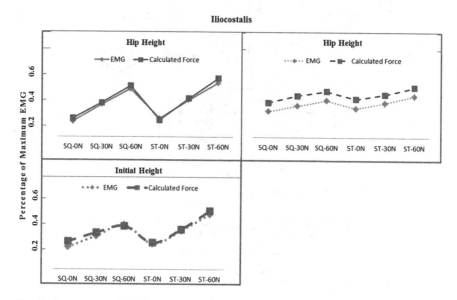

Fig. 5. Percentage of Maximum illiocostalis EMG RMS and Calculated Muscle of BKAs

4 Revised Modeling

There are two approaches currently for motion prediction: empirical statistical modeling and inverse kinematics or biomechanics. The first approach uses anthropometric data and motion patterns collected in the laboratory that are statistically analyzed to form a predictive regression model of posture with rule-based adjustments to accommodate the infinite motions possible. The second approach uses common inverse kinematics characterization to represent mathematically feasible postures. Inverse kinematics and optimization are used to assess the objective functions, such as joint limitations, physiology cost and thus generate the optimal posture/motion. In this paper, the mixture of the two approaches are applied to the algorithm of kinematic controller and dynamic controller to generate the comparative importance of each segment and optimize the posture functioned by the kinematic constraints and dynamic constraints (See Fig. 6).

Energy is the drive force of joint displacement while effort is a substitute to the changing posture from one point to another. Further optimization formulation is conducted to compute the factor of dynamic constraint for multi-FOD body segments.

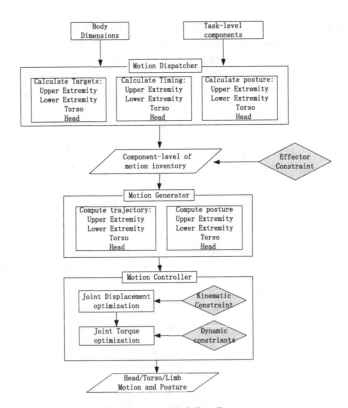

Fig. 6. Task Modeling Process

Joint Displacement Profile:

$$F\left(q'\right) = \sum_{i=1}^{n} w_i(q_i' - q_i)^2 \tag{1}$$

To minimize:

$$F(\tau) = \sum_{i=1}^{n} w_i' |\tau_i| \tag{2}$$

St: $F(q') \in F(q)$

$$\tau_i^L \le \tau_i \le \tau_i^U$$

w_i' is the deviation caused by the physical constraints relative importance of each joint in the motion. τ_i can be calculated as the following:

$$\tau_i = M_{ik}(q)\ddot{q} + \sum J(q_i)^+ m_{ik}g + \sum J(q_k)^+ F_k \tag{3}$$

$i = 1, 2, \ldots, n.$

$$M_{ik}(q) = \sum_{j=max(i,k)}^{n} Tr\left\{ \frac{\partial T_j(q)}{\partial q_k} I_j \left[\frac{\partial T_j(q)}{\partial q_i} \right] \right\} \tag{4}$$

$i, k, j = 1, 2, , \ldots, 3$

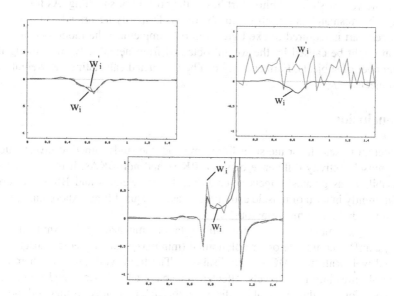

Fig. 7. The DOF weights of knee(a), L5/S1, and L3 over time. The red curve represents the value of wi and the green represents the value of w_i'.

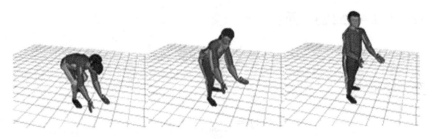

Fig. 8. Comparison of captured (yellow shirt) and modeled (blue shirt) task postures of the subject (Color figure online).

m_{jk} is the mass of link (i,k), $M_{ik}(q)$ is the mass inertia of link (i,k). F_k is the external force on the joint k. Joint i and k are the two joints on each side of the link (i,k).$\tau = \tau(t)$, $F_k = F_k(t)$, and $q = q(t)$.

The EMG trends and difference from calculated force in Sect. 3 were used to train neural network to get a satisfactory w_i and w_i'. The trained results of (w_i, w_i') are shown in Fig. 7.

Task simulation on one subject was used to explain the validity of the revised model. Manipulated by the weights at each corresponding time point, the model put out the optimization angles of 6 joints. The calculated result was put into Jack environment and a manikin was created, which was compared to another manikin only created by motion capture data. The matching results were shown in Fig. 8. As Fig. 8 shows, the yellow shirt is almost overlapped with blue shirt. The most obvious mismatching between the yellow shirt and blue shirt lies in the posture of squatting. As for the other postures, the mismatch is not observed obviously. Disparity occurs when the physical constrained part is required to exert great effort to implement the motion/posture. The variation might be caused by the weight obtained from neural network training from small number of subjects. Further study can be conducted calculating the weights with more subjects.

5 Conclusion

In an attempt to search for the safer lifting method, the study aimed to investigate the relative muscle activity difference between BKAs and non-BKAs. It is notably found that disability has greatest effects when lifting bigger weights and BKAs performed quite differently in term of muscle activities in case of squat lifting. Abdominal muscles reflected the difference most obviously.

Modeling examples shows that for lifting tasks simulated by the AnyBody Modeling System™, the infinite order polynomial (min/max) cannot predict muscle forces correlated well with the EMG due to disability. The framework proposed here reproduces disabilities into three levels: effecter, kinematic and physical, and optimize the position and force of the physical handicapped through motion controller and modified the calculated model. The results simulated in JACK shows good fidelity. The unsatisfactory part of the results lies in the validity of the weights and simplified kinematic model with limited FOD for each joint. The future work can focus on the enhancement of our weight based constraint model by enlarging more samples and set up a kinematic skeleton based on careful observation of the real motion which definitely require more FODs for each body link and joint.

References

1. Hidalgo, J., Genaidy, A., Karwowski, W., et al.: A comprehensive lifting model: beyond the NIOSH lifting equation[J]. Ergonomics **40**(9), 916–927 (1997)
2. Anderson, G.B.: Epidemiologic aspects on low-back pain in industry. Spine **6**(1), 53–60 (1981)
3. Hoogendoorn, W.E., Bongers, P.M., de Vet, H.C., Douwes, M.B.W.: Flexion and rotation of the trunk and lifting at work at risk factors for low back pain: results of a prospective cohort study. Spine **25**, 3087–3092 (2000)
4. Garg, A., Chaffin, D., Freivalds, A.: Biomechanical stresses from manual load lifting: a static vs dynamic evaluation[J]. IIE Trans. **14**(4), 272–281 (1982)
5. McGill, S.M., Hughson, R.L., Parks, K.: Changes in lumbar lordosis modify the role of the extensor muscles. Clin. Biomech. **15**, 777–780 (2000)
6. Garg, A., Herrin, G.D.: Stoop or squat, a biomechanical and metabolical evaluation. A.I.I.E Trans. **11**, 293–302 (1979)
7. Wright, E.J., Haslam, R.A.: Manual handling risks and controls in a soft drinks distribution centre[J]. Appl. Ergon. **30**(4), 311–318 (1999)
8. Ciriello, V.M., Snook, S.H.: Survey of manual handling tasks[J]. Int. J. Ind. Ergon. **23**(3), 149–156 (1999)
9. Chen, Y.L.: Changes in lifting dynamics after localized arm fatigue[J]. Int. J. Ind. Ergon. **25** (6), 611–619 (2000)
10. Thompson, D.D., Chaffin, D.B.: Can biomechanically determined stress be perceived? Proc. Hum. Factors Ergon. Soc. Annu. Meet. **37**(10), 789–792 (1993). SAGE Publications
11. El-Rich, M., Shirazi-Adl, A., Arjmand, N.: Muscle activity, internal loads, and stability of the human spine in standing postures: combined model and in vivo studies[J]. Spine **29**(23), 2633–2642 (2004)

Real-Time Static Gesture Recognition
for Upper Extremity Rehabilitation Using
the Leap Motion

Shawn N. Gieser[1]([✉]), Angie Boisselle[2], and Fillia Makedon[1]

[1] University of Texas at Arlington, Arlington, TX, USA
shawn.gieser@mavs.uta.edu, makedon@uta.edu
[2] Texas Scottish Rite Hospital for Children, Dallas, TX, USA
Angela.Boisselle@tsrh.org

Abstract. Cerebral Palsy is a motor disability that occurs in early childhood. Conventional therapy methods have proven useful for upper extremity rehabilitation, but can lead to non-compliance due to children getting bored with the repetition of exercises. Virtual reality and game-like simulations of conventional methods have proven to lead to higher rates of compliance, the patient being more engaged during exercising, and yield better performance during exercises. Most games are good at keeping players engaged, but does not focus on exercising fine motor control functions. In this paper, we present an analysis of classification techniques for static hand gestures. We also present a prototype of a game-like simulation of matching static hand gestures in order to increase motor control of the hand.

Keywords: Gesture recognition · Leap motion · Upper extremity rehabilitation · Gamification · Cerebral palsy

1 Introduction

Cerebral palsy (CP) is a condition directly related to a lesion in the brain that occurs early in the life of a child. Children with cerebral palsy (CP) have permanent issues with posture and movement that impact participation in daily activities. They may also experience musculoskeletal changes, cognitive impairment, communication and behavioral concerns [1]. There are several subtypes of cerebral palsy based on the type of muscle tone (spasticity, dyskinetic, hypotonia, and mixed tone) and location of impairment (quadriplegia, hemiplegia, diplegia, and others) [2]. Hemiplegia is a type of CP where the child experiences limitations in posture and movement on one side of the body. A child with hemiplegia does not use the impaired arm as often as the unaffected arm due to repeated experiences of failure in using that arm. Human computer interaction (HCI) is a method that supplement traditional rehabilitation therapy, such as occupational and physical therapy, to create experiences and environments to provide children with successful opportunities to promote the use of their affected hand or limb without feeling a sense of failure. Research has shown that the use of specially designed computer games can motivate and help children to enhance the use the affected limb while also strengthening the muscles involved and any related affected functionality [3–5].

© Springer International Publishing Switzerland 2015
V.G. Duffy (Ed.): DHM 2015, Part II, LNCS 9185, pp. 144–154, 2015.
DOI: 10.1007/978-3-319-21070-4_15

Introduction of low cost, off the shelf sensors, such as the Leap Motion [6], have increased the accessibility to and usability of equipment that was previously too expensive for many applications. The Leap Motion was specifically designed to detect hand motions and gestures. It operates over a small range and high precision due to its use of infrared optics. Rehabilitation therapists indicate that the Leap Motion has potential for rehabilitation and that it would be an effective motivational tool young people within a home environment without a therapist being present [7].

The purpose of this paper is twofold. First, we will compare three classification techniques, decision trees, Support Vector Machines (SVM) and k-nearest neighbors (KNN), to recognize and classify static gestures from the Leap Motion based on the position of the hand and fingers as well as the joint angles. Secondly, a game will be created to detect these gestures and will be evaluated by both student volunteers and occupational therapy experts in the field.

2 Background

Evidence for rehabilitation in the area of cerebral palsy has expanded in recent years due to new technologies and methodologies. Specific interventions have been researched to ensure efficacy, cost-effectiveness and safety [8]. In addition, the World Health Organization (WHO) has established the International Classification of Functioning, Disability, and Health (ICF) that is intended to serve as a collaborative global framework and scientific tool to measure health and disability. The ICF has shifted the focus from disability and impairment to that of function and participation within context of the social and physical environment [9]. It is for these reasons that it is important to develop rehabilitation interventions that are both evidence-based and consider contextual factors and participation.

Reference [8] completed a systematic review of smaller systematic reviews for interventions related to children with cerebral palsy. Therapeutic interventions that were found to have the strongest evidence included: bimanual training; Botulinum toxin (Botox) injections; context-focused therapy; goal-directed functional training using a motor-learning approach; therapeutic home programs; and Botox followed up by occupational therapy. Human computer interaction is an area within rehabilitation therapy that provides a new and innovative method for intervention. Virtual reality games are used in rehabilitation to promote movement and strengthening within a motivating environment [10]. Evidence is emerging to determine the efficacy of virtual reality and influence of functional outcomes related to children with cerebral palsy [11]. However, the principles of Virtual Reality (VR) support strong evidence because it can be designed to emphasize motor learning, bimanual training and goal-directed training within the home environment [10, 12]. The child's participation in rehabilitation through the use of highly motivational VR games within the context of their home also supports WHO initiatives.

Gaming systems such as the commercially-available gaming systems and robotic arm systems are most commonly used in the clinic setting. Children with CP are often unable to use commercially-available systems due to movement restrictions in the upper extremities. Additionally, they are not beneficial to the occupational therapist because they do not specifically measure small upper extremity movements such as finger extension, wrist extension, ulnar/radial deviation, and forearm supination [13].

3   Related Work

VR has been used in the treatment of CP with an increased success rate compared to conventional exercises. The authors of [4] show that children with and without CP found that VR exercises are more interesting than conventional exercises. These children also were able to hold exercises longer and showed an increased range of motion during VR exercises compared to conventional exercises. The parents for the children also noticed their children having more fun during VR exercises and believe that their children would continue the exercises at home. The authors of [14] also agree with this, stating that a VR training program has potential to improve reaching abilities and control in children with CP.

The Leap Motion controller has been used in game based physical therapy. Reference [7] evaluated the usefulness of the Leap Motion controller for a clinical environment by developing game-like versions of existing rehabilitation activities that were evaluated by clinicians. The results of their trial show that the Leap Motion does have potential to be used in place of some traditional techniques, especially in the home and for young people. Reference [15] focused on the responses from patients. The patients in this study said that the game presented to them was very engaging and addressing a need of practicing movements that are related to daily functions. Also, the patients said that they would play this game if provided as part of home therapy program.

Work has also been done with using the Leap Motion controller in terms of gesture recognition. Reference [16] shows classification techniques using the Leap Motion controller for both static and dynamic gestures. Reference [17] also presents a gesture recognition system using the Leap Motion control made for therapy applications, including a list of gestures created with the help of therapists. Both these systems, however, are lacking a game aspect to keep the patient involved. These present a good starting point, but missing the game component could lead to non-compliance similar to that of conventional therapy exercises.

4   Experimental Procedure

4.1   Equipment

This paper focuses on the use of the Leap Motion controller. As shown in Fig. 1, the Leap Motion consists of three infrared (IR) light emitters and two IR cameras. Since this system uses stereo vision, it can be categorized as an optical tracking system instead of depth based tracking system [18]. The Leap Motion controller provides detailed information about a user's hand, including the position of the wrist, palm, and finger digits in the Cartesian space, as well as the direction of the hand and finger digits.

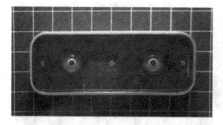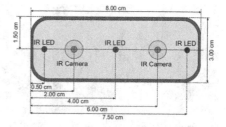

Fig. 1. A view of the real (left) and the schematic (right) of the leap motion controller

This information can be used to determine joint angles of the wrist and knuckles. The Leap Motion controller can also provide other information, such as what fingers are extended, the normal vector to the palm, information about the forearm and any tools being used within the Leap Motion controller's field of view.

4.2   Data Collection

A gesture library was created for this prototype with the help of an occupational therapist. The goal of this was to actually recognize gestures that are used as exercises. Figure 2 shows the gestures that were chosen for this library.

The training data for the various classification procedures was gathered by having student volunteers perform the gestures in a controlled environment. A visualization tool was developed using the Unity Game Engine [19] and the Leap Motion API.

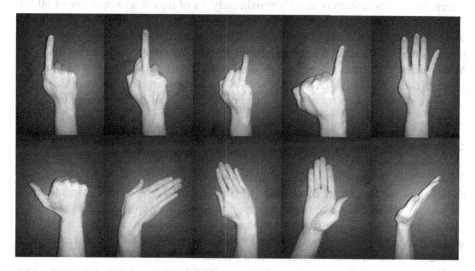

Fig. 2. Gesture library for the prototype. from top left corner to bottom right: extension of the index finger, extension of the middle finger, extension of the ring finger, extension of the pinky finger, extension of four fingers, extension of the thumb, ulnar deviation, radial deviation, supination of the forearm, extension of the wrist.

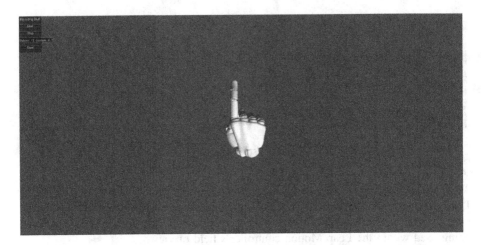

Fig. 3. View of the data collection program of extension of the index finger

UI tools were placed in the top left corner to allow the administrator of the data collection to easier start and stop data collection and save the data. Also, the volunteer can see a visualization their hand on the screen to allow the administrator and the volunteer to verify that the gesture is seen correctly by the Leap Motion Controller. Figure 3 shows this UI Design.

The volunteer was given photos of the gestures before data collection begun so they could know what they had to do. The volunteer then placed their right hand above the Leap Motion controller and made the first gesture. When it was shown correctly on the screen, the administrator collected approximately 5 s of data at a sample rate of 50 Hz and saved it. The volunteer then made the second gesture, and was recorded the same way. This task was repeated till all gestures were recorded, and the whole process was repeated two more times. We did not record all the data points produced by the Leap Motion control. Instead, we only recorded the features that were useful to determine the gesture. These included what fingers were extended, the direction of the forearm and the hand, the normal vector of the palm, and joint angles of the wrist and knuckles.

5   Analysis

We used three different methods of classification: Decision Tree, K-Nearest Neighbors (KNN), and Support Vector Machines (SVM). First, we had to determine what features are used to classify which gestures. For example, only the Supination of the Forearm gesture has the palm's normal vector in the positive Y direction. This feature can then be ignored for all other gestures in this gesture library. A full list of the features that were used to classify each gesture is shown in Table 1.

We made ten different decision trees to classify the ten different gestures. The reason for this was based on game play. During gameplay, we can assume what gesture someone is supposed to make by where they are in the game, since they would only make certian gestures at certian points. With this assumption, we can classify the

Table 1. List of feautres used to identify each gesture

Gesture name	Features used
Extension of the index finger	Extension values of the 5 fingers, angles of the metacarpophalangeal (MP), proximal interphalangeal (PIP), and distal interphalangeal (DIP) joints of the index finger
Extension of the middle finger	Extension values of the 5 fingers, angles of the MP, PIP, and DIP joints of the middle finger
Extension of the ring finger	Extension values of the 5 fingers, angles of the MP, PIP, and DIP joints of the ring finger
Extension of the pinky finger	Extension values of the 5 fingers, angles of the MP, PIP, and DIP joints of the pinky finger
Extension of four fingers	Extension values of the 5 fingers, angles of the MP, PIP, and DIP joints of the four fingers
Extension of the thumb	Extension values of the 5 fingers, angles of the MP and interphalangeal (IP) joints of the thumb
Unlar deviation	Direction of forearm and hand, angle of the wrist joint
Radial deviation	Direction of forearm and hand, angle of the wrist joint
Supination of the forearm	Palm's normal vector
Extension of the wrist	Direction of forearm and hand, angle of the wrist joint

gesture with a decision tree with fewer levels than a single tree that would classify all gestures at once. One of the decision trees is shown in Fig. 4. The tolerances for the joint angles and directional vectors were determined by looking at the training data to verify that a majority of the training data would be classified correctly, and to allow some error from any potential input from a game.

The KNN analysis was developed using the built in Matlab functions. The number of neighbors chosen was 294 as it still yielded a very low error. No other parameters were changed. This approach only used one model to classify gestures, unlike the decision tree approach mentioned above. We only used one model, because KNN can easily handle multiple classes without consuming too much time. This approach also was the only one to use all features collected to classify the gesture.

Lastly, we used 10 SVMs also developed using the built in Matlab functions using the Gaussian Radial Basis Function as the kernel function. We made 10 different SVMs for the same reason as mentioned with the decision trees. The feature vector for each SVM comes from the Table 1.

Table 2 shows a comparison between the 3 different methods. The method used to verify the classification models developed was resubstitution. Each model had the data samples that were supposed to match the model resubstituted back into the model to give the results below. As shown, KNN yielded the best results. Most of the decision tree models were above 90 %, and further modification on the tolerances for the middle, ring, and pinky finger extensions would help fix this.

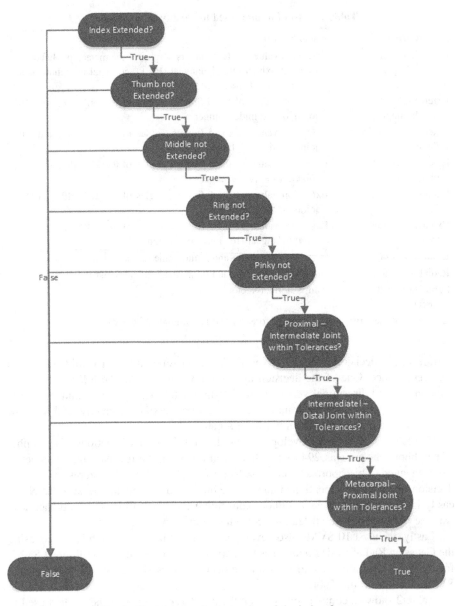

Fig. 4. Decision tree for extension of the index finger

Table 2. Classification results using resubstitution of training data

	Decision tree		KNN		SVM	
	Correct	Incorrect	Correct	Incorrect	Correct	Incorrect
Extension of the index finger	93.96 %	6.04 %	100 %	0 %	100 %	0 %
Extension of the middle finger	76.96 %	23.04 %	100 %	0 %	100 %	0 %
Extension of the ring finger	82.57 %	17.43 %	100 %	0 %	100 %	0 %
Extension of the pinky finger	89.09 %	10.91 %	100 %	0 %	100 %	0 %
Extension of four fingers	97.24 %	2.76 %	99.51 %	0.49 %	99.68 %	0.32 %
Extension of the thumb	100 %	0 %	100 %	0 %	100 %	0 %
Unlar deviation	96.7 %	3.3 %	100 %	0 %	99.91 %	0.09 %
Radial deviation	99.91 %	0.09 %	99.88 %	0.12 %	99.86 %	0.14 %
Supination of the forearm	100 %	0 %	100 %	0 %	100 %	0 %
Extension of the wrist	93.32 %	6.68 %	100 %	0 %	97.9 %	2.1 %

6 Game

For the game prototype development, we once again used the Unity Game Engine and the Leap Motion API. The game consists of two phases. The first is a fifteen second rest period. The player is not required to do anything during this phase. A picture of the next gesture is shown so that the player can prepare. During the second phase, the player is to match a gesture that is shown on the screen. Both a picture of the gesture and a visualization of the hand as seen from the Leap Motion are shown to players, so that they can see what they are doing with respect to real life and the Leap Motion itself. When the gesture is matched, the top left corner turns green, and red when it is not matched. The score increments by one for every second the gesture is held. A screen capture of this game is shown in Fig. 5. This is supposed to help strengthen the hand. We used the decision tree models for this game due to the lack of open source classification software readily available for Unity. The recognition of gestures did not seem to be affected by using decision trees in terms of response and recognizing most gestures. Certain gestures, however, did require more exact positioning than was expected by the authors.

Student volunteers played the game then filled out a three question survey afterwards. All but question was on a Likert Scale of 1–5 with 5 being the most positive and 1 being the most negative. The mean of the responses to the question "I feel the overall control interface is easy to use" was 3.67, but the mean of the responses to "I feel that with practice, I could become proficient in using the control interface" was 4.83. This shows that people feel that playing the game more would lead them to a higher score,

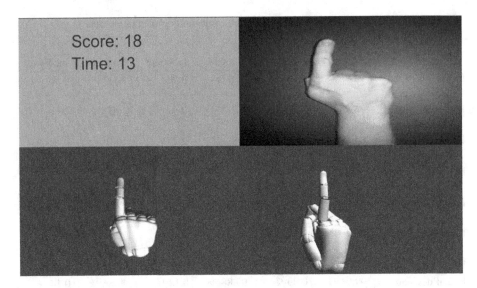

Fig. 5. Screen capture of the unity leap motion game

which would then improve range of motion. The mean of the responses to the question "The tasks presented on the screen are easy to understand" was 4.33. The only comment from the volunteers that one of the pictures was rotated from the Leap Motion model, which caused some confusion.

A video of one of the authors playing the game was made and sent out 2 area hospitals to be evaluated by physical and occupational pediatric therapists. This prototype got mixed reviews. The mean of "The Leap Motion appears easy to use" and "I feel that I could become proficient in using the Leap Motion" was 3.78, while the mean of "The tasks on the screen are easy to understand" was a 4. When asked about an improved version of the prototype, the most interesting response was to "I feel patients would be motivated to use an improved version of this prototype" which had a mean of 2.87. The comments provided by theses therapists said that the game needs to be more engaging, fun, and interactive to help hold a patient's attention.

7   Conclusion

In this paper, we have presented an analysis of classification techniques on data gathered from the Leap Motion controller. Decision trees provided over 90 % accuracy for the majority of gestures, but KNN and SVM provided much more accurate results. This is believed to be due to the tolerances chosen for the joint angles of the decision tree now allowing for a wide enough variance to properly classify certain gestures. Further adjustment of the tolerances should yield better classification results.

A game prototype also was presented. The reviews of the student volunteers playing this prototype said that the interface was easy to use and could easily become proficient in using it. Therapists viewing a demo of the game also had positive feedback in terms of using the Leap Motion controller and the way tasks were presented to the user. Therapists did comment on the engagement level of the game, saying that patients might not feel motivated to use the current or improved version of this prototype, saying that the game needs to have more features to keep the patient's attention so that they feel motivated to use the system. Based on the feedback from the student volunteers and the therapists, there is enough evidence to develop a new version of the game which incorporate other gestures and data modalities, as well as a more engaging interface.

8   Future Work

The next phase of this prototype is to expand on the gesture library. Adding gestures will increase the number of features to be viewed to distinguish gestures from each other. Gestures added could be either static or dynamic. This would then mean that more analysis of various gesture recognition algorithms would be needed to determine the best use for dynamic gestures using the Leap Motion.

Also, a therapist user interface will be added. This will allow therapists to view any important data gathered during gameplay sessions. This will also enable the potential for telerehabilitation, since the therapist can then view the data from sessions the patient does at home. This interface will also allow the therapist to control the exercises, such as the order of the gestures and the difficulty of the exercises, or how accurate the gesture has to be.

Lastly, a more engaging game will be developed. The current game is very basic, and therapists have commented on it. A more engaging game might help therapists feel that the patient would feel motivated to play this game, especially in pediatrics.

Acknowledgements. Special thanks to the students of the Heracleia Human Centered Computing Laboratory who volunteered to play the game and provide feedback. This work has been partially supported by the following NSF grants: CNS: 1338118, CNS: 1035913, and IIS: 1041637.

References

1. Rosenbaum, P., Paneth, N., Leviton, A., Goldstein, M., Bax, M., Damiano, D., Dan, B., Jacobsson, B.: A report: the definition and classification of cerebral palsy. Dev. Med. Child Neurol. **49**(supplement 109), 8–14 (2007)
2. Shevell, M., Dagenais, L., Hall, N.: The relationship of cerebral palsy subtype and functional motor impairment: a population based study. Dev. Med. Child Neurol. **51**(11), 872–877 (2009)
3. Aarts, P.B., Hartingsveldt, M., Anderson, P.G., Tillar, I., Burg, J., Geurts, A.C.: The pirate group intervention protocol: description and a case report of a modified constraint-induced movement therapy combined with bimanual training for young children with unilateral spastic cerebral palsy. Occup. Therapy Int. **19**(2), 76–87 (2012)

4. Bryanton, C., Bosse, J., Brien, M., Mclean, J., McCormick, A., Sveistrup, H.: Feasibility, motivation and selective motor control: virtual reality compared to conventional home exercise in children with cerebral palsy. Cyberpsychology Behav. **19**(2), 123–128 (2006)
5. Snider, L., Majnemer, A., Darsaklis, V.: Virtual reality as a therapeutic modality for children with cerebral palsy. Dev. Neurorehabil. **13**(2), 120–128 (2010)
6. Leap Motion Controller SDK. https://developer.leapmotion.com/
7. Charles, D., Pedlow, K., McDonough, S., Shek, K., Charles, T.: Close range depth sensing camera for virtual reality based hand rehabilitation. J. Assist. Technol. **8**(3), 138–149 (2014)
8. Novak, I., McIntyre, S., Morgan, C., Campbell, L., Dark, L., Morton, N., Stumbles, E., Wilson, S., Goldsmith, S.: A systematic review of interventions for children with cerebral palsy: state of the evidence. Dev. Med. Child Neurol. **55**(10), 885–910 (2013)
9. World Health Organization: International Classification of Functioning, Disability and Health. WHO, Geneva (2001)
10. Fluet, G.G., Qiu, Q., Kelly, D., Parikh, H.D., Ramirez, D., Saleh, S., Adamovich, S.V.: Interfacing a haptic robotic system with complex virtual environments to treat impaired upper extremity motor function in children with cerebral palsy. Dev. Neurorehabil. **13**(5), 335–345 (2010)
11. Yin, C.W., Sien, N.Y., Ying, L.A., Chung, S.F.M., Tan, M.L.: Virtual reality for upper extremity rehabilitation in early stroke: a pilot randomized controlled trial. Clin. Rehabil. **28** (11), 1107–1114 (2014)
12. Lewis, G.N., Rosie, J.A.: Virtual reality games for movement rehabilitation in neurological conditions: How do we meet the needs and expectations of the users? Disabil. Rehabil. **34** (22), 1880–1886 (2012)
13. Chen, Y., Caldwell, M., Dickerhoof, E., Hall, A., Odakura, B., Morelli, K., Fanchiang, H.: Game analysis, validation, and potential application of EyeToy play and play 2 to upper-extremity rehabilitation. Rehabil. Res. Pract. **2014**, 1–13 (2014)
14. Chen, Y., Kang, L., Chuang, T., Doong, J., Lee, S., Tsai, M., Jeng, S., Sung, W.: Use of virtual reality to improve upper-extremity control in children with cerbral palsy: a single subject design. Phys. Ther. **87**(11), 1441–1457 (2007)
15. Khademi, M., Hondori, H.M., McKenzie, A., Dodakian, L., Lopes, C.V., Cramer, S.C.: Free hand interaction with leap motion controller for stroke rehabilitation. In: Proceedings of the Extended Abstracts of the 32nd Annual ACM Conference on Human Factors in Computing Systems, pp. 1663–1668. ACM, New York (2014)
16. Nowicki, M., Pilarczyk, O., Wasikowski, J., Zjawin, K., Jaskowski, W.: Gesture Recognition Library for Leap Motion Controller. Bachelor thesis. Poznan University of Technology, Poland (2014)
17. Rahman, R,A.: Multimedia non-invasive hand therapy monitoring system. In: 2014 IEEE International Symposium Medical Measurements and Applications, pp. 1–5. IEEE Press, New York (2014)
18. Weichert, F., Bachmann, D., Rudak, B., Fissler, D.: Analysis of the accuracy and robustness of the leap motion controller. Sensors **13**(5), 6380–6393 (2013)
19. Unity Game Engine. http://unity3d.com/5

Experience Factors Influence on Motion Technique of "The Way of Tea" by Motion Analysis

Soutatsu Kanazawa[1], Tomoko Ota[2], Zelong Wang[3(✉)], Thodsaratpreeyakul Wiranpaht[3], Yuka Takai[4], Akihiko Goto[4], and Hiroyuki Hamada[3]

[1] Urasenke Konnichian, Kyoto, Japan
kanazawa.kuromon.1352.gentatsu@docomo.ne.jp
[2] Chuo Business Group, Osaka, Japan
Tomoko.ota@k.vodafone.ne.jp
[3] Advanced Fibro-Science, Kyoto Institute of Technology, Kyoto, Japan
simon.zelongwang@gmail.com
[4] Department of Information Systems Engineering, Osaka Sangyo University, Osaka, Japan
gotoh@ise.osaka-sandai.ac.jp

Abstract. In this paper, the difference technique of motion and process for "The way of tea" on were investigated. The expert and beginner's motion and trace were captured by High-speed camera system. In order to verify the correct motion technique, a tea master and three people were employed as expert and beginner, and two kinds of motion techniques and moving tracks were summarized and compared during the whole tea making process. The expert' motion can be considered as a good reference.

Keywords: The way of tea · Tea whisk · Bubble form · Japanese tea

1 Introduction

"The way of tea" is the Japanese tea ceremony, which is called "Chanoyu" or "Sadō", "Chadō" in Japan. It is a ritual process of preparing and serving "Matcha", a kind of green tea powder. As the same with other tea ceremony in East Asian, "The way of tea" is a special culture of judge tea and discusses tea, but also has distinct national characteristics and unique content and form. The history of "The way of tea" can be traced back to the 13th century, which was originally concentrated the mind by monks, and later developed into appreciating ceremony.

The most important mind in the ceremony of "The way of tea" is that all participator should pay attention into the predefined movements during the tea preparing. The whole process is not only drinking the tea, but also is enjoying the tea ceremony and feeling the tea making guest's heart. Each movement and gesture was always considered as an important part of ceremony. In additionally, tea-mixing movement process is the basic skill difficult to master with less progress, which was also the main content of this research.

In previous research, expert and beginner with different experience years were focused. The speed and frequency of the tea-mixing process of expert and beginner was

© Springer International Publishing Switzerland 2015
V.G. Duffy (Ed.): DHM 2015, Part II, LNCS 9185, pp. 155–163, 2015.
DOI: 10.1007/978-3-319-21070-4_16

Author Proof calculated and summarized. And the level of final teas made by expert and beginner were inspected and compared as well. It is deserved to find that expert's action quicker but accurate, focus longer but shift to next action without hesitation, which provided a beauty of the dependable environment for the guests rather than non-expert [1, 2, 3].

A good tea master can mix the green tea power into the hot water with a period of proper time, which ensures the mixed tea hold the optimal tasting temperature. As same with stirring speed and frequency, the movement skills and stirring track is also one of the most important features influence factors for master. In order to obtain a excellent cup of tea, master has to use the correct mix motion and stirring track to make a high level tea using experienced way.

In this research, one expert and three beginners were employed as the behavior subjects. During "the way of tea" performance, the expert and beginner's motion and trace were captured by High-speed camera system during the tea-mixing process. Base on the data from the High-speed camera system, each key gesture of expert and beginner were focused, motion feature affect on final teas were extracted and analyzed. It is deserved to find that expert's action quicker with high speed but accurate at first period. And changed gesture and stirred around with uniform speed at second period. The expert can make a delicious Japanese tea using this method, which provided a beauty of the dependable environment for the guests rather than beginner.

In a word, this study was focus on the stirring motion during the way of tea process between expert and beginner. Through High-speed camera system, expert's motional characteristics were summarized into two main parts and gave beginners as reference.

2   Experiment

2.1   Participants and Subjects

One Japanese tea masters and three beginners from Kyoto were employed as the participants. One of the participants had more than 20 years experience in "the way of tea", which was called as expert in this paper. Other participant had 20 years experience as called non-expert.

One classical type of Japanese tea whisks was selected for proceeding the experiment called as "Kankyuan" as shown in Fig. 2.

2.2   Experimental Process

The participants were required to whisk together green tea powder and hot water as shown in Fig. 1. 1.5 g of "Matcha" tea power and approximate 56 g of hot water were dumped into the bowl, and the moisture content of tea was controlled at approximately 97 % steadily. Two time stages including 100 % and 50 % of tea making finishing time were required and investigated for the tea made by expert and beginners called "First period" and "Second period". And 100 % and 50 % of tea-mixing processes of expert and beginners were clearly recorded by a high-speed camera (FASTCAM SA4 Photron CO. Ltd) from same angle as shown in Fig. 3. The shutter speed was 3600 frames per-second.

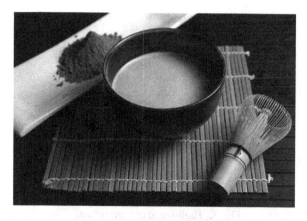

Fig. 1. The way of tea

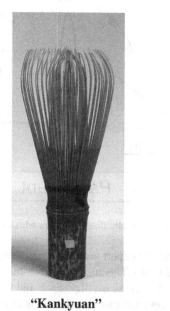

"Kankyuan"

Fig. 2. Japanese tea whisks

2.3 Analysis Processing

The three different markers were affixed to the participants' hand in order to make the further analysis by software as shown in Fig. 4. The coordinates of three markers in the x or y direction was captured and analyzed by TEMA 3.5 software (Photron CO. Ltd) as shown in Fig. 5. The angle B was calculated according to three markers coordinates by cosine law as called Finger-angle in this research.

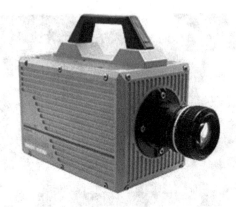

Fig. 3. High-speed camera system

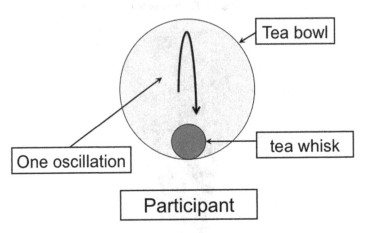

Fig. 4. The schematic diagram of tea whisk oscillate process

All movement elements of expert and beginners were counted and summarized by watching the High-speed video. The numbers of tea-mixing frequency was judged and summarized according to tea whisk oscillate back and forth as shown in Fig. 4.

The time of entire process was calculated accurately be given to two decimal places. The whole processes of expert and beginners divided into first period process and second period process were paid attention and contrasted with each other.

3   Results and Discussions

The tea-mixing motion of expert and beginner were categorized into two types and two tracks based on the High-speed camera data. The tea-mixing gesture was divided into two types depending on whether the fingers are moving or are holding slight as called "Type-1" and "Type-2". In case of "Type-1", the fingers kept moving during the tea-mixing process with slight power. And the tea whisk was moved like "A" shape as shown in Fig. 6. In other case of "Type-2", the fingers were held the tea-whisk tightly, and the

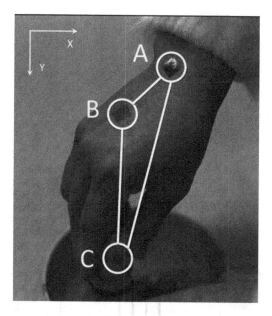

Fig. 5. Finger-angle

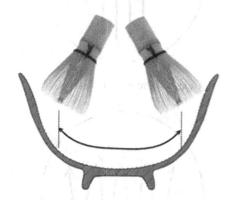

Fig. 6. The motion of "Type-1"

tea whisk was moved by elbow. The tea whisk was presented the horizontally moving as shown in Fig. 7.

The tea-mixing track of expert and non-expert also was divided into two types depending on tea whisk's moving trajectory as called "Track-1" and "Track-2". In case of "Track-1", the tea whisk was move back and forth as shown in Fig. 8 (Backwards and forwards moved). In case of "Track-2", the tea whisk was move back and forth and laterally as shown in Fig. 9 (Backwards, forwards and horizontally moved).

Based on the High-speed camera data, the feature of expert and beginners was summarized as shown in Table 1 The expert used the "Type-1" gesture and "Track-1" method to mix the tea powder and water at the first period. And used "Type-2" gesture and "Track-2"

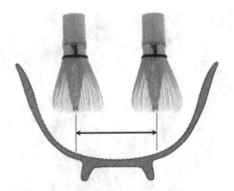

Fig. 7. The motion of "Type-2"

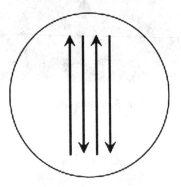

Fig. 8. The way of "Track-1"

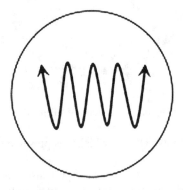

Fig. 9. The way of "Track-2"

method to break up the bubble on the surface of tea at the second period. The beginner used "Type-2" gesture and "Track-1" method to make the tea. It is easy to found that, used the "Type-1" gesture can obtain larger displacement by small fingers movement (Thumb, forefinger, and middle fingers) as shown in Fig. 6. Used the "Type-2" also can got faster speed, but it is difficult to obtain large displacement as shown in Fig. 7.

In previous research, the expert's method was considered that expert was able to perform high stirring speed during the first period in order to agitate the tea powder in hot water quickly, and control the suitable speed during the second period so that and mix agitated tea powder and presented the wider distribution of small bubbles finally, so that generate the beautiful tea in the end. In order to verify the motion characteristics of finger movement between expert and beginners, the "Finger-angle" of each participant was calculated and compared in Fig. 10. According to the result, the expert's finger angle was presented large standard deviation during the first period. It's mean that the expert's fingers was keeping move during the first period because the "Finger-angle" show the large change. The tea mixing speed also was calculated on the Fig. 11. The result explained that only the expert presented highest speed mixing during the first

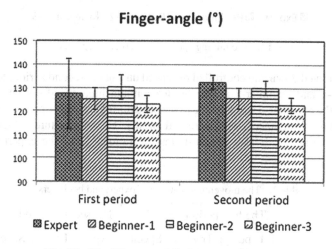

Fig. 10. The "Finger angle" of expert and beginners

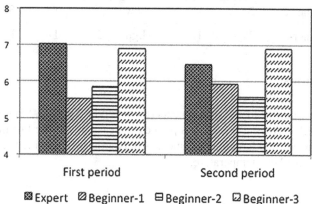

Fig. 11. The mixing speed of expert and beginners

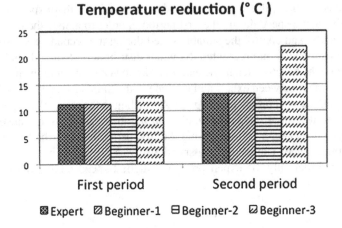

Temperature reduction (° C)

First period   Second period

⊠ Expert   ⊘ Beginner-1   ⊟ Beginner-2   ⊘ Beginner-3

Fig. 12. The mixing speed of expert and beginners

period, and slowed down and controlled the speed during the second period. Relatively, the beginner-1 and beginner-2 mixed the tea without high speed during the whole process. But the beginner-3 was kept the high speed during the whole process. However, the temperature of beginner-3 was decreased largely. The temperature reduction result was shown in Fig. 12. It also demonstrates the rationality of the expert's method (Table 1).

Table 1. The movement features of expert and beginners

	The first period			The second period		
	Type	Track	Speed	Type	Track	Speed
Expert	1	1	High	2	2	Slow
Beginner-1	2	1	Slow	2	1	Slow
Beginner-2	2	1	Slow	2	1	Slow
Beginner-3	2	1	High	2	1	High

4   Conclusions

In a word, it can be considered that the expert's method ("Type-1", "Track-1" on first period; "Type-2", "Track-2" on second period) can easy to achieve fast mixing speed with high frequency and large displacement. Afterwards, even mixing tea with appropriate speed so that keep temperature.

References

1. Tujimoto, N., Ichihashi,Y., Iue, M., Ota, T., Hamasaki, K., Nakai, A., Goto, A.: Comparison of bubble forming in a bowl of thin tea between expert and non-expert. In: Proceedings of 11 th Japan International SAMPE Symposium & Exhibiton (2009)
2. Goto, A., Endo, A., Narita, C., Takai, Y., Shimodeand, Y., Hamada, H.: Comparison of painting technique of Urushi products between expert and non-expert. In: Advances in Ergonomics in Manufacturing, pp. 160–167 (2012). ISBN: 978-1-4398-7039-6
3. Aiba, E., Kanazawa, S., Ota, T., Kuroda, K., Takai, Y., Goto, A., Hamada, H.: Developing a system to assess the skills of Japanese Way of tea by analyzing the forming sound: a case study. In: Human Factors and Ergonomics Society International Meeting (2013)

Study of Caregiver's Waist Movement Comparison Between Expert and Non-expert During Transfer Care

Mengyuan Liao[1(✉)], Takashi Yoshikawa[2], Akihiko Goto[3], Yoshihiro Mizutani[1], Tomoko Ota[4], and Hiroyuki Hamada[1]

[1] Advanced Fibro-Science, Kyoto Institute of Technology, Kyoto, Japan
Ada.mengyuanliao@gmail.com
[2] National Institute of Technology, Niihama College, Niihama, Japan
Yosikawa@mec.niihama-nct.ac.jp
[3] Department of Information Systems Engineering, Osaka Sangyo University, Daito, Japan
Gotoh@ise.osaka-sandai.ac.jp
[4] Chuo Business Group, Osaka, Japan
Tomoko.ota@k.vodafone.ne.jp

Abstract. As well know that caregivers employed in elderly nursing home suffer from low-back injuries/pain at a terrible rate worldwide, however there is little studies focusing on visual analysis of care works difference conducted by expert and non-expert caregivers. In current study, a 'hypothesis' elder was employed in both expert and non-expert caregiver's handling tasks. And two caregivers with different experience years were selected as subjects named as expert and non-expert, which were required to perform transfer care process for the same elder object. With three-dimensional motion analysis, non-expert's back pain cause was explained by waist up-down and horizontal plane movement, waist roundness, lower back bend angle and waist joint angle comparison to expert performance quantitatively. As a result, it could be concluded that expert kept straight upper body and stable waist motion in a smaller range during transfer care process which was considered as effective waist movement for back pain prevention in intensive heavy care works.

Keywords: Caregiver · Waist movement · Transfer care · Nursing home

1 Introduction

Due to the rapid improvement of economy, living standard and health care in Japan from "After World War II", Japanese longevity has boosted into a 80 years old "super ageing" era. In recent years, falling born ratio has resulted in a sharp reduce tendency of young population, on the contrary, the elderly population percentage accounts for total population has become larger and larger. By the end of 2014, the elder population over 65 years old has accounted for 26.8 % of total population, in which 13 % elders are over 75 years. According to the elderly population demographic and estimation reported in Japanese Ministry of Health, Labour and Welfare, current ageing situation

© Springer International Publishing Switzerland 2015
V.G. Duffy (Ed.): DHM 2015, Part II, LNCS 9185, pp. 164–173, 2015.
DOI: 10.1007/978-3-319-21070-4_17

is becoming serious year after year. Until 2035, elderly population over 65 years old will increase to 33.4 %, in other words, one elder must be contained in three citizen for imbalanced population structure. It is worth noting that the late over 75 age population proportion also reach for 20 %, in which more bedridden, dementia and elder required high nursing care level number are increasing.

Under such a crisis ageing issue, social factors such as generation size reduction, the improvement of women's employment opportunity and elderly care consciousness transition from family to social welfare facilities still brought some developing challenge and opportunities for Japanese nursing industry. Therefore, urgent requirement and demand of related elder nursing care welfare facilities and professional caregivers is increasing to a large scale significantly. In general, transfer care from wheel chair to port toilet was found to be an extremely toughness and frequent job among all of the nursing care works that had substantial danger of causing a low-back pain whether with multiple caregivers or assistant device [1]. Low back pain is a universally occupational disease troubling caregivers in nursing care industry, which may affect caregiver's care work efficiency and elder care service quality, moreover it leads to limitation and negative effect on shortening occupational year [2, 3]. In Japan, 60 %–70 % of caregivers in elderly nursing care industry have low back pain disease, which has become a realistic reason of the industry's turnover rate, even expert caregiver also has the same issue. Thus, in order to conduct safe transfer care process and prevent caregiver's low back pain situation in a long-term occupational period, it is very important to master proper nursing care gesture/technology and knowledge for beginner and non-expert caregivers.

By far, some researchers have reported some body loading comparison between assistant device and manual work in general. However, there is little paper focusing on the cause of low-back pain issue, limitation solution for the low back pain problem other than device substitution, quantitative description of expert and non-expert's waist motion effect on body burdening. In our previous study, expert and non-expert caregiver's lower limb utilization during transfer care process were investigated. It is clarified that expert's knee and joints angular acceleration is small and stable compared to non-expert, which resulted in little body loading for expert's transfer care process. As well known, up and down motion impact force for caregiver's head caused caregiver himself/herself body fatigue, and stable and slipping lifting transfer care process directly reflects head motion style. Referring to head movement, we also investigated expert and non-expert's motion characteristic in our previous research. It was considered that little impact power loaded for expert's head during whole transfer care process, which reflected a kind of care with small body burden. In general, low back pain symptom is origin from incorrect care gesture and concentrated force loaded in waist location. In this paper, continuing with previous study, waist movement track of caregivers with different experience years were focused. Afterwards, expert's waist movement characteristic was visual analyzed by waist moving velocity, accelerated velocity, waist bending angle and roundness discussion and comparison between expert and non-expert. In a word, this paper was aimed to give the feedback to elder nursing care occupational site, improve non-expert's awareness of correct care gesture and optimize their care skill finally.

2 Experiment

2.1 Participants

Two caregivers employed in the same Japanese nursing home (Asokaen) were considered as subjects for the whole study. One caregiver is 34 years old with 9 experience years for elder nursing care occupation referred as "Expert"; And the other one caregiver is 23 years old with only 4 month working experience referred as "Non-expert". Both of them have similar body weight and height with 50 kg and 161 cm respectively. A 'hypothesis' elder (a 80 kg co-operative female with 15 years of care occupation experience, assumed that the lower half body is paralyzed) was employed in both expert and non-expert caregiver's handling tasks. Additionally, the current study represented an "ideal" case scenario since the 'hypothesis' elder is a super expert (guider) could master good care motion skill with relatively heavy body. Thus, it is more conductive to evaluate both two caregiver's care gesture difference by guider's own comfort perception and get good knowledge of caregiver's body loading level during heavier object elder care task.

2.2 Experimental Preparation

Transfer care work from wheel chair to port toilet was predetermined for expert and non-expert's care job investigation process. One main and one assisted caregiver totally two caregivers (experts or non-experts) in a group were cooperated to carry out transfer care work for the same "hypothesis" elder, but only main caregiver was focused in this research. Prior to experimental process, both expert and non-expert caregiver subjects were required to attach 20 reflection markers throughout body positions as head top, head front, head left, head right, neck, back1, back2, waist, shoulder (left and right), elbow (left and right), hand (left and right), daitenshi (left and right), knee (left and right), ankle (left and right) and foot (left and right). And the whole process of caregiver's motion was recorded by infrared camera three-dimensional (3D) capture system with an interval of 100 frames per second.

2.3 Post Process

Firstly 20 detected markers on caregiver's body were fetched in coordinate by post process of cortex motion analysis system. Afterwards, all markers were jointed into human model to simulate and review caregiver's real care motion track in three-dimensional space. And next low back bending angle, waist joint angle (marker points back2-waist-knee) and waist roundness (marker points back1-back2-waist) were calculated and exported, which illustrated in Fig. 1. Due to the smooth movement could result in small physical JERK value with little impact of human perception, waist acceleration change (JERK) was also deduced by acceleration derivative with respect to time additionally. Furthermore, in order to discuss effective value of acceleration and JERK value of waist movement, both acceleration and JERK's root of mean square (RMS) were calculated.

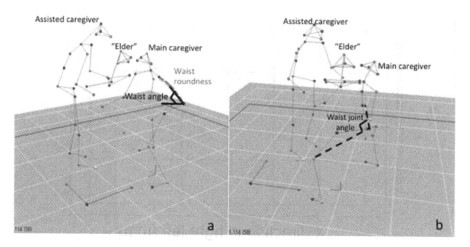

Fig. 1. Definition of waist roundness, waist angle and waist joint angle

3 Results and Discussions

3.1 Waist Movement Range

In Fig. 2, both expert and non-expert's waist movement in up-down direction was indicated. The whole transfer care process was separated into "lift-up", "turning" and "moving" three stages. It is clearly to find that expert caregiver's waist moved more stable during "turning" period with nearly 700 mm height, and "lift-up" and "sit" stages indicated a comparable larger movement range in up-down direction than non-expert. Expert's stable waist movement during turning stage resulted in smooth transfer care

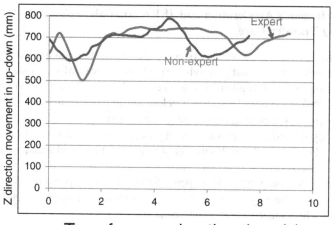

Fig. 2. Waist movement in up-down direction

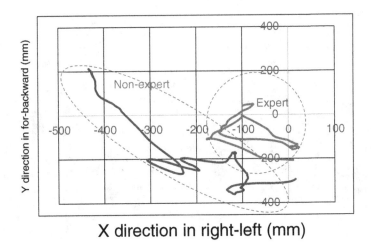

Fig. 3. Waist movement in horizontal plane

process and also able to eliminate elder's uneasy feeling. Referring to "lift-up" and "sit" stages, expert's waist moved owing to whole body movement with knee's flexion and extension.

In Fig. 3, both expert and non-expert's waist movement tracks during transfer care behavior in horizontal plane were illustrated. As showed in Fig. 3, it is deserved to find that non-expert caregiver's waist moved in horizontal plane in a wider region, which showed around 3 times longer distance than expert performance in both for-backwards and right-left directions. Thus, non-expert's transfer care process was considered to have heavier loading on her waist region which easily lead to low back pain with a larger space movement.

3.2 Waist Region's Acceleration and JERK Analysis During Transfer Care

In previous discussions, we have understood expert's waist region narrow movement in three-dimensions. Here, waist's moving acceleration was also compared between expert and non-expert caregiver. As showed in Fig. 4, it is notified to find that non-expert's shake composed rotation acceleration of three-dimensions during whole transfer care process with numbers of huge large wave peaks. However, expert displayed a steady rotated acceleration inferring a continuous and smooth motion among varied stages. For further detail discussion of non-expert's pausal transfer care process, composed acceleration of waist in horizontal plane during "turning" stage was extracted in Fig. 5. Comparing with expert's behavior, non-expert existed a super large acceleration peak in turning moment, which means there were some difficulties in waist rotation from wheel chair to port toilet position.

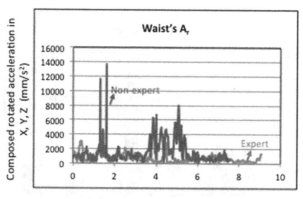

Fig. 4. Composed rotated acceleration of waist in X, Y and Z direction

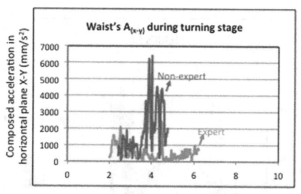

Fig. 5. Composed acceleration of waist in horizontal plane during "turning" stage

In Figs. 6 and 7, both expert and non-expert's effective acceleration and JERK value of waist movement were computed and compared. According to Fig. 6, expert's care process could be explained as quicker lift-up, slower turning and sit stages than non-expert, during which stable turning process and comfortable sitting process other falling feeling were also understood. JERK is the change of acceleration, where also characterize action force at minimum time interval. As showed in Fig. 7, comparing with expert's care behavior, non-expert displayed more than 2 times of action force on waist region during whole process. Consuming energy value is a kind of indicator to define body burden or caregiver's fatigue situation after care process. As well know that energy could be calculated by product-term of applied force and movement distance. Therefore, it could draw a conclusion that non-expert has more possibility to suffer from low back pain with larger waist energy cost during care process.

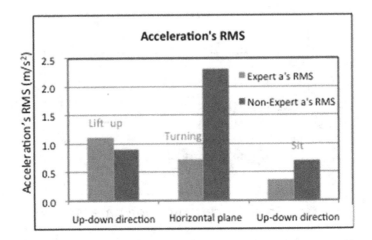

Fig. 6. Acceleration's RMS value during transfer care process

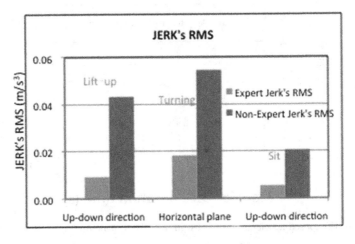

Fig. 7. JERK's RMS value during transfer care process

3.3 Waist Roundness, Bending Angle and Waist Joint Angle Discussion

In Fig. 8, expert and non-expert's waist roundness comparison during transfer care were summarized. It is found that expert kept a comparative straight back line with nearly 170° waist roundness. However, non-expert performed a wide range of waist motion and back extension along with different stages of transfer care process. Waist angle (back bend) of caregiver was also plotted in Fig. 9. It was easy to found that expert displayed sharper increase of waist angle when lifting-up elder in shorter time duration. And comparing with non-expert's wider range of waist extension angle, expert caregiver kept nearly vertical straight upper body gesture during turning stage in care process.

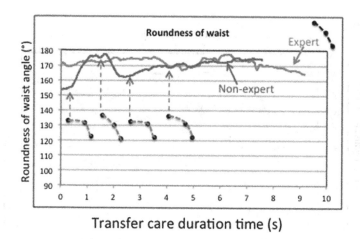

Fig. 8. Comparison of expert and non-expert's waist roundness during transfer care

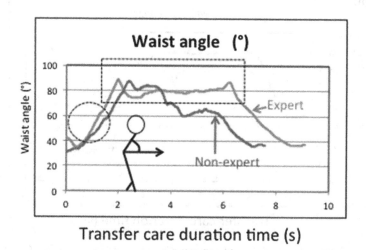

Fig. 9. Comparison of expert and non-expert's waist bending angle during transfer care

Both right and left waist joint angles were compared between expert and non-expert in Fig. 10a and b respectively. It is obvious to detect that non-expert's right and left waist joint angles were smaller than expert especially during turning stage with 20°, which visually explained non-expert's waist fatigue loading by bending forward style.

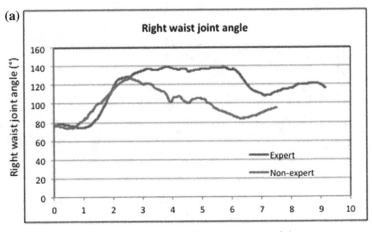

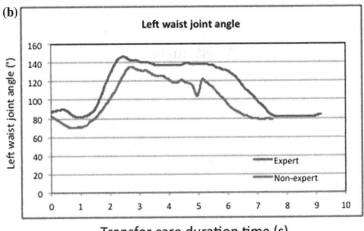

Fig. 10. (a) Comparison of expert and non-expert's right waist joint angle (b) Comparison of expert and non-expert's left waist joint angle

4 Conclusions

In this research, caregiver's waist movement comparison between expert and non-expert during transfer care was studied by visually analysis based on three-dimensional coordinate system. Through comparing waist movement range, waist bending angle, roundness and waist joint angle with expert caregiver, non-expert's waist region was found to suffer from larger force during care process in larger space movement. Consequently, it could be concluded that expert kept straight upper body gesture with less bending and stable waist motion in a smaller range during transfer care process, which was considered as effective waist movement for back pain prevention in intensive heavy care works.

References

1. Marras, W.S., Davis, K.G., Kirking, B.C., Bertsche, P.K.: A comprehensive analysis of low-back disorder risk and spinal loading during the transferring and repositioning of patients using different techniques. Ergonomics **42**(7), 904–926 (1999)
2. Coenen, P., Kingma, I., Boot, C.R., Bongers, P.M., van Dieën, J.H.: Cumulative mechanical low-back load at work is a determinant of low-back pain. Occup. Environ. Med. **71**(5), 332–337 (2014). doi:10.1136/oemed-2013-101862. Epub 27 Mar 2014
3. Ito, M., Endo, A., Takai, Y., Yoshikawa, T., Goto, A., Kuwahara, N.: Study on kind transfer assistance between wheelchair and bed in the case of eye movement analysis. In: Proceeding of 5th International Conference on Applied Human Factors and Ergonomics (AHFE 2014)

Effect of Care Gesture on Transfer Care Behavior in Elderly Nursing Home in Japan

Mengyuan Liao[1(✉)], Takashi Yoshikawa[2], Akihiko Goto[3], Tomoko Ota[4],
and Hiroyuki Hamada[1]

[1] Advanced Fibro-Science, Kyoto Institute of Technology, Kyoto, Japan
Ada.mengyuanliao@gmail.com
[2] National Institute of Technology, Niihama College, Niihama, Japan
Yosikawa@mec.niihama-nct.ac.jp
[3] Department of Information Systems Engineering, Osaka Sangyo University, Daito, Japan
Gotoh@ise.osaka-sandai.ac.jp
[4] Chuo Business Group, Osaka, Japan
Tomoko.ota@k.vodafone.ne.jp

Abstract. In this paper, care gesture effect on elder transfer care behavior between bed and wheelchair was investigated. A 'hypothesis' elder (a 80 kg co-operative female with 15 years of care occupation experience, assumed that the lower half body is paralyzed) was employed in both expert and non-expert care-giver's handling tasks. Both expert and non-expert's care gestures during transfer care process (hold up, turning, lower down) were recorded by three-dimensional motion capture system. In order to extract expert and non-expert care gesture's feature difference, motion analysis of caregiver's body exertions was also summarized by body gravity movement track, knee's flexion/extension, low-back bending situation. As a result, it could be concluded that expert master optimal care gesture to accomplish the transfer care work with reduced body loading and limited energy by taking full advantage of lower half body exertion.

Keywords: Care gesture · Transfer care · Nursing home

1 Introduction

Nowadays, Japan has evolved from "ageing society" to "aged society". The ageing of Japan, indeed of any other country, is invariably presented in wholly negative birth rate and increasing number of bedridden or dementia elders. Ageing is not just a question of what happens to the old, but a crucial issue for society and family. Japanese working-age population is shrinking so quickly that by 2050 it will be smaller with four out of ten Japanese over 65. Unless Japan's productivity rises faster than its workforce declines, which seems unlikely, its economy will shrink. In other words, Japanese "ageing" issue has affected the size of the working population or advanced on a prolonged working age for whole society. By far, caregiver's working age in most Japanese nursing home tended to older and older, and extensive care work also resulted in caregiver's increasing

© Springer International Publishing Switzerland 2015
V.G. Duffy (Ed.): DHM 2015, Part II, LNCS 9185, pp. 174–183, 2015.
DOI: 10.1007/978-3-319-21070-4_18

demission rate. Therefore, it is urgent to develop some high quality level care system with reduced body burden.

Transfer care behavior is a common and frequent nursing care motion for elder's daily care life. Even if some mechanical lift assist devices were applied during specific care movement, but in general transfer care work is mainly charged by human power (manual handling). Transfer care behavior is conducted by complicated interaction force between caregiver and elder with short action duration time. Heavy care work usually brings out low-back injuries or other body 2 damage suffering, especially for beginner and non-expert caregiver with incorrect or improper care gesture [1, 2, 3]. However, until now there is limited research works quantifying the difference of this specific movement performed by the expert and non-expert elder caregiver. In previous Marras et al. study [1], comprehensive evaluation system (low-back disorder risk model) and theoretical model (biomechanical spinal loading model) were applied to evaluate for 17 participants performing several patient's handling tasks. Tomioka K et al. also conduct a study to develop better ways of patient transfer which reduce and prevent low-back pain, low back loads and operation time during transfer care by comparing mechanical lift (Lift) and manual handling (handling) assistance, which suggested transfer by lift is a valid way of reducing the burden on caregiver's low back but required 10 times operation time than handling. Additionally, they also demonstrate the importance of proper procedure observation and self-skill levels raising during transfer.

In general, caregiver's transfer care work was found to be an extremely hazardous job, which had substantial risk of causing a low-back injury whether with one or two caregivers. The urgent task for caregiver beginner was to master valid transferring techniques for actual body motion performance with minimized energy consumption and body loading effect. Therefore, in current study, expert and non-expert's care gesture effect on elder's daily basic transfer care behavior between bed and wheelchair was investigated. A 'hypothesis' elder (a 80 kg co-operative female with 15 years of care occupation experience, assumed that the lower half body is paralyzed) was employed in both expert and non-expert caregiver's handling tasks. Both expert and non-expert's care gestures during transfer care process (hold up, turning, lower down) were recorded by three-dimensional motion capture system. In order to extract expert and non-expert care gesture's feature difference, motion analysis of caregiver's body exertions was also focused on body gravity movement track, knee's flexion/extension, low-back bending situation. Furthermore, expert and non-expert caregiver's transfer care motions were also clarified by quantitative evaluation. As a result it could be concluded that expert master optimal care gesture to accomplish the transfer care work with reduced body loading and limited energy by taking full advantage of lower half body exertion.

2 Experiment

2.1 Participants

Two caregivers employed in the same Japanese nursing home (Asokaen) were considered as subjects for the whole study. One caregiver is 34 years old with 9 experience years for elder nursing care occupation referred as "Expert"; And the other one caregiver is 23 years old with only 4 month working experience referred as "Non-expert". Both of them have similar body weight and height with 50 kg and 161 cm respectively. A 'hypothesis' elder (a 80 kg co-operative female with 15 years of care occupation experience, assumed that the lower half body is paralyzed) was employed in both expert and non-expert caregiver's handling tasks. Additionally, the current study represented an "ideal" case scenario since the 'hypothesis' elder is a super expert (guider) could master good care motion skill with relatively heavy body. Thus, it is more conductive to evaluate both two caregiver's care gesture difference by guider's own comfort perception and get good knowledge of caregiver's body loading level during heavier object elder care task.

2.2   Experimental Preparation and Setting

Transfer care work from wheel chair to port toilet was predetermined for expert and non-expert's care job investigation process. One main and one assisted caregiver totally two caregivers (experts or non-experts) in a group were cooperated to carry out transfer care work for the same "hypothesis" elder, but only main caregiver was focused in this research. And the real experimental site and process were showed in Fig. 1. Prior to experimental process, both expert and non-expert caregiver subjects were required to attach 20 reflection markers throughout body positions as head top, head front, head left, head right, neck, back1, back2, waist, shoulder (left and right), elbow (left and right), hand (left and right), daitenshi (left and right), knee (left and right), ankle (left and right) and foot (left and right), which as showed in Fig. 2. And the whole process and caregiver's motion were recorded by infrared camera three-dimensional (3D) capture system with an interval of 100 frames per second.

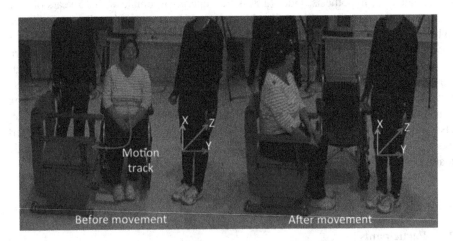

Fig. 1. Experimental site and process

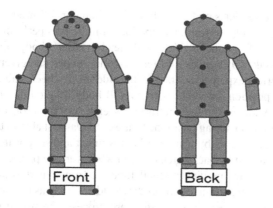

Fig. 2. 20 Markers location attached throughout caregiver's body

2.3 Post Process

First 20 detected markers on caregiver's body were fetched in coordinate by post process of cortex motion analysis system. Afterwards, all markers were jointed into human model to simulate and review caregiver's real care motion track in three-dimensional space. In order to calculate caregiver's body gravity location during care work motion, a serious of body segments inertia property ratios/coefficients reported by Hai-pengTang et al. were applied. And consequently caregiver's body gravity three-dimensional coordinates (x, y, z) were synthesis by Eq. 1.

$$Gravity_x = \frac{\sum_{i=1}^{n} m_i x_i}{\sum_{i=1}^{n} m_i}; \; Gravity_y = \frac{\sum_{i=1}^{n} m_i y_i}{\sum_{i=1}^{n} m_i}; \; Gravity_z = \frac{\sum_{i=1}^{n} m_i z_i}{\sum_{i=1}^{n} m_i}; \tag{1}$$

14 rigid body segments in subject's body (head, trunk, upper arm, fore arm, hand, thigh, crus and foot) were supposed as rigid system and employed to estimate the body gravity location.

3 Results and Discussions

3.1 Transfer Care Process Analysis and Comparison

The whole transfer care process conducted by expert and non-expert were separated into "hold", "lift-up", "move" (turning) and "sit" important moments and illustrated from Figs. 3, 4, 5 and 6 in sequence. In Fig. 3, it is deserved to find that elder's body was held by expert more steady with her lower forward body posture. However, non-expert only kept upper body bending forward to hold elder as a standby, which is easier to cause low back fatigue and slipping possibility. Important lift-up moment comparison between expert and non-expert was also clarified in Fig. 4. As the same with weight-lifting player, expert caregiver took elder's body weight on her shoulder followed by exerting lower limb's strength to lift elder upward. Comparing with expert's performance, non-expert just held elder in her front chest which easily lead to elder's body slipping downside, what's more, that sink body trend would aggravate non-expert caregiver's lifting weight. During "move" period, expert could transfer the elder from wheel chair side to port toilet direction once in position smoothly with overall body rotation due to stable gravity supporting point by knees. On the contrary, it seems very hard for non-expert to turn elder's body to port toilet sitting position. Non-expert was just able to turn elder's body to some certain angle mainly by waist part's movement and supporting, thus low back pain was easily produced by back extension and whole turning process was longer with one more footpace. After moving a small footpace, non-expert could adjust elder's sitting position correctly and finally lower down elder's body as the same with expert's performing. According to expert's transfer care process, the whole process tips and motion essential could be summarized as following 4 points: (1) Drop body gravity and forward to hold the elder by close body contact; (2) Put elder body's weight on the shoulder, hold up elder body using the leg power by knee's extension; (3) Turn elder's body to port toilet side by rotating body with feet as driving shaft and keep upper body straight; (4) Slower down elder's location and support elder's bottom with hand.

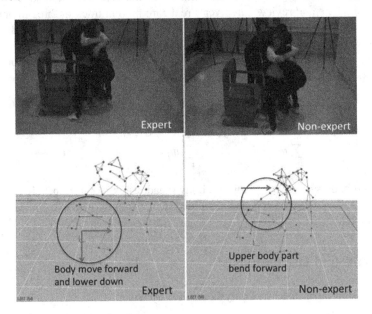

Fig. 3. Pictures of holding moment by expert and non-expert caregiver

3.2 Transfer Care Working Distance and Range

In Figs. 7 and 8, both expert and non-expert's body gravity movement tracks during transfer care behavior of lifting up elder object from wheel chair to sitting on the port toilet

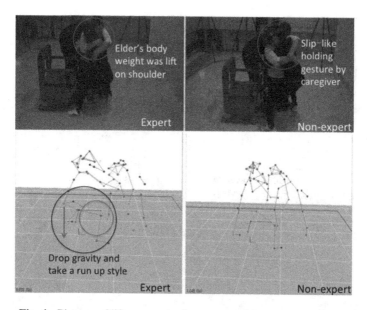

Fig. 4. Pictures of lift-up moment by expert and non-expert caregiver

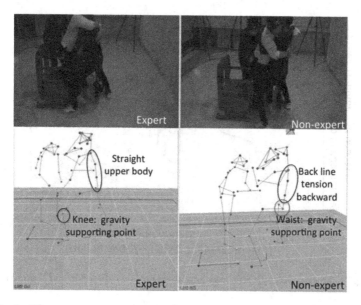

Fig. 5. Pictures of moving (turning) moment by expert and non-expert caregiver

were indicated. Plotting numerical data in up-down and horizontal (left-right and for-backward) move was offset by different caregiver's body build index, which was normalized movement range by caregiver's height. As showed in Fig. 7, it is deserved to find that expert caregiver's body moving in up-down direction in a large scale (0.12) compared with non-expert (0.11) with 16 cm difference. Referring to the whole

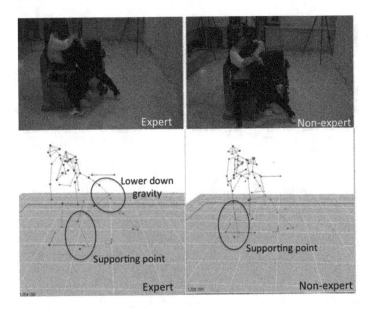

Fig. 6. Pictures of sitting moment by expert and non-expert caregiver

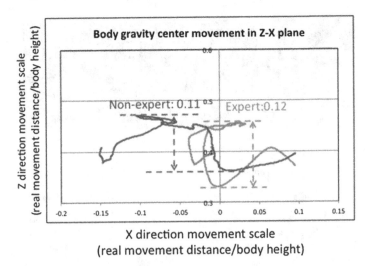

Fig. 7. Tracks of caregiver's body gravity on up-down direction and X direction

movement process, expert's body gravity displayed lower position than non-expert. Working range on horizontal plane was also illustrated in Fig. 8. It is very clear to note that non-expert move in left-right and for-backward direction with a longer working range of 0.24 and 0.26 respectively, which displayed nearly 2 times of expert. According to the integration of three directions working distance, it is obvious to understand non-expert conducted a longer and wider working range than expert. Therefore, expert's transfer gesture was inferred to produce the smallest body burden with short working distance.

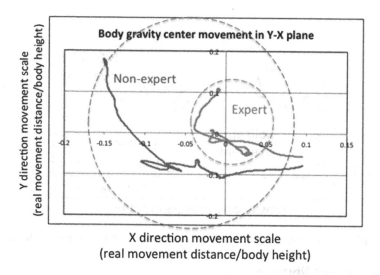

Fig. 8. Tracks of caregiver's body gravity on horizontal plane

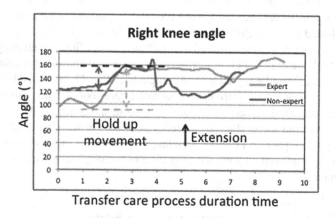

Fig. 9. Comparison of expert and non-expert's right knee angle during transfer care

3.3 Knee's Angle During Lower Limb Exertion

In previous transfer care gesture process analysis, we had detected that expert hardly bent her low back but mainly depended on knee's flexion and extension to accomplish "lift-up" and "sit" care task. Figures 9 and 10 illustrated both expert and non-expert's right and left knee angle change during transfer care process. It is clarified that expert's knee angle variation is larger in lift-up and sit-down situations, and that variation range is around 2 times of non-expert with 60°. Based on this data supporting, it is considered that expert made full advantage of low limb power to lift up elder during transfer care process, thus it was effective to protect the waist location and prevent low back pain by less waist bend action.

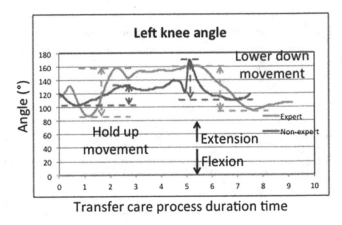

Fig. 10. Comparison of expert and non-expert's left knee angle during transfer care

3.4 Foot Distance Discussion

One of important element for transfer care behavior is keeping body steady and eliminating elder's uneasy feeling during care process. In previous care process analysis, expert was found to complete "turning" work breezily once in place, but non-expert showed incoherence actions with one additional foot pace to adjust herself body position. In order to evaluate expert and non-expert moving steady ability quantitatively, foot distance were considered a key factor and compared in Fig. 11. It is notable to find that expert caregiver kept a comparative constant and larger foot distance value than non-expert, which supported a more stable standing gesture and contributed to a wide range of angle rotation from wheel chair to port toilet position. On the other hand, non-expert applied smaller foot pace as a standby standing gesture for transfer care process, therefore non-expert displayed a longer working time in "turning" step with one small foot pace adjustment.

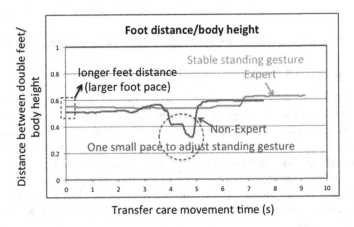

Fig. 11. Comparison of expert and non-expert's foot distance during transfer care

4   Conclusions

In this research, expert and non-expert caregiver's transfer care behavior from wheel chair to port toilet were investigated by three-dimensional motion analysis. Through comparing the moving process, body gravity track range and lower limb exertion, expert and non-expert's gesture effects on their body loading were clarified. It demonstrated that expert applied proper gesture during transfer care process in a narrow working range with short working distance. Furthermore, expert caregiver put lower limb's strength as more as possible in lift-up, turning and sit stages with knee's flexion and extension, which reduce the low back loading by waist bending motion. In a word, expert's proper care gesture made a positive effect on preventing low back pain issue in extensive transfer care works.

References

1. Marras, W.S., Davis, K.G., Kirking, B.C., Bertsche, P.K.: A comprehensive analysis of low-back disorder risk and spinal loading during the transferring and repositioning of patients using different techniques. Ergonomics **42**(7), 904–926 (1999)
2. Coenen, P., Kingma, I., Boot, C.R., Bongers, P.M., van Dieën, J.H.: Cumulative mechanical low-back load at work is a determinant of low-back pain. Occup. Environ. Med. **71**(5), 332–337 (2014). doi:10.1136/oemed-2013-101862. Epub 27 Mar 2014
3. Ito, M., Endo, A., Takai, Y., Yoshikawa, T., Goto, A., Kuwahara, N.: Study on kind transfer assistance between wheelchair and bed in the case of eye movement analysis. Proceeding of 5th International Conference on Applied Human Factors and Ergonomics (AHFE 2014)

Balancing Power Consumption and Data Analysis Accuracy Through Adjusting Sampling Rates: Seeking for the Optimal Configuration of Inertial Sensors for Power Wheelchair Users

Tao Liu, Chuanwei Chen, Melicent King, Gang Qian, and Jicheng Fu[(✉)]

Department of Computer Science, University of Central Oklahoma, Edmond, OK, USA
jfu@uco.edu

Abstract. Smartphones have already been used to capture wheelchair maneuvering data to analyze a wheelchair user's activity level, which is directly related to his/her quality of life. Typically, the inertial sensors (e.g., accelerometer and gyroscope) in a smartphone are used for data collection. However, the limited battery life of the smartphone has become a major barrier to effective data collection. The sampling rate, as a primary configurable parameter of an inertial sensor, may have important impact on power consumption. Presumably, a lower sampling rate would consume less battery power. However, it may compromise the accuracy of data analysis. In this study, we investigate how the sampling rate of inertial sensors impacts the battery power consumption as well as the accuracy of data analysis. The four pre-defined sampling rate settings of the Android OS were evaluated for their impact on the smartphone's power consumption. Additionally, we also measured the accuracy differences of the four sampling settings by comparing the sensor data-derived wheelchair maneuvering distances with the actual distances. The experimental results showed that it is possible and practical to balance the power consumption and data analysis accuracy by switching between appropriate sampling rate settings.

Keywords: Smartphone · Inertial sensors · Power wheelchair · Power consumption · Sampling rate

1 Introduction

Physical activity is associated with a decrease of depression and anxiety effects while enhancing the psychological well-being of individuals [1]. Unfortunately, only 15 percent of Americans achieved the recommended level of physical activity [2]. For wheelchair users, the situation is even worse since they face a higher risk of certain serious diseases due to their limitation of physical activities. For instance, a wheelchair user with spinal cord injury (SCI) suffers a significant higher rate (225 %) of mortality due to the coronary heart disease than normal people [3].

Nowadays smartphones have found the way into our daily lives. Smartphones are usually equipped with a rich set of sensors, e.g., accelerometers, gyroscope, compass,

© Springer International Publishing Switzerland 2015
V.G. Duffy (Ed.): DHM 2015, Part II, LNCS 9185, pp. 184–192, 2015.
DOI: 10.1007/978-3-319-21070-4_19

GPS, etc. [4]. Due to its prevalence and functionality, smartphones can be an ideal choice for wheelchair users to monitor their daily activities and collect wheelchair maneuvering data for the subsequent analysis [5, 6]. It is then possible to quantify the wheelchair users' physical activities and motivate them to be more active and healthier to improve their quality of life [7].

A problem of using smartphones for activity monitoring is that they have only limited battery life, which will be a serious barricade between high accuracy and the service time. When a smartphone's inertial sensor is working at a high sampling rate, it will generate a large volume of data and consequently cause heavy workload on networks and/or system storage, which can drain the battery rapidly. On the other hand, if a low rate setting is applied, it may yield unsatisfying accuracy in data analysis. In this study, we aim to investigate the effect of sensor sampling rates on the power consumption as well as how to configure the inertial sensors to collect acceptable accurate data while consuming relatively low energy.

This paper is organized as follows. Section 2 introduces the related research works, and limitations on smartphone inertial sensors and the power consumption. Section 3 presents our evaluation method on power consumption of the 4 pre-defined sampling rate settings. Section 4 shows the experimental results and discussion of the evaluation. Section 5 concludes the paper with our consideration on balancing power consumption and analysis accuracy. We also identified our contributions to researches in similar areas.

2 Related Works

In order to address the balancing issue between energy and accuracy, a lot of works need to be done on smartphone network connection, operating system (e.g. Android, iOS), programming and configuration [8–11].

A recent research in [12] evaluated some major inertial sensors on a Google Nexus 4 smartphone for accuracy, sampling frequency, sampling period jitter and power consumption of two pre-defined sampling rate settings. The authors demonstrated that the inertial accelerometers and gyroscope could offer reliable readings and the "Normal" setting consumed 25 %–28.6 % less power than the "Fastest" setting during one hour. The authors did not present further data analysis for other sampling settings or practical applications. In order to see the impact of power efficiency of each subsystem and/or app running on a smartphone, Gordon et al. developed a power monitoring app [13] to directly demonstrate and record the battery usage status. This app can collect consumed power data for the major system components on a smartphone. However, currently this app mainly works for HTC G1, G2 and Nexus One phones and may only obtain rough results on other phones [13]. Another app related to smartphone energy consumption is a benchmark suite [14], which provided energy evaluation for smartphone platforms by executing a series of representative applications. This benchmark suite can evaluate mobile systems from architectural aspects and mainly focused on the application cores, memory and storage subsystem.

For power saving approaches, Qiu et al. proposed an algorithm [9] based on dynamic voltage scaling (DVS) to reduce the total energy consumption for smartphones for up to 34.2 %. The algorithm focused on CPU voltage and OS concerns, but did not consider the inertial sensors. For the GPS sensor in [15], a power efficient touring scheme (PETS) is presented for smartphone power saving. This scheme adjusts the sampling rate of GPS dynamically to keep yielding accurate positioning for pedestrians with 45 % less power consumption. Another way for energy management is to switch between working and sleeping mode. A mode, namely, O-Sleep was given in [16], which could make a smartphone UI to sleep when no meaningful output was detected. The authors reported that it could save 37 % of the power consumption in the experiments for some key applications, e.g., Internet browsing, email sending, Facebook accessing of different scenarios. Network connection type is a crucial concern for cloud and mobile computing. Hence, a measurement was taken in [17] included Wi-Fi, 2G and 3G networks on Samsung Galaxy SII and SIII phones. The Wi-Fi connection is found to consume by far the least energy for the same uploading task. Additionally, the author also proposed an energy consumption model, which can help decide whether to migrate computational tasks to the cloud or take a local processing.

In this paper we tried to find out a solution to balance the power consumption and data analysis accuracy. To the best of our knowledge, this is the first study that aims to investigate the impact of sensor sampling rates on battery power consumption and data analysis accuracy.

3   Method

We have developed an Android app to capture and transmit wheelchair maneuvering data to a cloud computing environment for storage and analysis [5] as shown in Fig. 1.

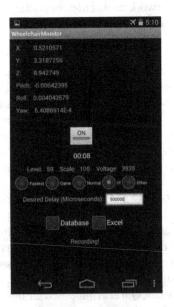

Fig. 1. The Android app for this study

This app controls the accelerometer and gyroscope in a smartphone for data collection. Specifically, it captures accelerations in 3 axes (x, y and z) with the accelerometer and collects angular velocities (yaw, pitch and roll) with the gyroscope, as shown in Fig. 2. In addition, this app can monitor power consumption by periodically recording battery voltage and percentage. The Android system predefines four sampling settings, namely, Fastest, Game, Normal and UI. We tested two LG Nexus 5 smartphones and found that the actual sampling rates ranged from 4–134 Hz for these predefined settings. As shown in Fig. 1, our app allows users to either select sampling setting or define the sampling rate by themselves. The recorded power consumption data is saved in a local file on the smartphone. The purpose is to save battery power by alleviating the network load, i.e., only wheelchair maneuvering data is transmitted to the cloud.

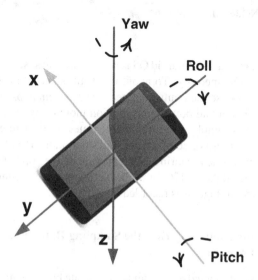

Fig. 2. Three axes of a smartphone

The Android app was designed to be easy-to-use. The user can simply click the button in the center of the interface, and then the app will start to collect and transmit data to the cloud. The app also offers the option of storing wheelchair maneuvering data locally on the phone (i.e., by selecting the "Excel" option).

3.1 Experiments for Evaluating How the Sampling Rate Impacts Power Consumption

In the Android OS context, the sensor reading is event-driven, i.e., a data item is read whenever the sensor detects a change. We have conducted an experiment to investigate how the sampling rates impacts battery power consumption. Table 1 illustrates and explains the four predefined settings of sampling rates for an inertial sensor supported by the Android SDK [18]. Since the sampling rate for each setting is not fixed, but falls within a range, the smartphone app also keeps the time when a data item is read, i.e., the timestamp for each data item.

Table 1. Sampling settings of inertial sensors (unit: Hz)

Option	Sampling rate		Description
	Accelerometer	Gyroscope	
SENSOR_DELAY_FASTEST	127-134	46 - 49	get sensor data as fast as possible
SENSOR_DELAY_GAME	46 - 49	46 - 49	suitable for games
SENSOR_DELAY_UI	14 - 16	14 - 16	suitable for the user interface
SENSOR_DELAY_NORMAL	14 - 16	4 - 6	suitable for screen orientation changes

Considering the fact that the Android OS is a multi-tasking system, it allows different applications to run simultaneously. To avoid the disturbance from other applications, we performed a factory-reset and only kept necessary system apps. Then, we installed our app for data collection and power consumption monitoring. The same experiment was performed for each sampling setting for five times in order to guarantee a sturdy result. To ensure the fairness of comparisons, the smartphone (LG Nexus 5) was fully charged before any experiment. During each experiment, the app kept collecting accelerometer and gyroscope data for 120 min. The battery power consumption, in terms of battery percentage and voltage, was recorded every 10 min.

3.2 Experiments for Evaluating How the Sampling Rate Impacts Data Analysis Accuracy

In this experiment, we conducted experiments to evaluate how the sampling rate impacts data analysis accuracy. Particularly, we use wheelchair maneuvering distance as the evaluation metrics for analysis accuracy. During the experiments, we still used the LG Nexus 5 smartphone, which was installed on the left armrest of a wheelchair and was oriented with its Y-axis aligned to the driving direction as shown in Fig. 3.

Additionally, we attached an ActiGraph sensor on each side of the wheels to obtain referential distances [19, 20]. The maneuvering data was collected inside an academic building for 20 trials for each of the 4 predefined sampling rate settings. During a trial, the wheelchair would be driven for a distance of 60.855 ± 1.847 meters and would make four 90-degree and one 180-degree turns. Hence, the trials included major wheelchair maneuvers for the user's daily activities.

After data is collected, we performed noise reduction and distance calculation using the approach we proposed in [21]. We developed a k-nearest neighbors (KNN) algorithm that could classify fine-grained wheelchair maneuvers. First, the wheelchair maneuvers were classified into 8 classes, namely, idle, acceleration, deceleration, constant speed, left turn, right turn, spot turn to left, and spot turn to right. The training samples for KNN were setup by pre-collected data. Since the Y axis of the smartphone was oriented to the

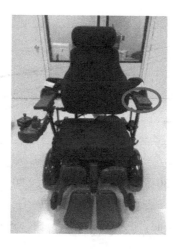

Fig. 3. The smartphone and the wheelchair

driving direction, acceleration data in the Y axis was used for classification. The data sequence was divided into data segments, with each segment containing 10 consecutive data elements. We used 40 training samples for each class of the wheelchair maneuvers (totally 320 samples for 8 classes). The maneuvering class was determined by the majority of the nearest neighbors. To determine the nearest neighbors, the Euclidian distance was used for measuring the distance between the testing data and each of the training samples. Once the maneuvering class was obtained, we used the trapezoidal rules [22] to calculate distances for the moving maneuvers individually. The overall distance was obtained by summing up the individual distances. As a result, the accumulated errors were significantly reduced.

4   Results

Figure 4 illustrates the experimental results for battery power consumption which was introduced in Sect. 3.1. The smartphone indeed consumed the most battery power with the "Fastest" setting: after 120 min, the smartphone consumed 50 % of the total battery power. When it worked with the "Normal" setting, it only consumed 28 %. Moreover, the "UI" and "Normal" settings had very close power consumption due to their similar sampling rates for accelerometers.

Table 2 displays the distance calculation accuracy. The "Fastest" setting had the smallest average error, while the "Normal" setting had the largest. Furthermore, statistical significance existed only between the "Fastest" and "Normal" settings (p = 0.024). Thus, we will not experience significant accuracy loss if we configure the app to collect data with a lower sampling rate, such as the "UI" or "Game" setting.

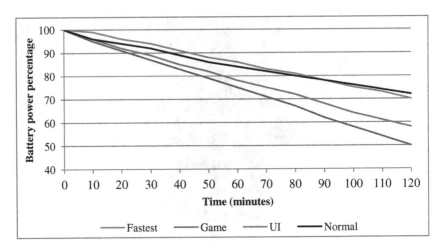

Fig. 4. The battery power drop percentage for different sampling

Table 2. Relative error of distance calculation on different rates (unit: %)

	Fastest	Game	UI	Normal
Min. error	0.73	0.08	5.49	6.23
Max. error	28.6	34.05	27.39	31.71
Avg. error	9.86	13.00	13.09	14.82

5   Discussion and Conclusions

In this study, we aimed to investigate how to balance the battery power consumption of smartphones and data analysis accuracy through adjusting inertial sensors' sampling rates. Correspondingly, we conducted two types of experiments to evaluate how the sampling rate of inertial sensors impacts battery power consumption as well as data analysis accuracy. Experimental results confirmed that higher sampling rates indeed consumed more battery power. As shown in Fig. 4, the battery power was consumed almost linearly as time elapsed. The higher sampling rate corresponded to a steeper slope. Hence, to save battery power, a lower sampling rate is preferable. In addition, the experiment for evaluating data analysis accuracy demonstrated that higher sampling rates achieved relatively better analysis accuracy (as shown in Table 2). It appears that a higher sampling rate is preferred if we desire to achieve good analysis accuracy. The good news is that the accuracy differences are not statistically significant between "Fastest" and "Game", and between "Fastest" and "UI". Hence, the sampling rates of "Game" or "UI" may be a good tradeoff, which balances battery power consumption without significantly decreasing data analysis accuracy.

Based on information obtained from this study, we will develop a context-aware algorithm in our future work, which can adjust the sampling rate of an inertial sensor based on the actual context, e.g., stationary, moving, etc., to achieve efficient power consumption while maintaining satisfactory data analysis accuracy.

Study limitations exist in this study. First, we only tested the LG Nexus 5 smartphone. Different smartphones may demonstrate different power consumption patterns. Second, we only used the wheelchair maneuvering distance as the metric to evaluate the impact of inertial sensor's sampling rates. In the next step, we will test other brands of Android smartphones to evaluate more metrics that are related to wheelchair users' activities, such as maneuvering time, number of bouts [23], etc.

In summary, the approach proposed in this study and the experimental results may generate immediate benefits to researchers, who use Android smartphone sensors in research.

Acknowledgement. This study was supported by the National Institute of General Medical Sciences of the National Institutes of Health through Grant Number 8P20GM103447.

References

1. Wendel-Vos, G.C.W., Schuit, A.J., Tijhuis, M.A.R., Kromhout, D.: Leisure time physical activity and health-related quality of life: Cross-sectional and longitudinal associations. Qual. Life Res. **13**, 667–677 (2004)
2. Healthy people 2010: Understanding and improving health, Washington, DC, November 2000
3. Jacobs, P.L., Nash, M.S.: Modes, benefits, and risks of voluntary an delectrically induced exercise in persons with spinal cord injury. J. Spinal Cord Med. **24**, 10–18 (2001)
4. Lane, N.D., Miluzzo, E., Lu, H., et al.: A survey of mobile phone sensing. IEEE Commun. Mag. **48**, 11 (2010)
5. Fu, J., Hao, W., White, T., Yan, Y., Jones, M., Jan, Y.K.: Capturing and analyzing wheelchair maneuvering patterns with mobile cloud computing. In: Conference proceedings: IEEE Engineering in Medicine and Biology Society, vol. 2013, pp. 2419–2422 (2013). PMID: 24110214
6. Hiremath, S.V., Ding, D., Cooper, R.A.: Development and evaluation of a gyroscope-based wheel rotation monitor for manual wheelchair users. J. Spinal Cord Med. **36**, 347–356 (2013)
7. Tolerico, M.L., Ding, D., Cooper, R.A., Spaeth, D.M., Fitzgerald, S.G., Cooper, R., et al.: Assessing mobility characteristics and activity levels of manual wheelchair users. J. Rehabil. Res. Dev. **44**, 561–571 (2007)
8. Anastasi, G., Bacioccola, A., Cicconetti, C., Lenzini, L., Mingozzi, E., Vallati, C.: Performance evaluation of power management for best effort applications in IEEE 802.16 networks. In: 14th European Wireless Conference, 2008. EW 2008, pp. 1–6 (2008)
9. Meikang, Q., Zhi, C., Yang, L.T., Xiao, Q., Bin, W.: Towards power-efficient Smartphones by energy-aware dynamic task scheduling. In: 2012 IEEE 14th International Conference on High Performance Computing and Communication and 2012 IEEE 9th International Conference on Embedded Software and Systems (HPCC-ICESS), pp. 1466–1472 (2012)
10. Mizouni, R., Serhani, M.A., Benharref, A., Al-Abassi, O.: Towards battery-aware self-adaptive mobile applications. In: 2012 IEEE Ninth International Conference on Services Computing (SCC), pp. 439–445 (2012)
11. Alawnah, S., Sagahyroon, A.: Modeling Smartphones Power. In: EUROCON, p. 6. IEEE (2013)

12. Ma, Z., Qiao, Y., Lee, B., Fallon, E.: Experimental evaluation of mobile phone sensors. In: Signals and Systems Conference (ISSC 2013), 24th IET Irish, p. 8, 20–21 June 2013

13. Gordon, M., Zhang, L., Tiwana, B.; A Power Monitor for Android-Based Mobile Platforms 9 October 2011. http://ziyang.eecs.umich.edu/projects/powertutor/instructions.html

14. Pandiyan, D., Lee, S.-Y., Wu, C.-J.: Performance, energy characterizations and architectural implications of an emerging mobile platform benchmark suite – MobileBench, pp. 133–142 (2013)

15. Chung-Ming, H., Chao-Hsien, L., Wei-Shuang, C.: A power efficient pedestrian touring scheme based on sensor-assisted positioning and prioritized caching for smart mobile devices. In: 2013 21st International Conference on Software, Telecommunications and Computer Networks (SoftCOM), pp. 1–5 (2013)

16. Jungseok, K., Hyunwoo, J., Hyungshin, K.: O-Sleep: Smartphones' output-oriented power saving mode. In: 2012 IEEE 15th International Conference on Computational Science and Engineering (CSE), pp. 334–340 (2012)

17. Segata, M., Bloessl, B., Sommer, C., Dressler, F.: Towards energy efficient smart phone applications: energy models for offloading tasks into the cloud. In: 2014 IEEE International Conference on Communications (ICC), pp. 2394–2399 (2014)

18. Android developers reference (Android 4.4 r1 ed.). http://developer.android.com/reference/android/hardware/
SensorManager.html#registerListener(android.hardware.SensorEventListener)

19. Actigraph. (2013). GT3X + and wGT3X + Device Manual (v2.0.0 ed.). http://dl.theactigraph.com/GT3Xp_wGT3Xp_Device_Manual.pdf

20. Sonenblum, S.E., Sprigle, S., Caspall, J., Lopez, R.: Validation of an accelerometer-based method to measure the use of manual wheelchairs. Med. Eng. Phys. 34, 781–786 (2012)

21. Jicheng, F., Tao, L., Jones, M., Gang, Q., Yih-Kuen, J.: Characterization of wheelchair maneuvers based on noisy inertial sensor data: a preliminary study. In: 2014 36th Annual International Conference of the IEEE Engineering in Medicine and Biology Society (EMBC), pp. 1731–1734 (2014)

22. Tallarida, R.J., Murray, R.B.: Area under a curve: Trapezoidal and Simpson's Rules. In: Tallarida, R.J., Murray, R.B. (eds.) Manual of Pharmacologic Calculations, pp. 77–81. Springer, New York 1987

23. Sonenblum, S.E., Sprigle, S., Harris, F.H., Maurer, C.L.: Characterization of power wheelchair use in the home and community. Arch. Phys. Med. Rehabil. 89, 486–491 (2008)

MoCap-Based Adaptive Human-Like Walking Simulation in Laser-Scanned Large-Scale as-Built Environments

Tsubasa Maruyama[✉], Satoshi Kanai, and Hiroaki Date

Graduate School of Information Science and Technology, Hokkaido University,
Sapporo 060-0814, Japan
t_maruyama@sdm.ssi.ist.hokudai.ac.jp,
{kanai,hdate}@ssi.ist.hokudai.ac.jp

Abstract. Accessibility evaluation to enhance accessibility and safety for the elderly and disabled is increasing in importance. Accessibility must be assessed not only from the general standard aspect but also in terms of physical and cognitive friendliness for users of different ages, genders, and abilities. Human behavior simulation has been progressing in crowd behavior analysis and emergency evacuation planning. This research aims to develop a virtual accessibility evaluation by combining realistic human behavior simulation using a digital human model (DHM) with as-built environmental models. To achieve this goal, we developed a new algorithm for generating human-like DHM walking motions, adapting its strides and turning angles to laser-scanned as-built environments using motion-capture (MoCap) data of flat walking. Our implementation quickly constructed as-built three-dimensional environmental models and produced a walking simulation speed sufficient for real-time applications. The difference in joint angles between the DHM and MoCap data was sufficiently small. Demonstrations of our environmental modeling and walking simulation in an indoor environment are illustrated.

Keywords: Walking simulation · Laser-scanning · Accessibility evaluation · Motion capture

1 Introduction

Accessibility evaluation to enhance accessibility and safety for the elderly and disabled is increasing in importance. Accessibility must be assessed not only from the general standard aspect specified by International Organization for Standardization [1] but also in terms of physical and cognitive friendliness for users of different ages, genders, and abilities. Conversely, human behavior simulation has been progressing in crowd behavior analysis and emergency evacuation planning [2], and there is a high possibility that the simulation can be applied to the accessibility evaluation. In human behavior simulation, the activities of a pedestrian model in indoor and outdoor environments are predicted. Moreover, human behavior simulation using kinematic digital human models (DHMs) even in a three-dimensional (3D) environmental model has become possible because of recent advances in computer performance [3]. However, in the previous human behavior simulation [2, 3], an environmental model represents only

© Springer International Publishing Switzerland 2015
V.G. Duffy (Ed.): DHM 2015, Part II, LNCS 9185, pp. 193–204, 2015.
DOI: 10.1007/978-3-319-21070-4_20

"as-planned" situations, in contrast to "as-built" or "as-is" environments. In addition, a pedestrian model cannot generate detailed articulated movements of specific groups of people such as the elderly, children, males, and females.

Our research aims to develop a virtual accessibility evaluation by combining realistic human behavior simulation using DHMs with as-built environmental models. As shown in Fig. 1, our research group has developed a prototype system of environmental modeling and walking simulation for a kinematic DHM to achieve this goal [4]. In our system, the kinematic DHM can walk autonomously with different strides and turning angles adapted to walking environments such as stairs and slopes. However, the kinematic DHM cannot necessarily recreate human-like articulated walking motion of various types of people. Motion-capture (MoCap) data of an individual person's walk enables the DHM to generate human-like walking motion. However, it is still difficult to acquire a large collection of MoCap data from many people with various strides and turning angles in different walking environments such as stairs and slopes.

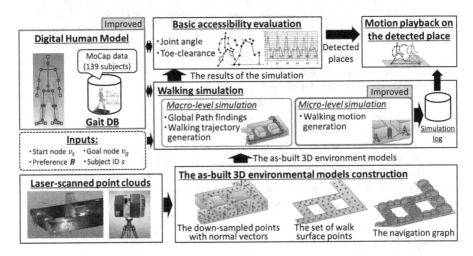

Fig. 1. Overview of the research

Therefore, in this research, we developed a new algorithm that adaptively recreates a human-like DHM walking motion using only one MoCap data reference in different flat indoor environments. As the first stage of the research, a walking simulation algorithm is proposed that enables a DHM to walk autonomously, while adapting its strides and turning angles to different as-built and flat indoor environments by combining inverse kinematics (IK) with interpolation of reference MoCap data of flat walking. Modeling and simulation efficiency and accuracy are evaluated.

2   Related Work

This research relates primarily to three areas, human behavior simulation, 3D environmental modeling from laser-scanned point clouds, and digital human modeling for walking simulation.

In human behavior simulation, studies have been conducted on crowd behavior analysis or emergency evacuation planning [2]. For example, Helbing [5] proposed a two-dimensional (2D) human behavior simulation based on a social force model. However, its simulation algorithm still remains in 2D as-planned environments. Recently, Kakizaki [6] proposed an evacuation-planning simulator that enables kinematics-based walking simulation in a 3D environmental model. However, this work used "as-planned" 3D computer-aided-design (CAD) data of a building as the environmental model. In a simulation by Pettre [7], a navigation graph representing a free space and environmental connectivity can be generated automatically from a 3D mesh model. However, Pettre used a simple-shaped 3D mesh model that was too rough to capture the detail of as-built environments.

3D as-built environmental modeling from massive laser-scanned point clouds has been actively studied. Algorithms can automatically extract floors and walls [8], household goods [9], and a constructive solid geometry model of environments [10] from massive laser-scanned point clouds. However, these researches focus only on general object recognition, without necessarily aiming for human walking navigation in the environmental models. Moreover, the algorithms cannot model small barriers on a floor as the environmental model, which is an important factor for accessibility evaluation.

Many algorithms have been developed in digital human modeling for walking simulation. Among them, a variety of human walking patterns can be synthesized using principal component analysis (PCA) [11]. Although such simulation systems can generate human-like walking motion, they still require a large collection of MoCap data in advance. Therefore, many researchers focus on estimating and generating an arbitrary human motion only from a small number of existing MoCap data. Motion synthesis and editing [12], motion rings [13], and machine learning [14] are typical examples. However, they still require a small number of MoCap data to adapt DHM strides and turning angles to walking environments. In addition, it is generally difficult to persuade elderly persons, the main targets of accessibility evaluation, to join prolonged MoCap data collection efforts. Conversely, human-like walking motions have been generated in recent physics-based walking simulation using motion controllers and game-engines [15, 16]. However, naturalness of the walking motion is sensitive to the motion controller parameters. Recently, Rami [17] proposed a motion-retargeting algorithm in which joint positions relative to the walking surface can be adapted to changes in the walking environments. However, the resultant motion is not evaluated. In addition, there is no guarantee that human-like articulated movements can be generated on slopes and stairs, because the algorithm does not use real motion data for the adaptation.

In contrast to previous research, our walking simulation algorithm

- generates human-like walking motion using only one MoCap data reference,
- adapts the DHM stride and turning angle to different as-built and flat indoor environments,
- provides fast and autonomous walking simulation directly in the point clouds-based environmental models,
- provides a sufficiently small difference in joint angles between the DHM and MoCap data.

3 3D Environmental Modeling from Laser-Scanned Point Clouds

Figure 2 shows an overview of the 3D environmental modeling and the walking simulation of the DHM. For the DHM walking simulation, first, the 3D environmental models are constructed automatically from the 3D laser-scanned point clouds of the as-built environments [4]. As shown in Fig. 2, a 3D environmental model consists of two point clouds (the down-sampled points with normal vectors and the set of walk surface points) and the navigation graph. Processing overviews are described in the following sub sections.

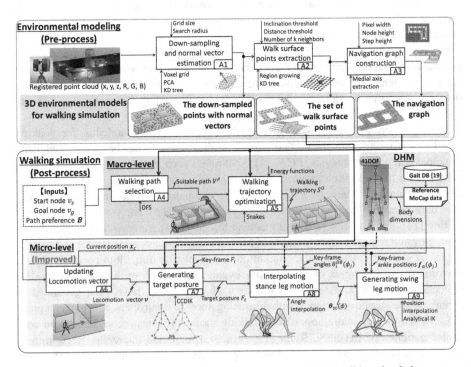

Fig. 2. Overview of 3D environmental modeling and DHM walking simulation

(A1) Down-sampling and normal vector estimation. Multiple laser-scanned point clouds are first merged to make one registered point clouds. This registered point clouds contain many points; hence; it is down-sampled using a voxel grid. In this study, around 1,000 points per square meter is sufficient for modeling and simulation.

Then, normal vectors at the down-sampled points are estimated using PCA on the locally neighboring points [18]. These point clouds with normal vectors $Q^D = \{(\boldsymbol{q}_i, \boldsymbol{n}_i)\}$ are used as a part of the 3D environmental model to express the geometry of the entire environment.

(A2) Walk surface points extraction. The walk surface points, representing walkable surfaces such as floors and stair-steps, are automatically extracted from the down-sampled points Q^D.

First, as shown in Fig. 3(a), if the angle between a normal vector n_i at a point q_i and a vector $v = [0, 0, +1]$ is smaller than the threshold ε (we set $\varepsilon = 20$ deg.), then the point is added into horizontal points $Q^H = \{q_j^H\}$ placed on a horizontal plane.

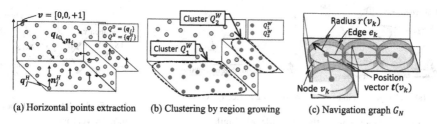

(a) Horizontal points extraction   (b) Clustering by region growing   (c) Navigation graph G_N

Fig. 3. 3D environmental modeling from 3D laser-scanned point clouds

Then, as shown in Fig. 3(b), the horizontal points are clustered into a set of walk surface points $W = \{Q_k^W\}$ using a region growing algorithm based on k-nearest search [4].

(A3) Navigation graph construction. Finally, we generate a navigation graph representing the environmental pathways for navigating the DHM during walking simulation. To generate a navigation graph from laser-scanned point clouds, we extend the algorithm of Pettre [7], which generates navigation graphs from a simple-shaped 3D mesh model. As shown in Fig. 3(c), the navigation graph $\langle G_N = V, E, c, t \rangle$ comprises a set of graph nodes V and a set of edges E. Each node $v_k \in V$ represents free space of the environment. It has a position vector $t(v_k)$ and an attribute of a cylinder $c(v_k)$, whose radius $r(v_k)$ and height h represent the distance to the wall and the walkable step height, respectively. Each edge e_k represents connectivity of the environment and is generated between two nodes with a common region [4].

4 MoCap-Based Adaptive Walking Simulation in as-Built Environments

After environmental modeling, a walking simulation of the DHM is performed directly in the point clouds-based environmental models. To generate human-like walking motion, we use only one reference MoCap data of flat walking in a gait database (DB) containing the data of 139 subjects provided by the National Institute of Advanced Industrial Science and Technology (AIST) [19].

As shown in Fig. 2, our DHM has 41 degrees of freedom (DOF) totally and the same body dimensions as the subjects in the gait DB. The walking simulation consists of both macro- and micro-level simulations. Details are described in the following sub sections.

4.1   Macro-Level Simulation

As shown in Fig. 4(a), in the macro-level simulation, first, a set of DHM walking paths $V^W = \{V^i\}$ is found automatically using depth-first search over the navigation graph G_N. Each path V^i consists of a set of graph nodes and edges from the user-defined start node v_s to goal node v_g. Next, a suitable walking path $V^P \in V^W$ is selected automatically from V^W based on the path cost and user's path preference [4].

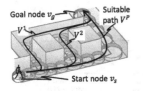
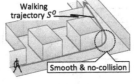

(a) Global path findings   (b) Walking trajectory generation

Fig. 4. Overview of the macro-level simulation

Fig. 5. Updating next locomotion vector

Then, as shown in Fig. 4(b), the DHM walking trajectory $S^O = \{s_i\}$ tracing a time sequence of the DHM pelvis position s_i, is generated automatically. An optimization algorithm is applied to make the trajectory S^O more natural and smooth, while avoiding contact with the walls [4].

4.2   Micro-Level Simulation Based on MoCap Data

After the walking trajectory S^O is determined, one-step DHM walking motion along the trajectory S^O is generated in the micro-level simulation. Variable stride and turning angle during the walk can be achieved while estimating footprint positions automatically using reference MoCap data of flat walking selected from the gait DB [19]. As shown in Fig. 2 (A6–A9), one-step walking motion is generated according to the following processes.

4.2.1   Updating Locomotion Vector (A6)

As shown in Fig. 5, when the DHM passes through the trajectory point $s_k \in S^O$, the system determines a sub goal position x_t as $x_t = s_{k+2}$, which serves as a temporary target position during the simulation. The sub goal position x_t is continuously updated as the DHM walks along the trajectory S^O. Then, the next locomotion vector v is determined using $v = (x_t - x_c)/ \parallel x_t - x_c \parallel$, where x_c represents the current DHM pelvis position.

Then, as shown in Fig. 6, the next footprint point x_f is determined on the walk surface points W. To this end, a cylindrical search space C_F is generated centered at a point p_f placed ahead of the current heel position x_{hs} by the stride length w. Next, a subset of the walk surface points W_S with the maximum point number inside of C_F is extracted from W. Finally, the next footprint point x_f is determined as a centroid of W_S.

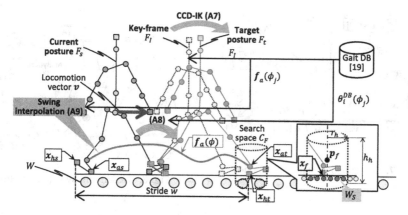

Fig. 6. Overview of the micro-level simulation

Note that any user-defined stride length w that is different from the original stride length of the reference MoCap data in the gait DB can be used.

4.2.2 Generating Target Posture (A7)

As shown in Fig. 6, to achieve the next footprint point x_f, a DHM target posture F_t is generated using cyclic-coordinate-descent inverse kinematics (CCDIK) [20]. First, aey-frame posture F_I, representing the full-body posture at the initial contact frame in the next walking step is obtained from among a set of frames in the reference MoCap data selected from the gait DB. Then, we apply a CCDIK method, an iterative inverse kinematics (IK) solver for redundant link-mechanisms, to the key-frame posture F_I to determine the 14 DOF leg posture of the DHM. To obtain a plausible target posture F_t, we introduce a range of motion (ROM) and symmetric hip joint angles as CCDIK constraints.

4.2.3 Interpolating Stance Leg Motion (A8)

As shown in Fig. 6, once a target posture F_t is obtained, as described in 4.2.2, the stance leg motion is interpolated so that the motion finally satisfies F_t at the end of the interpolation. Figure 7 shows the interpolation algorithm. In Fig. 7, $\theta_i^{DHM}(\phi)$, $\theta_i^{DB}(\phi)$, $\phi \in [0,1]$ represent the ith joint angle of the DHM's stance leg, the corresponding joint angle obtained from the reference MoCap data, and the normalized walking phase, respectively.

First, the specific key-frame angle $\theta_i^{DB}(\phi_j)$ of the ith joint at ϕ_j is loaded from the reference MoCap data. We assume that the angles of the stance leg at the middle stance phase changed less against strides, and we select angles $\theta_i^{DB}(\phi_j)$ at $\phi_j \in \{0.4, 0.5, 0.6\}$ as the key-frame angles to be left unchanged. Then, the stance leg angles $\theta_i^{DHM}(\phi)$ are interpolated using a cubic spline curve, so that they coincide with the key-frame angles $\theta_i^{DB}(\phi_j)$ at $\phi_j \in \{0.4, 0.5, 0.6\}$. The angles $\theta_i^{DHM}(0)$ and $\theta_i^{DHM}(1)$ and the angular velocities $\dot{\theta}_i^{DHM}(0)$ and $\dot{\theta}_i^{DHM}(1)$ at the current and target postures F_s and F_t, respectively, are also used as boundary conditions. The angular velocity $\dot{\theta}_i^{DHM}(0)$ is estimated

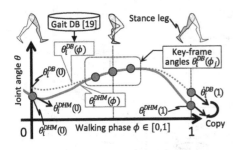

Fig. 7. Interpolating stance leg motion

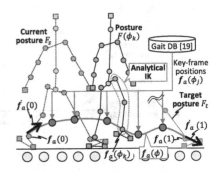

Fig. 8. Generating swing leg motion

by fitting a cubic polynomial curve locally to the DHM joint angles. And $\dot{\theta}_i^{DHM}(1)$ is also estimated similarly by fitting a cubic polynomial curve locally to the reference MoCap data.

If a turning or steering motion is required on the floor, the internal or external angle of the stance leg hip joint is increased gradually in each frame during one-step walking until the rotation angle θ^{rot} is reached. θ^{rot} represents the angle between the current locomotion vector v and the locomotion vector v^{pre} at the previous one-step walking.

4.2.4 Generating Swing Leg Motion (A9)

Applying the generated stance leg angles $\theta_i^{DHM}(\phi)$ to the DHM automatically determines the DHM pelvis position. As shown in Fig. 8, the swing ankle position trajectory $f_a(\phi)$ is then interpolated using a cubic spline curve, so that they coincide with the key-frame ankle positions $f_a(\phi_j)$ at $\phi_j \in \{0.2, 0.4, 0.6, 0.8, 0.9\}$. The positions $f_a(0)$ and $f_a(1)$ and the velocities $\dot{f}_a(0)$ and $\dot{f}_a(1)$ at the current and target postures F_s and F_t, respectively, are also used as boundary conditions. As in stance interpolation (Sect. 4.2.3), the velocities $\dot{f}_a(0)$ and $\dot{f}_a(1)$ are estimated by fitting a cubic polynomial curve locally to the reference MoCap data.

Finally, all of the joint angles of the swing leg are determined by solving IK analytically to achieve the interpolated ankle position trajectory $f_a(\phi)$ in each frame. In this simulation, walking phase ϕ is increased by 0.01 in each frame, and the one-step DHM motion is interpolated by 100 frames.

5 Simulation Results

We validated our modeling and simulation algorithm in a laser-scanned indoor environment. The 3D point clouds were acquired using a terrestrial laser scanner (FARO Focus^{3D} S120) and have seven million points. Figures 9(a), (b) and (c) show the entire point clouds, walk surface points, and navigation graph, respectively. As shown in Fig. 9(b), the walk surface points represent walkable surfaces such as floors and stairs.

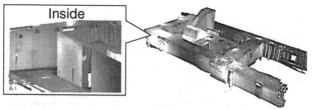

(a) Point clouds of an indoor environments

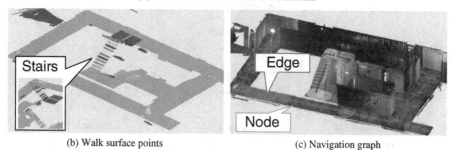

(b) Walk surface points   (c) Navigation graph

Fig. 9. 3D environmental model construction

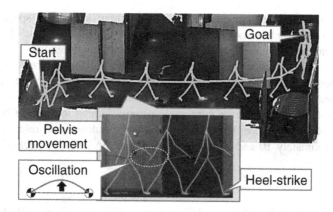

Fig. 10. Walking simulation in a corridor in case of a subject males, age 22

Moreover, as shown in Fig. 9(c), the navigation graph represents the free space and its connectivity even in stairs.

5.1 Walking Simulation Results in the 3D Environmental Models

Figure 10 shows a walking simulation result in a corridor with corners. The DHM was able to walk along the pathway automatically step by step. In addition, the proposed simulation algorithm could plausibly recreate the oscillation of the pelvis that has been

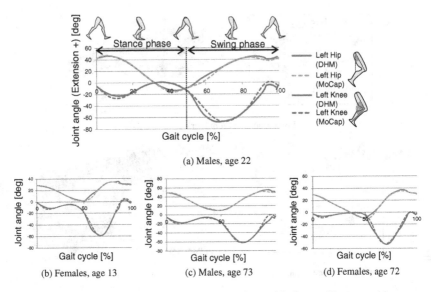

(a) Males, age 22

(b) Females, age 13

(c) Males, age 73

(d) Females, age 72

Fig. 11. Comparisons of DHM walking motions with those of human subjects

observed as a feature of human walking [21] without any direct specification or interpolation of the pelvis movements. This shows the effectiveness of generating human-like walking motion while respecting human walking features.

In addition, Fig. 11 shows a comparison of DHM walking motions with those of human subjects of different ages and genders. The DHM motions were estimated using a limited number of MoCap data frames from corresponding subjects. As shown in Fig. 11, the DHM could generate joint angle patterns similar to those of human subjects. The maximum angle differences between the simulation and reference MoCap data are approximately 10 and 5 deg in the knee and hip joints, respectively.

Table 1. Elapsed time of modeling and simulation (CPU: Intel(R) Core(TM) i7 3.30 GHz, Memory: 32 GB, GPU: GeForce GTX 560 Ti)

Processing			Time [s]
Pre-process	Laser scanning		(5 h)
	Registration of point clouds		(1 h)
	As-built environmental model construction		5.48
Post-process	Macro-level simulation		0.001-0.02
	Micro-level simulation	Updating locomotion vector	0.001
		Generating target posture	0.2
		Interpolating stance leg motion	0.001
	Generating one-step walking motion (100-frame interpolation)		0.271

5.2   Modeling and Simulation Performance

Table 1 shows the elapsed time of the 3D environmental model construction from the original point clouds and of the walking simulation. The Point Cloud Library (PCL) [22] was partly used for point cloud processing, and OpenGL was used for rendering. The 3D environmental model construction required approximately 6 s for approximately seven million points, significantly faster than manual modeling.

The elapsed time for the macro-level simulation, a preparation for beginning the micro-level simulation, was less than 0.1 s, and the elapsed time for one-step walking motion simulation with 100-frame interpolation in the micro-level simulation required approximately 0.3 s, less than that of a human walking. This shows the possibility of real-time walking simulation for one DHM.

6   Conclusions

In this study, we developed a new algorithm for generating human-like walking motion for a DHM using one MoCap data reference of flat walking selected from a gait DB. The DHM could walk autonomously, while adapting its stride and turning angle to as-built environmental models automatically constructed from laser-scanned point clouds. The simulation results were validated through comparison with original MoCap data. It was confirmed that the DHM could walk autonomously in the environmental model, while respecting the walking motions of various types of people of different ages and genders. The elapsed time for modeling and simulation was suitable for practical application.

As future work, we aim to develop walking simulations for more complex environments. An algorithm for stairs and slope walking would significantly advance the field of the virtual human accessibility evaluation.

References

1. ISO21542: Building construction –Accessibility and usability of the built environment (2011)
2. Thalmann, D., Musse, S.R.: Crowd Simulation, pp. 3–4. Springer, London (2007)
3. Kakizaki, T., Urii, J., Endo, M.: Post-Tsunami evacuation simulation using 3D kinematic digital human models and experimental verification. J. Comput. Inf. Sci. Eng. **14**(2), 021010-1–021010-9 (2014)
4. Maruyama, T., Kanai, S., Date, H.: Simulating a walk of digital human model directly in massive 3D laser-scanned point cloud of indoor environments. In: Duffy, V.G. (ed.) HCII 2013 and DHM 2013, Part II. LNCS, vol. 8026, pp. 366–375. Springer, Heidelberg (2013)
5. Helbing, D., Farkas, I., Vicsek, T.: simulating dynamical features of escape panic. Nature **407**, 487–490 (2000)
6. Kakizaki, T., Urii, J., Endo, M.: A three-dimensional evacuation simulation using digital human models with precise kinematics joints. J. Comput. Inf. Sci. Eng. **12**(3), 031001-1–031001-8 (2012)

7. Pettre, J., Laumond, J.-P., Thalmann, D.: A navigation graph for real-time crowd animation on multi-layered and uneven terrain. In: Proceedings of 1st International Workshop on Crowd Simulation (V- CROWDS 2005), pp. 81–90 (2005)

8. Nüchter, A., Hertzberg, J.: Towards semantic maps for mobile robots. Robot. Auton. Syst. 56(11), 915–926 (2008)

9. Rusu, R.B., Marton, Z.C., Blodow, N., Dolha, M., Beetz, M.: Towards 3D point cloud based object maps for household environments. Robot. Auton. Syst. 56(11), 927–941 (2008)

10. Xiao, J., Furukawa, Y.: Reconstructing the world's museums. Int. J. Comput. Vision 110(3), 243–258 (2014)

11. Troje, N.F.: Decomposing biological motion: a framework for analysis and synthesis of human gait patterns. J. Vis. 2(5), 371–387 (2002)

12. Min, J., Liu, H., Chai, J.: Synthesis and editing of personalized stylistic human motion. In: Proceedings of the 2010 ACM SIGGRAPH Symposium on Interactive 3D Graphics and Games, pp. 39–46 (2010)

13. Mukai, T.: Motion rings for interactive gait synthesis. In: Proceedings of ACM Symposium on Interactive 3D Graphics and Games, pp. 125–132 (2011)

14. Grochow, K., Martin, S.L., Hertzmann, A., Popovic, Z.: Style-based Inverse Kinematics. ACM Trans. Graph. 23(23), 522–531 (2004)

15. Yin, K., Loken, K., van de Panne, M.: SIMBICON: simple biped locomotion control. ACM Trans. Graph. 26(3), 105 (2007)

16. Coros, S., Beaudoin, P., van de Panne, M.: Generalized biped walking control. ACM Trans. Graph. 29(4), 130 (2010)

17. Al-Asqhar, R.A., Komura, T., Choi, M.G.: Relationship descriptors for interactive motion adaptation. In: Proceedings of the 12th ACM SIGGRAPH/Eurographics Symposium on Computer Animation, pp. 45–53 (2013)

18. Rusu, R.B.: Semantic 3D Object Maps for Everyday Robot Manipulation. Springer, Heidelberg (2013)

19. Kobayashi, Y., Mochimaru, M.: AIST Gait Database 2013 (2013). https://www.dh.aist.go.jp/database/gait2013/

20. Pan, H., Hou, X., Gao, C., Lei, Y.: A method of real-time human motion retargeting for 3D terrain adaptation. In: Proceedings of 13th IEEE JICSIT, pp. 1–5 (2013)

21. Perry, J., Burnfield, J.M.: GAIT ANALYSIS Normal and Pathological Function, 2nd edn. SLACK Inc., New Jersey (2010)

22. PCL –Point Cloud Library. http://pointclouds.org/

Electromyography Measurement of Workers at the Second Lining Pounding Process for Hanging Scrolls

Yasuhiro Oka[1]([⊠]), Yuka Takai[2], Akihiko Goto[2],
Hisanori Yuminaga[3], and Kozo Oka[1]

[1] Kyoto Institute of Technology, Kyoto, Japan
okayas@mac.com, oka@bokkodo.co.jp
[2] Osaka Sangyo University, Osaka, Japan
{takai,gotoh}@ise.osaka-sandai.ac.jp
[3] Kansai Vocational College of Medicine, Osaka, Japan
yuminaga@kansai.ac.jp

Abstract. Hanging scrolls are a traditional Japanese form of binding and displaying artwork or calligraphy. The scrolls are rolled up from the bottom up and stored in a box, or hung on a wall for display. It is important for the scroll to be able to roll up smoothly without causing any creases when on display. Several layers of Japanese *washi* paper attached to the back of the scroll make these two functions possible. Wheat starch glue, a weak form of adhesive used to fortify the back, is combined with a technique called "pounding" with the use of a pounding brush, to promote adhesion. In this research, we attached an electromyograph on two subjects – an expert and non-expert binder – to study the movement of their muscles in 9 locations when pounding. Results of this study are expected to help contribute to the acquisition of the binding technique.

Keywords: Electromyograph · Hanging scroll · Pounding brush · Aged glue

1 Introduction

Hanging scrolls are among the most recognized of the many forms of binding and displaying Japanese paintings and calligraphy (Fig. 1).

Scrolls are unique in that they are hung on a wall or in an alcove only during viewing, and stored in a box otherwise. When the scrolls are rolled up for storage, the artwork faces inside, protecting it from exposure to light and air to minimize damage. This binding method is garnering attention even within the area of preserving cultural assets for its ability to preserve artwork in the long-term.

The scroll has to be able to roll up smoothly without causing any creases. And, when hung for viewing, the scroll has to hang straight without curling up. To enable this, the back of the scroll is typically lined with 3–4 layers of Japanese *washi* paper. The *washi* is attached to the back with the wheat starch. The second layer of *washi* and beyond, in particular, requires wheat starch with weak adhesive to keep the backing from hardening after it's dried. This adhesive is what makes the smooth and creaseless scrolling possible. However, in order to withstand frequent handling, the *washi* needs

© Springer International Publishing Switzerland 2015
V.G. Duffy (Ed.): DHM 2015, Part II, LNCS 9185, pp. 205–215, 2015.
DOI: 10.1007/978-3-319-21070-4_21

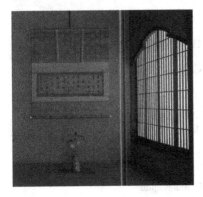

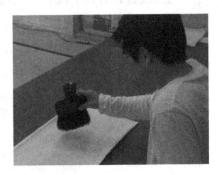

Fig. 1. A scroll hanging in an alcove

Fig. 2. Pounding in action

sufficient adhesion. This is where the surface of the *washi* is pounded down with a brush to enhance adhesion (Fig. 2). This technique is called pounding.

Pounding with too much force can damage the surface of the backing, but also potentially the artwork that lies several layers beneath. Pounding with too little force, on the other hand, makes for ineffective adhesion.

This pounding technique requires repetitive tapping with the right amount of force evenly across a wide area. The acquisition of this technique is said to require a lot of training. Much like other traditional Japanese techniques with a high degree of difficulty, "watch and learn" is currently considered the main correct method of acquiring this skill.

For this research, we had two subjects, one an expert and another a non-expert, perform the pounding technique with their right arm, which we hooked up to an electromyograph to study the muscle activities involved with the work. We hope the results of this research will deepen our understanding of the pounding technique, a skill that takes a long time to learn, and help contribute to the acquisition of this skill.

2   Structure and Material of the Hanging Scroll

Hanging scrolls consist of several layers, starting with the main sheet, which would be a painting or calligraphy, followed by the first, second, third and the final linings. The washi paper used for each layer differs slightly in terms of where and how they were made. Each washi layer contributes to the aforementioned rolling and unfurling possible, providing the scroll with sufficient strength. To attach the first lining, wheat starch is turned into paste and used as adhesive. The wheat starch is heated in a large pot for about 50 min, then cooled off naturally overnight to produce wheat starch glue with strong adhesion. This is used to attach the first layer of washi to the main sheet. This first sheet serves as the main sheet's backing. However, using this adhesive for the second lining and beyond will only harden the layer more than necessary after the starch dries and prevent the scroll from rolling and unfurling smoothly. Which is why, for the second layer and beyond, an adhesive referred to as aged glue, with a weak adhesive strength, is used. To make aged glue, wheat starch powder is heated, turned into paste, then poured into a large jar and sealed with a wooden lid. After sitting in a cool and dark place for 10 years, the glue is ready. Aged glue has low adhesive strength compared with regular wheat starch glue. Long-term storage causes the starch to deteriorate and lose molecular weight, and because the microorganisms metabolize enzymes in lower volume compared with regular wheat starch glue, aged glue has weaker bonding power. Figure 3 shows the cross-sectional view of a hanging scroll.

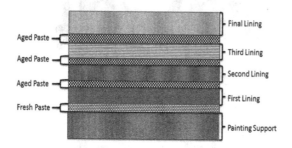

Fig. 3. Abbreviated diagram of the cross-section of a hanging scroll

3 Experimental Method

3.1 Subjects

The electromyograph experiment was performed on a 22-year expert and a 6-year non-expert. Details about each subject are shown in Table 1. The expert is acclaimed for his ability to deliver a quality product with his pounding technique. The non-expert, on the other hand, had received regular warning from the expert about pounding too strongly, and is yet to receive permission to begin pounding work. Furthermore, during an interview conducted before the experiment, we learned that the expert can perform pounding work continuously for more than several hours without feeling tired, whereas the non-expert begins to feel fatigue after 30 min of continuous pounding.

Table 1. Data about the subjects

Subject (Age)	Years of experience	Height (cm)	Weight (kg)	Sex	Interviewer
Expert (40)	22	171	72	M	R
Non-expert (27)	6	170	54	M	R

3.2 Method of Experiment

The subjects were asked to begin pounding work after gluing on a second lining on a plain sheet of silk measuring 40 square cms already backed with a first lining. Each subject's muscular movements will be measured in the process. The pounding action is to begin at front right, moving to the left in even and continuous motion to adhesion enhancement. The number of times the backing is pounded and the amount of time spent pounding differ by subject. Which is why, we measured the muscular movements of just the right arm. The parts we measured are shown in Fig. 4. There are 9 locations, which are listed below.

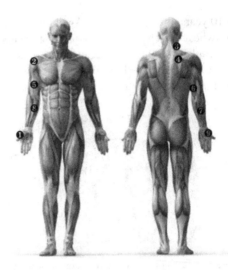

Fig. 4. Locations that were tracked.

❶Abductor pollicis brevis, ❷Deltoid middle, ❸Upper trapezius, ❹Middle trapezius, ❺Biceps brachii, ❻Triceps brachii, ❼Extensor carpi radialis brevis, ❽Flexor carpi radialis, ❾Interossei dorsales.

Electrodes (Nihon Kohden, web-1000) that were attached to the subjects' arms measured muscular activity while they performed their pounding work in an environment similar to the one they usually work in. The sampling rate was set at 1000 Hz. Two cameras – one in the front and another to the right – captured them at work.

4   Measurement Results

Results of each subject's muscle activity in the 9 locations are shown. From the overall results, we will look at which muscles were being used during the pounding action, then pinpoint which muscles were used per one pounding motion for each of the 9 muscles.

4.1   Muscles that Worked During Pounding

Figure 5 shows the expert's muscle activity as expressed in raw waveforof the EMG; Fig. 6, that of the non-expert. Of the 9 locations monitored, the biggest difference between the expert and non-expert was in their ❶abductor pollicis brevis activities. On the expert's graph, a big wave could be seen immediately following his movements, but after that, there were no large waves until after the work was completed. The big wave created by the abductor pollicis brevis immediately after monitoring begins relates to the expert's movements before pounding work is about to begin – a wave generated by the gripping action his abductor pollicis brevis makes when re-adjusting the pounding brush in his hands. On the other hand, the non-expert's abductor pollicis brevis creates big waves throughout the monitoring period that becomes more dramatic especially in the last-half of the pounding process. This indicates the non-expert is using force with his thumbs during the work to stabilize his grip.

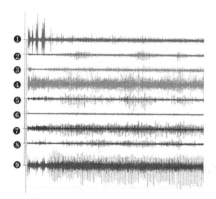

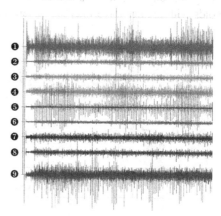

Fig. 5. Results of the rest on the expert   **Fig. 6.** Results of the test of the non-expert

We were able to confirm waves from the expert's chart in the following muscle groups: ❹the middle trapezius, ❼extensor carpi radialis brevis, ❾and interossei dorsales. But when juxtaposed with the video, for most the muscle movements, we found that the biggest waves were formed right after the pounding, when the pounding brush was being lifted. Furthermore, we were not able to detect any regular waves in the ❻triceps brachii.

As for the non-expert, we detected large waves occurring in most muscle groups, compared with the expert in areas other than the aforementioned ❶abductor pollicis brevis. Also, the waves tended to get larger toward the last half of the process. When matched up against the video, we were able to confirm the occurrence of large waves right after the pounding motion, which is much like the expert, but also when he is bringing the pounding brush down. We confirmed that the non-expert was consistently using all 9 monitored muscles to a greater degree than the expert.

4.2   Activity Per Muscle Group of the Expert and Non-expert

Here, we can find the type of activity that takes place in each muscle group for each pounding motion by smoothing the data.

Abductor Pollicis Brevis. The abductor pollicis brevis is activated during the palmar abduction of the thumb to grasp an object. It is also a functional position used by the expert. This muscle attaches itself to the scaphoid bone and the retinaculum of flexor, to the sesamoid bone, abductor proximalis. The graph shows that the expert uses very little of this muscle, which makes it clear that he does not hold the brush firmly in his hands. Furthermore, we can say that he pounds without creating tension in his arms. If anything, he is relaxed. His actions are well timed without any waste. Because of this, the timing of the pounding, the force he applies to the brush and even the intervals are well balanced. For the non-expert, on the other hand, high muscle activity and use of first joint can be seen. This is most likely due to his firm grip on the brush, which he holds with greater force than his expert counterpart. This is shown in Fig. 7.

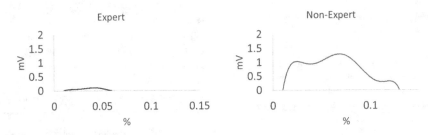

Fig. 7. Abductor Pollicis Brevis

Deltoid Middle. The deltoid originates at the lateral side of the clavicle, the acromion, and the spine of the scapula,and attaches to the deltoid tuberosity. Its function is to abduct the shoulders. The middle fibers of the deltoid, in particular, extends from the acromion to the deltoid tuberosity and is the main muscle to help the shoulders abduct. When compared against the non-expert, the expert's muscle activity while pounding tended to be long and intense. This is because the expert, more so than the non-expert, uses his middle deltoid fibers to keep the arm slightly abducted while working. We believe this action contributes to stabilization of the shoulder joins. On the other hand, the non-expert was considered incapable of stabilizing his shoulder joint and continuing his work. Furthermore, we were able to see that the non-expert's upper arm was actively lifted at about the same time that he was pounding with the brush. This means increased muscle activity was likely due to the shoulder abduction while he was lifting his arm. This is shown in Fig. 8.

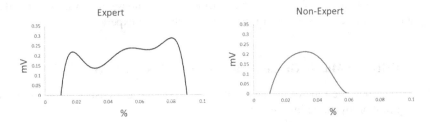

Fig. 8. Deltoid middle

Upper Trapezius. The upper trapezius connects from the lateral end of the clavicle, the acromion and the spine of scapula to the occipital external protuberance, nuchal ligament and the spinous processes of C1-C7. This muscle is responsible for preventing scapular depression. Between the expert and non-expert, muscle activity is overwhelmingly high but for a short duration for the expert. The non-expert, on the other hand, differs from the expert in that his muscle activity is low, but for a longer duration. This indicates that one action of an expert is completed in a shorter amount of time, and muscle activity per action is more intense. This is because when moving the brush up and down, the expert fully engages his upper trapezius when lifting his arm, stabilizing the surface of his shoulder blades. This movement with the brush is called pounding, but more accurately, the moment the brush hits the target, the expert lifts his arm to move on to the next action. The non-expert's data showed less action in this movement, which was insufficient to stabilize the shoulder blades, unlike the expert, and resulted in a difference in the quality of the work. When performed by the expert, the lifting action in the arm was swift, while the non-expert barely raised his arm – all of which became evident after smoothing the data. This is shown in Fig. 9.

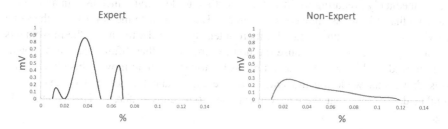

Fig. 9. Upper trapezius

Middle Trapezius. The middle fibers of the trapezius muscle are connected from the upper portion to the middle of the spine of the scapula and adducts the shoulder blades. When comparing activity in this muscle between the expert and non-expert, data shows a very high level of prolonged activity for the non-expert, whereas the opposite was true for the non-expert in both activity and duration. It became clear that when working, the expert actively engages the middle fibers of the trapezius without adducting them. This finding was unexpected. Ordinarily, when performing an action, the shoulder blades need to be stabilized, which is why, with regards to the expert, we were anticipating that the data would show an active engagement of the middle fibers of the trapezius. But the results indicated otherwise, showing low key activity in that area. This points to the fact that while working, the expert doesn't allow his shoulder blades to adduct. This was evident even when observing his movements. The shoulder blades were rather in a state of abduction, and upward rotation, enabling him to work with just a moderate amount of muscle activity. We believe the non-expert adducted his shoulder blades and over-exerted while working. This is shown in Fig. 10.

Biceps Brachii. The two-headed biceps brachii originate at two locations: the supraglenoid tubercle and the coracoid process of the scapula, and insert into the radial tuberosity and the bicipital aponeurosis to the fascia on the medial side of the forearm. They flex the elbow and the shoulders and supinate the forearm. With the expert, the

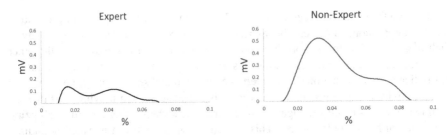

Fig. 10. Middle trapezius

movements were bimodal, indicating an increase in the start of the activity, while the non-expert's results were trimodal, showing an increase in bimodal activity. Activity was much less and shorter compared with the non-expert's. This means the expert's movements were shorter than the non-expert's. By bringing the pounding brush down and immediately preparing to lift it, the expert's muscle activity increases in an instant, showing that it is an instantaneous movement. However, with the non-expert, the same activity takes place longer and with more intensity. And the timing of the movements are slightly slow. This is because the non-expert, rather than lifting the brush, potentially moved his biceps at the same time as his triceps without moving his elbow joint. This shows that while the movements of the expert and the non-expert may appear similar, data shows that their movements are completely different. This is shown in Fig. 11.

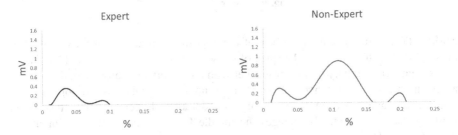

Fig. 11. Biceps brachii

Triceps Brachii. The triceps originate in the infraglenoid tubercle and attaches to the olecranon. They are responsible for extending the elbow and, when activated together with the biceps brachii, fixate the elbow joint. They also aid secondarily in fixating the shoulder joint. Results were bimodal for both the expert and non-expert. With the expert, muscle activity was light and short. For the non-expert, muscle activity was high and very long. This showed that the non-expert was using force to pound the brush on the washi paper, while keeping his biceps and elbow joints fixated. Activity was low-key for the expert, and what the bimodal indicated was that compared with the non-expert, he didn't exert much force and used the least amount of muscularity. Furthermore, the bimodal results also showed that in the picture of the overall movement, he extended his elbow, and in the last half, flexing the elbow served as a sort of brake on the action.

Results for the non-expert were bimodal like those of the expert, but the timing differential with the biceps brachii activated the triceps, then the biceps after that, followed by both the triceps and the biceps. Results indicated that the non-expert's biceps and triceps were working in excess, compared with the expert. See Fig. 12.

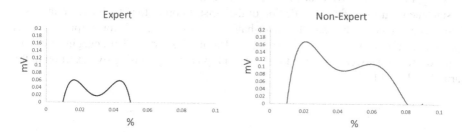

Fig. 12. Triceps

Extensor Carpi Radialis Brevis. For this research, we focused on the extensor carpi radialis brevis and the flexor carpi radialis muscles as the main muscles of the forearm. The extensor carpi radialis brevis originates at the lateral epicondyle of humerus and inserts into the posterior base of the third metacarpal. These are muscles that extend and abduct the hands at the wrists. Furthermore, they work together with the palm muscles to help stabilize the wrist. This study showed unimodal results for both the expert and the non-expert. The expert's activity in this muscle was comparable to that of the non-expert, but the duration of his muscle activity was considerably shorter. We can see from this study that he was dorsally extending and radially flexing his wrist instantaneously. Viewing the timing of the expert's movements, activity heightens in the latter half. We can see from this that he engages his extensor carpi radialis brevis to lift the pounding brush for an instant after pressing down into it. The non-expert, however, that muscle is continuously activated, resulting in a difference in work quality. This is showin in Fig. 13.

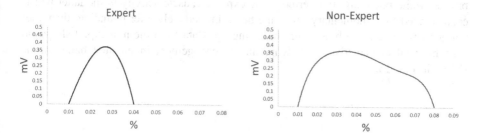

Fig. 13. Extensor **carpi radialis brevis**

Flexor Carpi Radialis. One can say that muscle activity involving the flexor carpi radialis and the extensor carpi radialis brevis defines the muscle activity of the forearm. They do not indicate independent muscle movement, but rather the flexing and extending activities of the forearm. The muscle originates on the medial epicondyle of the humerus and inserts on the anterior aspect of the base of the second metacarpal. The flex and abduct the wrist and help stabilize the joint. The extension of the flexor carpi radialis can contribute to the radial flexion of the wrist. The results are bimodal for both the expert and the non-expert, but the non-expert's muscle activity in the latter part is low. Engagement in the flexor carpi radialis triggered a volar flexion in the wrist, causing a reflexive movement in the extensor carpi radialis brevis that resulted in the instantaneous dorsal and radial flexion of the wrist. In order to put a brake on the wrist movement, it could be that the latter-half activation of the flexor carpi radialis is preventing a dorsal extension in the wrist. The non-expert is also engaging the dorsiflexor, which is overly fixating the wrist joint, potentially causing overexertion in the arm. See Fig. 14.

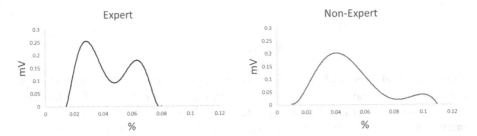

Fig. 14. Flexor carpi radialis

First Dorsal Interosseous Muscle. We've called attention to the first dorsal interosseous muscle and the abductor pollicis brevis as the extrinsic hand muscles. The first dorsal interosseous originates at the the first metacarpal and the radial side of the second metacarpal bone and inserts into the base of the second proximal phalanx. The first dorsal interosseous assists in thumb adduction and is activated when gasping. Research results differed for the two subjects, with the expert's data being bimodal, unlike the non-expert's. When comparing the timing, the muscles were engaged when the brush was being pounded. This indicates that the subjects were gripping their brushes while pounding. Furthermore, the expert's muscle activity in the latter half is characterized by a momentary lift in the brush immediately after pounding, then after that activity to stop the brush from bouncing up. Data from the non-expert shows no such bimodal characteristics, showing mostly engagement in the first half. This is shown in Fig. 15.

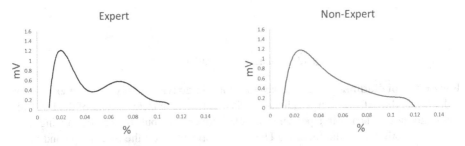

Fig. 15. First dorsal interosseous muscle

5   Conclusion

For our research, we smoothed out data from the electromyograph to extract the characteristics of each muscle activity. The result was that overall, the amount and duration of muscle activity of the non-expert was considerably higher than those of the expert. Data smoothing revealed that this caused excess tension in the non-expert's arm while he pounded. It was consistent with the non-expert's statement during the interview portion of the research that he was exhausted after just a short amount of time. By contrast, the expert rarely used force, and was relaxed through the shoulders. The only muscle the expert engaged to a greater degree and for a longer duration than the non-expert was the middle fibers of the deltoid middle. We interpreted this to mean that the deltoid abducted the shoulder joints and held them in that position throughout the duration of the action. Then, the trapezius would depress momentarily from the first-half, but rise up again after that to form a trimodal pattern. In order to move the shoulder, elbow and wrist joints rhythmically the middle section of the shoulder joints have to be stable, which show up in the results of this study. Additionally, a dramatic increase in activity was seen in the expert's upper fibers of the trapezius which, seen that it was accompanied by a sudden lift in the pounding brush, indicates a well-timed act of mid-scapular stabilization. Going forward, we would like to study and compare the timing of each muscular action and consider their implications.

Acknowledgments. This research was made possible due to a grant from JSPS Research Grant 25350327.

References

1. Hayakawa, N., Kigawa, R., Kawanobe, W., Higuchi, H., Oka, Y., Oka, I.: Basic research of the physical properties and chemical compositions of aged paste. Conserv. Sci. **41**, 15–28 (2002)
2. Hayakawa, N., Kimijima, T., Kusunoki, K., Oka, Y.: Effects of the Pounding Brush as an Adhesive. Conserv. Sci. **43**, 9–16 (2004)
3. Nishiura, T.: Adhesive Effects of Pounding by Brush. The Science of Picture Framing, 99–107 (1997)
4. Hayakawa, N., Kigawa, R., Nishimoto, T., Sakamoto, K., Fukuda, S., Kimishima, T., Oka, Y., Kawanobe, W.: Characterization of Furunori (Aged Paste) and preparation of a polysaccharide similar to furunori. Stud. Conserv. **52**(3), 221–232 (2007)
5. Inaba, M.: Conservation Science Primer for Cultural Assets Chapter 2, 4th Clause "Paper," 63 (2002)
6. Ishii, N.: The mechanism of muscles, encyclopedia of mechanisms (2013)
7. Kizuka, T., Masuda, T., Kiryu, T., Sadoyama, T.: Electromyogram (2006)

EMG Activity of Arms Muscles and Body Movement During Chucking in Lathebetween Expert and Non-expert

Porakoch Sirisuwan[1]([⊠]), Hisanori Yuminaga[2], Takashi Yoshikawa[3], and Hiroyuki Hamada[1]

[1] Advanced Fibro-Science, Kyoto Institute of Technology, Kyoto, Japan
p-sirisuwan@hotmail.com, hhamada@kit.ac.jp
[2] Department of Physical Therapy, Kansai Vocational College of Medicine, Osaka, Japan
yuminaga@kansai.ac.jp
[3] Mechanical Engineering, Niihama National College of Technology, Ehime, Japan
yosikawa@mec.niihama-nct.ac.jp

Abstract. The subjects were three men differential experience of lathe processing such as 87,500 h, 6,300 h and 384 h on 87, 32 and 40 years old respectively. The attendees were affixed fourteen reflective markers for motion analysis and ten surface electrodes on the muscles of arms. The chucking movement did not leaned the body and used the center of the body to be a center of movement characterized the muscle contraction of expert on bilateral muscle of Flexor carpi radialis and Triceps bracii and then they still used the right Extensor carpi radialis longus, right Biceps brachii and left Deltoid. The abnormal twisting movement by bending the body to the left side and leaned the left knee down indicated the experts still contracted the muscle as like the first movement. The muscle energy usages of the experts had higher than the non-expert whom took a muscle continuously contraction along time.

Keywords: Arms muscles contraction · Center of gravity movement · Body twisting movement · Chucking movement

1 Introduction

Lathe is one of the machine tools most well used. It is a machine tool used principally for shaping pieces of metal, wood, or other materials by causing the work piece to be held and rotated by the lathe while a tool bit is advanced into the work causing the cutting action. A lathe chuck is a special kind of clamp used on a lathe. These chucks hold objects that are cylindrical, radial, or irregularly shaped, gripped by what are called lathe chuck jaws. They hold steady the objects to be worked on. The Fig. 1 showed the lathe chuck jaws which have been usually tightened into place on the work-piece using a chuck key, a t-shaped wrench.

The chuck has either three or four jaws and mounts on the end of the main spindle. The universal scroll chuck usually has three jaws, which move in unison as an adjusting pinion rotated. The advantage of the universal scroll chuck is its ease of operation in centering the work for concentric turning. This chuck is not as accurate as the independent chuck but,

© Springer International Publishing Switzerland 2015
V.G. Duffy (Ed.): DHM 2015, Part II, LNCS 9185, pp. 216–226, 2015.
DOI: 10.1007/978-3-319-21070-4_22

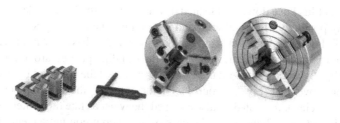

Fig. 1. Chuck jaw and chuck key

when in good condition, it will centre the work automatically to within 0.003 of an inch. In addition, the universal scroll chuck is capable of holding and automatically centering round or hexagonal work-pieces. However, this chuck is unable to effectively to hold square, octagonal, or irregular shapes. The independent chuck includes four jaws that are adjusted individually on the chuck face by means of adjusting screws. The jaws of the independent chuck may reverse so that the steps face in the opposite direction; thus, work-pieces capable grip either externally or internally. The independent chuck can uses to hold square, round, octagonal, or irregular shape work-pieces in either a concentric or an eccentric position due to the independent operation of each jaw. Because of its versatility and capacity for fine adjustment, the independent chuck is commonly to use for mounting work-pieces that require extreme accuracy. The jaws of the universal scroll chuck and the independent chuck have a series of teeth that mesh with spiral grooves on a circular plate within the chuck. This plate is rotated by the chuck-key inserted in the square socket [1]. The objective of this study would like to observation the effect only the three jaw chuck gripping.

Even if the chucking performance of the lathe worker include two characteristics as loose and tighten the jaws tooth of chuck with the work-piece but the mistake of force gripping on the work-piece surface indentations have occurred by chuck jaws gripping as like Fig. 2 that always have found on the chucking movement of the non-expert.

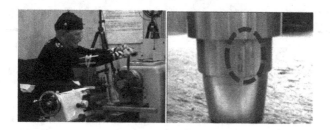

Fig. 2. The work-piece indentation by jaws gripping

The research of the differences of chucking behavior on the expert and the non-expert in lathe processing showed there were two characteristic of chucking behavior of them within the two standing posture and two hand holding position on chuck key. The characteristic of standing posture and the hand holding position on chuck key of the expert worker have not influenced on movement pattern of body along the vertical movement.

He has not bent his knee down and leaned down the body to the left side. Anyway, the hand holding positions: right and left hand hold on the handle, only left hand hold on the shank of chuck key but right hand hold on the handle: have not influenced on the activities pattern of horizontal movement. On the standing posture around in front of a chuck that slightly stood at the left, the expert always used the center of body as like the axial rotation movement (Fig. 3-Group 1). On the contrary, the standing posture at the right side of the chuck indicated he always fixed the waist as like the center for twisting the body (Fig. 3-Group 2 and 3). In the case of the uncommon movement of the non-expert who has stood slightly at the left side of chuck and both left and right hand have held on the handle always showed he have swung the body together with bent the knee down by using the left hand as the center rotation (Fig. 3-Group 4).

In addition, the experiment of effect of chucking movement with the indentation on the work-piece surface in chuck jaws gripping of a lathe between an expert and a non-expert that had imitation the both activity on first experiment by three novice students

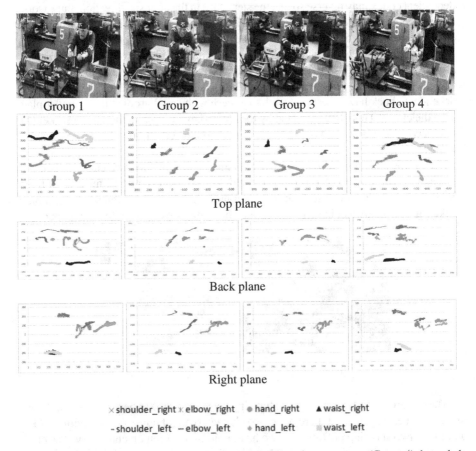

Fig. 3. Chucking activity on an expert (Group 1, 2 and 3) and a non-expert (Group 4) depended on standing posture and hand holding position. An expert has worked on the lathe processing more than 70 years but a non-expert has worked only 1 years experience on lathe.

of lathe experience on Niihama National College of Technology explained the strain value on chuck jaws gripping varied amongst four movement. There were the tendency of strain sequence similarly pattern although the subjects have been a variously personality. It was clearly confirmed that the chucking imitation mobility of the attendees on the non-expert movement pattern (Fig. 3-Group 4) have been the highest in terms of apparent strain average value on chuck jaws gripping. This power grip strength was higher than any event of the expert movement pattern (Fig. 3-Group 1, 2 and 3) second half, double and four times respectively. All resultants analysis have confirmed that the chucking behavior of the non-expert worker whom could not keep the balance movement, always leaned the body to the left side and bent the left knee while he was beginning twisted the chuck key cause of the indentation on work-piece surface [2]. The torque on the chucking behavior of the non-expert was excessive and affect to the compression of jaw teeth.

2   Methods

2.1   Participants

The subjects were three males differential experience of lathe processing such as 87,500 h, 6,300 h and 384 h on aged 87, 32 and 40 years and 155, 180 and 170 cm height respectively. Furthermore, Table 1 still showed the differential data of hand griping strength. The first one has worked at Takayoshi Company Limited in Ehime prefecture and the others have been a technical staff at Mechanical Engineering in Niihama National College of Technology, Japan.

Table 1. Three male Subjects characteristics and lathe experience

Subject	Age	Weight (Kg)	Height (cm.)	Hand grip strength (Kg) (Average)		Experi-ence (Hours)
				Left	Right	
1	85	52.7	155	26.75	28.35	87,500
2	32	62.2	180	48.25	54.2	6,300
3	40	64.8	170	44.4	48.6	384

2.2   Apparatus

This study focused the relationship between the direction patterns of body movement by using the Motion analysis measurement with the muscles activity investigated by EMG. The participants were concentrated on fourteen reflective markers position for motion analysis such as a bilateral body part of shoulder, elbow, wrist, hip, knee, ankle and foot (Fig. 4). In addition, ten muscles responsible for arm motion were studied namely a bilateral muscle of Deltoid, Biceps brachii, Triceps bracii, Flexor carpi radialis and Extensor carpi radialis longus (Fig. 5).

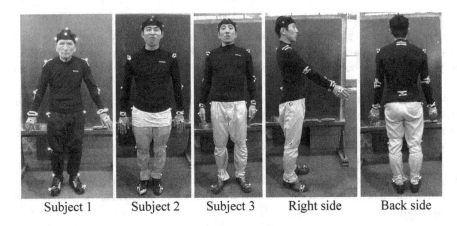

Subject 1   Subject 2   Subject 3   Right side   Back side

Fig. 4. Reflective markers placement of each subject

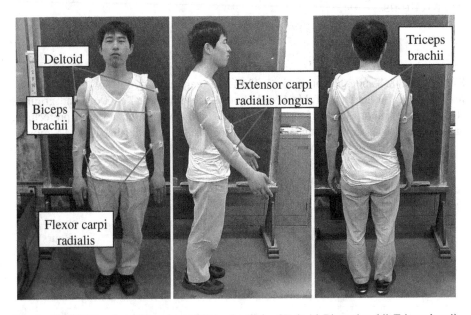

Fig. 5. Ten EMG surface electrodes on bilateral muscle of Deltoid, Biceps brachii, Triceps bracii, Flexor carpi radialis and Extensor carpi radialis longus.

As equipment of Motion analysis is three dimensional motion capture system (Mac3D Motion analysis) consisted of 7 infrared cameras and 2 video cameras captured the reflective markers of each subject. The machine telemeter system WEB-1000(NIHON KOHDEN Co.) and the sampling frequency rate of 1,000 Hz are the electromyography devices of EMG system which are used as the record condition (Fig. 6).

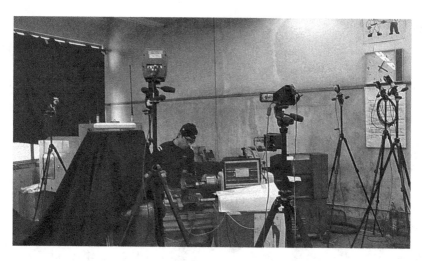

Fig. 6. The experiment setup for recording the motion of chucking movement and muscular activity.

3 Results and Discussions

3.1 Participants Characteristics of Chucking Motion Analysis

This experimental measurement of chucking motion captured on the actually working behavior without movement control. It illustrated the chucking movement only two groups in Figs. 7 and 8. Figure 7 showed the movement characteristic on slightly standing at the right side moreover left and right hand holding position on the handle of chuck key. The pattern movement of all subject on Fig. 7 showed they did not lean the body to the left side and not bend the left knee. They used the center of vertical axial as like the center of body twisting. It has caused of distance movement similarly occurrence between left and right side. For reliability and validity data, there were six time of chucking capture on subject 1 but only one time of this one showed the chucking activity which moved the body to the left side as like the non-expert movement on the first experiment. The other chucking performance of subject 1 still had similarly pattern movement with the expert. Three time of chucking movement observation on subject 2 disappeared the leaning the body to the left side and bending the left knee. However, four time of subject 3 indicated that he often moved the body to the left side by bending the left knee. This resultant analysis identified that the subject 1 and 2 who have worked many year of lathe experience always kept the controllable balance of the body movement. The observation on the left elbow movement showed the subject 1 and 2 always jerked this part down meanwhile this activity was invisible on subject 3.

Figure 8 showed only subject 1 and subject 3 have not the capability to control the body balanced of twisting. However, as above-mentioned described that only one time of six times on subject 1 had uncommon pattern movement. This Figure demonstrated they used their hands as like the center of rotation and bent the left knee while they began

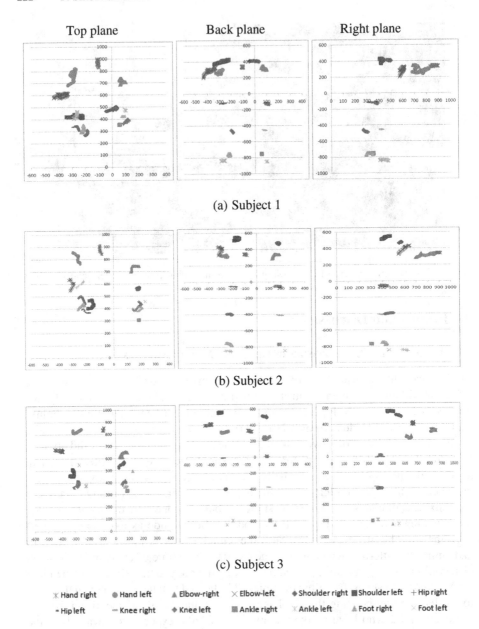

(a) Subject 1

(b) Subject 2

(c) Subject 3

✕ Hand right   ● Hand left   ▲ Elbow-right   ✕ Elbow-left   ◆ Shoulder right ■ Shoulder left ＋ Hip right

– Hip left   — Knee right   ◆ Knee left   ■ Ankle right   ✕ Ankle left   ▲ Foot right   ✕ Foot left

Fig. 7. The pattern of chucking movement which the subjects capable of being controlled the balance of body.

twisting the chuck key. The body trajectory movements were a curve line and had a lot of distance movement that were invisible on the controllable chucking performance on Fig. 7.

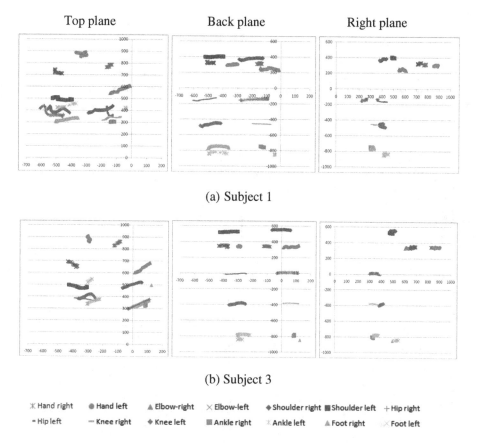

(a) Subject 1

(b) Subject 3

| ✕ Hand right | ● Hand left | ▲ Elbow-right | ✕ Elbow-left | ◆ Shoulder right | ■ Shoulder left | ✛ Hip right |
| ▪ Hip left | ━ Knee right | ◆ Knee left | ■ Ankle right | ✕ Ankle left | ▲ Foot right | ✕ Foot left |

Fig. 8. The uncommon chucking activity by bending the left knee and moving the body down to the left side while twisting the chuck key.

3.2 EMG Processing Analysis

The comparison of EMG activity during the muscle of arms contractions among subject 1, 2 and 3 who had differential experience of lathe processing on Figs. 9 and 10 indicated although there were the similarly pattern movement in chucking process on these subject but the arms muscles activity of them have differed. On the muscle activity of the tighten gripping in chucking process that the subjects stand slightly on the right side of the chuck which left and right hand holding on the handle which disappeared the bending of body down to the left side explained the muscle activity using between subject 1 and 2 on Fig. 9 were quite similarly pattern. They always used the bilateral muscle of Flexor carpi radialis(L and R-FCR) and Triceps bracii(L and R-TB) and then they still used the right Extensor carpi radialis longus(R-ECRL), right Biceps brachii(R-BB) and left Deltoid(L-D). There were just a little using a muscle of left Extensor carpi radialis longus(L-ECRL), Biceps brachii(L-BB) and right Deltoid(R-D). Although the chucking performance of subject 1 had more like a muscle jerk of subject 2 but the period term muscle using of subject 2 were shorter than the subject 1. The duration of arms muscle contraction while

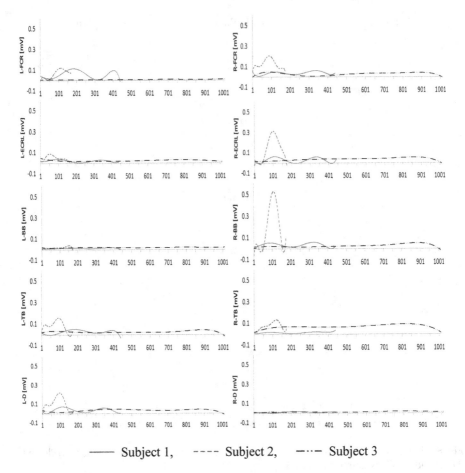

Fig. 9. The differential muscle activity on the subjects who capable controlled the body balance which did not bend the knee down and lean the body to the left side.

chucking on subject 1, 2 and 3 were 0.44 s, 0.2 s and 1.01 s respectively. In addition, subject 2 had a lot of the power exertion of arms muscle than the others and he had a high force of arms jerk only 1 time for chucking. The arms jerk on subject 1 was visible on 2 times. However, the subject 3 has continued to use the muscle of arms but it had not more muscle activity and did not obtain the arms jerk. All of arms muscle performances of subject 3 were on approximately 0 mV.

The EMG muscle of arms contraction of Fig. 10 which included the muscle performance not only the subject 1 who had a 1 time for bending the left knee down and leaned the body to the left side but also the subject 3 who very often bent the left knee down together with leaned the body to the left side. Even if these 2 subjects changed the pattern of chucking movement from the body balanced controlling to uncommon body movement but the arms muscle contraction of later movement were still similarly performance with the former. The subjects still contracted the bilat-

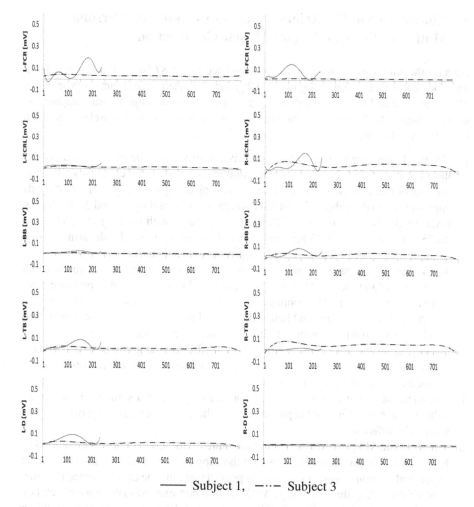

Fig. 10. The differential muscle activity on the subjects who bent the knee down and leaned the body to the left side.

eral muscle of Flexor carpi radialis(L and R-FCR) and Triceps bracii(L and R-TB) and then they still used the right Extensor carpi radialis longus(R-ECRL), right Biceps brachii(R-BB) and left Deltoid(L-D). Nevertheless, there was a differential muscle power using on the subject 1. The comparison between the first character-istic of chucking movement and the second one showed the second pattern activity affected the increasing of arms muscle contracting that it occurred only the subject 1. All of arms muscle performances of subject 3 kept in almost exactly on 0 mV. Conversely, the period of the arms muscle contraction while chucking on the subject 1 and subject 3 have decreased to 0.24 s and 0.8 s respectively.

4 Conclusions of the Relation Among the Subjects Personality, Motion Activity and Arms Muscle Contraction

Because the attendees on this experiment consisted of the 87,500 h, 6,300 h and 384 h therefore, the subjects were categorized in 2 group depended on the hours of experience. The subject 1 and 2 have assumed an expert workers and the subject 3 was supposed to be the non-expert. The result of chucking motion analysis and arms muscle contraction explained as a below;

1. The hands grip strength data of all subjects confirmed that the strength of this parts have not effected of the arms muscle using while twisting the chuck key. Because the data of them on Table 1 have showed the subject 2 got the grip strength of hands approximate to the subject 3; left hand 48.25, 44.4 kg and right hand 54.2, 48.6 kg respectively; but the strength of the first one differed with the subject 1; left hand 26.75 and right hand 28.35 kg; around double times. Conversely, the arms muscle using of the subject 1 was similarly pattern only the subject 2.
2. The age and height have not influenced both chucking movement, arms muscle using characteristic and the jerk direction of left elbow but the hours of experience have more effected of them. The confirmation test indicated on Table 1 the group of the expert that had a lot of age and height differential but the body movement pattern of chucking and the arms muscle activities still were correspondent. However, the age has impact on the arms muscle strength [3, 4]. Beside the group of expert always jerked the left elbow down when they were twisting the chuck key on the body balancing movement pattern.
3. Although the group of the expert and the non-expert had a similarly of the body balance controlling movement pattern even so the arms muscle exertion of both were positively different.
4. The arms muscle performance on the movement characteristic by bending the left body and leaning the left knee down on the subject 1 and 3 who were assumed the expert and the non-expert consecutively proved that only the expert exerted the arms power for twisting the chuck key. As the non-expert exerted to twist the chuck key by swinging the body to the left side together with he has used the arms as like a power transmitter from the body twisting.

References

1. Army Institute for Professional Development: Lathe Operation, Edition 8, pp. 30–33 (1988)
2. Yoshikawa, T., Ito, R., Tsujinaka, T.: Stance of chucking by the Takumi on Lathe Working. In: Proceeding, The Japan Society of Mechanical Engineering, Japan, pp. 517 (2012)
3. Hiroshi, Y., Morihiko, O., Toshiaki, O., Satoko, N., Tomomi, S., Tomohiro, K., Shinya, K., Tadashi, M.: Effects of aging on EMG variables during fatiguing isometric contractions. J. Hum. Ergol. **29**, 7–14 (2000)
4. Laxman U.S., Januaria, M.: Pinch Grip, Power Grip and Wrist Twisting Strengths of Healthy Older Adults 3(2), 77–88 (2004). www.gerontechjournal.net

Process Analysis of the Hand Lay-Up Method Using CFRP Prepreg Sheets

Toshikazu Uchida[1(✉)], Hiroyuki Hamada[2], Koji Kuroda[2], Atsushi Endo[2],
Masakazu Migaki[2], Junpei Ochiai[1], Tadashi Uozumi[3], and Akihiko Goto[4]

[1] UCHIDA Co., Ltd., Fukuoka, Japan
{Uchida,j-ochiai}@uchida-k.co.jp
[2] Kyoto Institute of Technology, Kyoto, Japan
hhamada@kit.ac.jp, Koji_splash_kuroda@jcom.home.ne.jp,
{Shootingstarofhope30,iloveseta}@gmail.com
[3] Gifu University, Gifu, Japan
uozumi@gifu-u.ac.jp
[4] Osaka Sangyo University, Daito, Japan
gotoh@ise.osaka-sandai.ac.jp

Abstract. The autoclave molding method is performed by stacking CFRP prepreg sheets in a mold; this method is widely used in airplanes and by the automobile industry. Most three-dimensional-shaped parts are manually produced by the hand lay-up stacking sequence method. Because of this, mechanical properties such as shape accuracy and strength vary depending on the worker's skill. This is the major issue when tackling the difficulty of quality control in hand lay-up molded products. In order to alleviate these quality management difficulties, ideally, all workers are provided operation manuals and obtain the sufficient skills to prevent individual differences from occurring in the hand lay-up process. In this study, we aim to establish qualification criteria and standardize the work process of this method. We discuss how the differences in the hand lay-up work process influence the mechanical performance of molded products, based on the workers' skill.

Keywords: Hand Lay-Up · CFRP · Modulus · Tensile strength · Process analysis · Mechanical performance

1 Introduction

The autoclave molding method is performed by stacking CFRP prepreg sheets in a mold; this method is widely used in airplanes and by the automobile industry. Most three-dimensional-shaped parts are manually produced by the hand lay-up stacking sequence method. Because of this, mechanical properties such as shape accuracy and strength vary depending on the worker's skill. This is the major issue when tackling the difficulty of quality control in hand lay-up molded products. In order to alleviate these quality management difficulties, ideally, all workers are provided operation manuals and obtain the sufficient skills to prevent individual differences from occurring in the hand lay-up

© Springer International Publishing Switzerland 2015
V.G. Duffy (Ed.): DHM 2015, Part II, LNCS 9185, pp. 227–236, 2015.
DOI: 10.1007/978-3-319-21070-4_23

process. However, there is no efficient curriculum to support workers in acquiring these skills and no assessment system to establish skill level. Moreover, there is no useful literature to explicitly explain the hand lay-up method and the molding tools used in this process; no reports verifying how working process variations influence the performance of molded products currently exist. In this study, we aim to establish qualification criteria and standardize the work process of this method. We discuss how the differences in the hand lay-up work process influence the mechanical performance of molded products, based on the workers' skill.

2   Experimental Method

As shown in Fig. 1, we used a tray-shaped square mold measuring 405 mm on each side; the edge height was 30 mm.

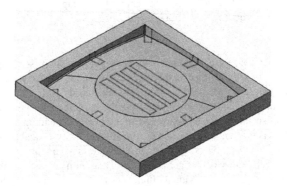

Fig. 1. Mold

2.1   Experimental Materials

We used carbon fiber T-300 3 K plain woven fabric epoxy prepreg sheet (produced by Toho Tenax Co., Ltd.) as the reinforcing material.

2.2   Experimental Method

Carbon cloth prepreg was stacked in three layers in this mold. Based on the square mold's sides we set the fiber orientation of carbon cloth; the first layer was 0 degrees, the second at 45 degrees, and the third 90 degrees. The following processes required the hand lay-up method to be applied to this mold. The subjects were allowed to decide the process order and choose molding tools for themselves. Subject A had 12 years of professional experience, Subject B had 2 years, and Subject C only had 11 months. In order to analyze this method we recorded the hand lay-up work process performed by each subject with a video camera; their postures and motions while working are shown in Table 1. We compared the process order, molding tools, and time needed for each process, as well as their overall body posture.

Table 1. Requirements and purpose for stacking

	Requirements and purpose
Inspection before stacking	Mold confirmation
	Envisioning the stacking process
	Cleaning
Stacking sequence	Material confirmation
	Stacking positioning
	Repeating the stacking process
Bagging	Positioning the release film
	Positioning the breather cloth
	Vacuum drawing

2.3 Molding Method

While the motion by the expert, Subject A, was very smooth as shown in Fig. 2, Subject C's motions were very awkward. When considering working posture, Subject A's body was tilted forward; he bent his head and was closer to the mold than subject C. We will verify these details in further analysis.

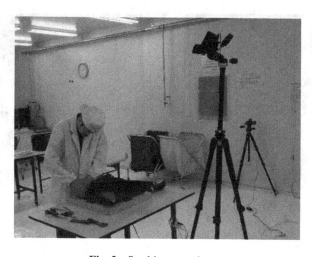

Fig. 2. Stacking experiment

The appearances of the molds processed by Subjects A and C were compared. While there were no wrinkles on Subject C's mold's bottom surface, a wrinkle was observed on the mold processed by Subject A. The original carbon fiber alignment also remained in the corner of Subject C's mold. Moreover, in order to examine the accuracy of the mold shapes performed by each subject, we bisected the molds and measured the thickness at the corners plus the bending radius for comparison.

2.4   Specimens and Evaluation Method

For the tensile test, we cut rectangular specimens 30 mm x 20mm in size from the bottom surface of the mold shown in Fig. 1. For the results shown in Fig. 3 and Table 2, we clarified how the differences in the working processes influenced shape accuracy and mechanical properties of the finished mold; we also illuminated the fundamental working process of the hand lay-up method and displayed the instructions for this process.

Table 2. Process analysis evaluation method

	Requirements and purpose
Process analysis	Working-time analysis
	Use of tools
	Working posture comparison
Property analysis	Product shape differences
	Weight comparison
	Section analysis

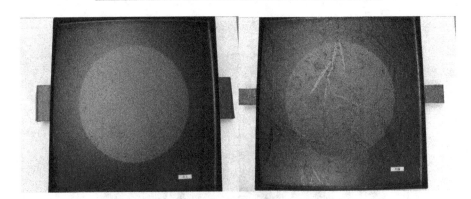

Fig. 3. Wrinkles

3 Experimental Results and Discussion

There are three major elements in the mold designated for this study – it is flat and smooth surface, with corner R, and deep edges in the four corners. It looks typically-shaped, but was designated to require a great deal of skill to use. Thus, significant difference appeared in expert and non-expert's mold's mechanical properties. In order to verify the details, we will repeat this study on a constant basis with more subjects. The amount of time required for stacking as well as bagging are clearly shown in Fig. 4. The amount of time required to apply several layers was almost the same; however, in the bagging process, with the difference of making wrinkles as small as possible in the bagging film and release film, and preventing wrinkles from occurring, it was clear through analysis and just by looking that the parts that were rich in resin had been successfully made as small as possible.

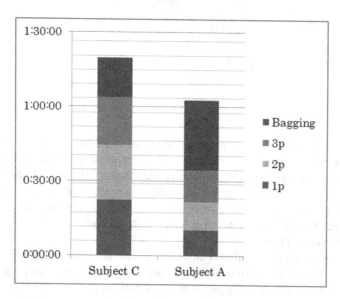

Fig. 4. Processing time

In Fig. 5, it is apparent that subject C often spent most of his time using the tools repeating the same actions, while Subject A clearly distinguished the roles of the scissors and Stanley knife used on one side of the cut to use the tools in as minimal a process as possible. Thus, he adopted two of the three different ways to use a chisel, separated the fiber from the chisel holding down angle R and his fingertips, and had become familiar with the pattern of repeating the process for the third layer, eliminating wasted time. It is clear that by increasing and decreasing the strength applied to the fingertip on the bamboo chisel in the bagging process, the auxiliary raw materials that gather on the inside of the wrinkles in the bagging film are made smaller.

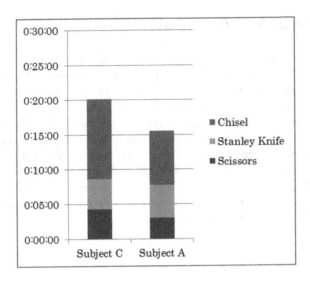

Fig. 5. Time using the materials

We analyzed the 19 different processes involved in molding the three layers, as is shown in the process analysis graph in Fig. 6. By expressing the entire process from preparations before stacking until completing the stacking, the axis for the amount of time that Subject C required to repeat each action is made even clearer. In particular, the actions that were repeated in the process of molding angle R are heavily represented, and for subject A, apart from time spent on angle R and corner R on the first side, it is a speedy allocation of time.

The process analysis has also been arranged into the chart in Table 3 to further clarify from a finer point of view. Because Subject A was clear on the purpose of the process, he was able to quickly setup his next actions and execute the task while using both hands evenly and looking at all of the corners. However, because of repeated movements that cause wrinkles due to the gathering of wrinkles and uneven application of strength in his actions, Subject C's inability to make decisions and lack of awareness of the purpose affected his actions. Furthermore, working postures of the two subjects were clearly different. Subject A had stable body movements, while Subject C's neck had bent his neck towards the desk and at a right angle, and his body was askew when working.

The cross-section analysis shown in Fig. 7 is the cross-section that was closest to a right angle. The other three sides clearly showed cross-sections of corners that are not shown in the estimated results or actual results. However, in contrast to Subject A's smooth cross-section between lawyers, for Subject C, the cross-section of the fiber and uneven resin, and the thickness of the unevenness and the cross-section are also uneven. Furthermore, Subject C's other angle Rs were confirmed to

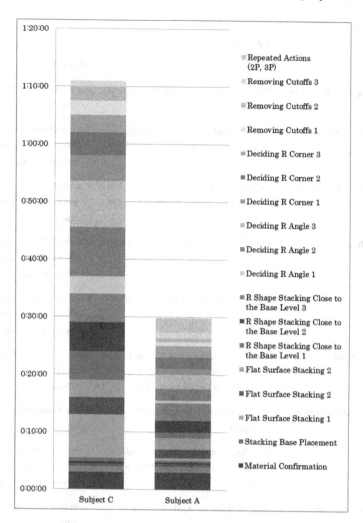

Fig. 6. Process list

have gaps and wrinkles. Thus, the technical ability to an angle R that is close to a right angle is required.

It is clear from the test specimen results on the underside of the mold that the effects on the mechanical properties are similar, as is shown in Fig. 8. Because the need for tracking from the underside is low, we have plotted angle R's need for tracking.

Table 3. Process analysis results

Process	Subject C	Subject A
Positioning the release film	Put it into the mold while making wrinkles	Put it into the mold without making wrinkles
Arranging the breather cloth (Securing)	Set the breather from the stacking surface's position	Turned the mold upside down and pushed the breather down
Placing inside the bagging film	Repeatedly made wrinkles in both sides numerous times before turning the template over	Placed the mold in the film and quickly closed it with tape
Vacuum drawing	Pulled it 4 times, pulled it back 3 times	Checked whether it was okay after pulling 5 times and checking once
Checking for leaks	Repeated the task in all of the corners	Carefully checked places which appear at risk of having problems
Process comparison	Often made checks and repeated actions; attitude for not being able to make it durable stood out	Sensed with his fingertips and tools and applied the square scale
Working time comparison	Was overly conscious and often repeated tasks	Did not unnecessarily repeat tasks
Use of tools	Divided the application of strength into three steps; use of the chisel was uneven	Used only when needed; used the chisel on a wide number of sections
Comparing even part stacking	Repeated the tasks on each side	Repeated the tasks on each side
Comparing corner part stacking	Uneven application of strength and unnecessary repetition of tasks; Had his body in bent position instead of moving his hand to a different position or even the mold	Put it in by sensing with his fingertips and with the pressure from the chisel
Working posture comparison	Had his neck bent at 90° which looked painful; was confused as to how his body should be positioned	Had no shakiness in his stance

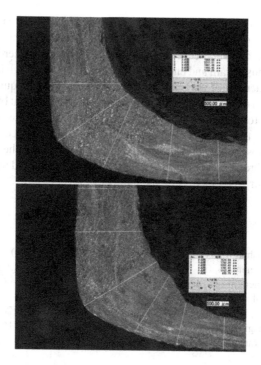

Fig. 7. Examining the angle R cross-sections

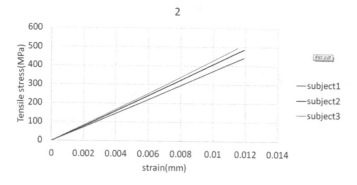

Fig. 8. Pull test results

4 Conclusion

By specifying the requirements and purpose in the initial molding conditions, we could clarify the differences between experts and non-expert workers in the selection of molding tools, working postures, time needed, and the overall working process. This helped us understand the need to standardize the hand lay-up method using CFRP prepreg sheets, which has been recently gaining popularity; these are the origins related to the basic elements of mass-production robot work. Because of this, we will continuously explore the fundamental concepts inherent in the plane, corner R, and edge, and the need to continuously train and encourage workers to obtain a high level of expertise. It is clear from the actions of our subjects that they are able to act quickly by planning what to do next based on their level of experience and that the amount of strength applied to the fingertips and tools creates an effect. Despite the conditions they were given being the same, the ability to transition between setting-up different processes and maintain concentration are closely linked to your body's muscle memory. The next challenge is to clarify this with three-point bending tests and durability tests, and determine whether any differences occur when increasing the number of layers.

References

1. Ogasawara, T., Yoshikawa, N.: JSME Annual Meeting **8**, 37–38 (2010)
2. Matsumoto, T., Minemura, T., Masago, J., Hayashikawa, T., He, X.: Theory application dynamics lecture memoirs **58**, 42–42
3. Nishikawa, Y., et al.: Materials **54**, 494–499
4. Hirano, Y., Kusano, H., Aoki, Y.: Compos. Sci. Technol **40**, 153–159 (2014)
5. Suzuki, N., Koyanagi, J., Arikawa, S.: Compos. Sci. Technol. **40**, 160–169 (2014)
6. Yoneyama, S., Koyanagi, J., Arikawa, S.: Compos. Sci. Technol. **40**, 35–43 (2014)

Human Modeling in Transport and Aviation

Hybrid BFO-PSO and Kernel FCM for the Recognition of Pilot Performance Influenced by Simulator Movement Using Diffusion Maps

Jia Bo[1]([✉]), Yin-Bo Zhang[2], Lu Ding[1], Bi-Ting Yu[1], Qi Wu[1], and Shan Fu[1]

[1] School of Aeronautics and Astronautics, Shanghai Jiao Tong University,
800 Dongchuan Road, Minhang District, Shanghai 200240, China
icesea137@163.com
[2] Shanghai Aircraft Design and Research Institute, Shanghai, China

Abstract. This paper proposed a novel data reduction and classification method to analyze high-dimensional and complicated flight data. This method integrated diffusion maps and kernel fuzzy c-means algorithm (KFCM) to recognize two types of simulator modes at different tasks. To optimize the unknown parameters of the KFCM, a hybrid bacterial foraging oriented (BFO) and particle swarm optimization (PSO) algorithm was also presented in this paper. This algorithm increased the possibility of finding the optimal values within a short computational time and avoided to be trapped in the local minima. By using the proposed approach, this paper obtained meaningful clusters respecting the intrinsic geometry of the standard data set, and illustrated the phenomenon that the pilots vestibular influenced pilot performance and control system under the Manual departure task.

Keywords: Flight simulator · Vestibular · Diffusion maps · Bacterial foraging oriented · Particle swarm optimization · Kernel fuzzy c-means algorithm

1 Introduction

Recent papers showed that pilots utilized many different cues to control aircraft. Central visual and peripheral visual can help pilots to get flight instruments and position information. Vestibular and cockpit motion also have influences on sensory perception [1]. In some investigations, multi-channel models, shown in Fig. 1, were developed to describe various sensory channels' affection on pilot control behavior in distinguished conditions.

However, the multi-channel models are not unchangeable all the time. Human sensory system should be studied to make sure which sensing path affects human's behavior under certain circumstance. Whether the pilot performance is different is essential for human sensory model research. This paper aimed to find a reliable method to recognize whether the performance is different when the sensing path has changed. In the experiment, same tasks were carried out at

© Springer International Publishing Switzerland 2015
V.G. Duffy (Ed.): DHM 2015, Part II, LNCS 9185, pp. 239–247, 2015.
DOI: 10.1007/978-3-319-21070-4_24

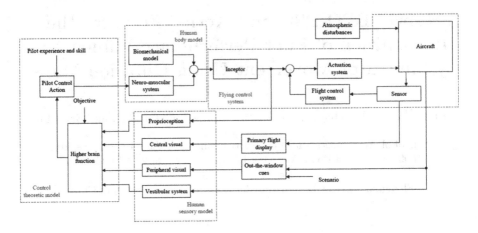

Fig. 1. Block diagram representing the pilot-vehicle-system under manual control

two simulator modes (static and dynamic). Because the flight data was hard to be distinguished by using traditional cluster methods. Our goal was to classify these complicated data precisely and quickly.

2   Feature Extraction and Classifier

2.1   Wavelet Based Feature Extraction

To classify pilot performances of controlling the flight simulator efficiently, features should be extracted from both time-domain and frequency-domain. Wavelets are versatile harmonic analysis tools which combine time and frequency representations into localized waveforms. Given a segment of experimental data, the wavelet transform convolves a selected series of local waveforms with the data to identify correlated features. The resulting set of wavelet coefficients can be interpreted as multidimensional correlation coefficients. Features of shape, size, and location are naturally characterized by these waveforms and related coefficients [2]. As a result, besides common features such as mean value and standard deviation, we extract features using wavelet transform.

2.2   Classifier Based on Hybrid Diffusion Maps and Kernel FCM

The construction of the proposed classify method based on diffusion maps and KFCM is shown as Fig. 2. First, using diffusion maps, the complicated and high dimensional set turned into an arbitrary set. This obtained arbitrary set represents the distribution of the original data and its inner connection. On the basis of diffusion maps, kernel FCM is used to classify the patterns, which cluster centroid is optimized by the new technique BFO-PSO. After the optimal cluster block the minimum object function are calculated. The final result is the cluster when the object function is minimal.

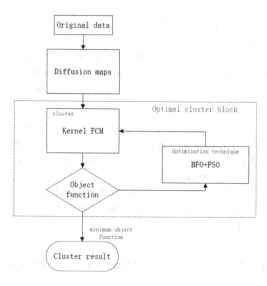

Fig. 2. The process of the hybrid cluster algorithm

Diffusion Distances. The ambition of diffusion distance is to define a distance metric on an arbitrary set that reflects the connectivity of the points within the set. Points within regions of high density (defined as groups of nodes with a high degree in the graph), will have a high connectivity. The connectivity is furthermore decided by the strengths of the weights in the graph. The diffusion framework was put into the context of eigenmaps, dimensionality reduction, and Markov random walk learning on graphs and it first appeared in [3].

Let $G = (\Omega, W)$ be a finite graph with n nodes, where the matrix $W = \{w(x, y)\}_{x,y \in \Omega}$ satisfies the following conditions:

symmetry: $W = W^T$

and points positivity: $w(x, y) \geq 0$ for all $x, y \in \Omega$

$w(x, y)$ should represent the degree of similarity or affinity of x and y.

The graph G with weights W represents our knowledge of the local geometry of the set.

We are mainly concerned with the following idea: For a fixed but finite value $t > 0$, we want to define a metric between points of Ω which is such that two points x and z will be close if the corresponding conditional distributions $p_t(x, .)$ and $p_t(z, .)$ are close. A similar idea appears in [4], where we consider the L^1 norm $\|p_t(x, .) - p_t(z, .)\|$. However, as shown below, the L^2 metric between the conditional distributions has the advantage that it allows one to relate distances to the spectral properties of the random walk and thereby connect Markov random walk learning on graphs with data parameterization via eigenmaps. As in [5], we will define the "diffusion distance" D_t between x and y as the weighted L^2 distance

$$D_t^2(x, z) = \|p_t(x, .) - p_t(z, .)\|_{1/\phi_0}^2 = \sum_{y \in \Omega} \frac{(p_t(x, y) - p_t(z, y))^2}{\phi_0(y)} \tag{1}$$

where the "weights" $\frac{1}{\phi_0(x)}$ penalize discrepancies on domains of low density more than those of high density.

This notion of proximity of points in the graph reflects the intrinsic geometry of the set in terms of connectivity of the data points in a diffusion process. The diffusion distance between two points will be small if they are connected by many paths in the graph.

Kernel FCM. As an enhancement of classical FCM, the KFCM maps the data set X from the feature space or the data space $\Xi \subseteq R^p$ into a much higher dimensional space H (a Hilbert space usually called kernel space) by a transform function $\varphi : \Xi \rightarrow H$. In the new kernel space, the data demonstrate simpler structures or patterns. According to clustering algorithms, the data in the new space show clusters that are more spherical and therefore can be clustered more easily by FCM algorithms [6–8].

3   The Parameters Optimization of the Proposed Classifier

In clustering algorithm, the grouping is identified by randomly placing the cluster centroids and grouping of records with minimum distance. The algorithm faces several challenges in effectiveness and efficiency. Similarly, KFCM algorithm is also modified including spatial information and kernel [9]. Then, optimization algorithms are introduced for clustering parameters setting. Based on the similar kind of procedure, genetic algorithm (GA) [10], Particle Swarm optimization (PSO) [11], bacterial foraging optimization (BFO) [12] and simulated annealing [13] are applied for clustering.

PSO is a stochastic search technique and BFO is a new type of bionic optimization algorithm. In this paper, the random variable of BFO is replaced by the particle swarm algorithm. By this way, the bacteria with poor position could soon gather in a good region, and the bacteria with good position search in the neighborhood region. It also aims to avoid from being trapped in local minima as PSO.

3.1   Bacterial Foraging Optimization

BFO is an evolutionary optimization technique, introduced by Passino, based essentially on the social foraging behavior of Escherichia Coli (E. Coli) bacteria present in human intestine. The selection behavior of bacteria improves successful foraging strategies and suppresses those with poor foraging. A foraging animal seeks to maximize the energy obtained per unit time spent foraging. E. Coli bacteria has a chemotactic action behavior that enables it to search for food and avoid noxious substances. In bacterial foraging process, E. Coli bacteria undergo four stages: chemotaxis, swarming, reproduction, elimination and dispersal.

3.2 Particle Swarm Optimization

PSO is a stochastic computation technique developed by Eberhart and Kennedy, inspired by the social behavior of fish schooling or bird flocking, more exactly, the collective behaviors of simple individuals that interact each other on one hand and with their environment on the other hand. PSO is a population-based optimization technique, in which the system is initialized with a population of random candidate solutions called particles and searches for the best solution by updating generations. Each particle has a position represented by a vector X_k^i (i is the index of the particle) and velocity V_k^i that directs its flying in the multidimensional search space. Every particle remembers its own best position P_{LBest}^i corresponding to its lowest fitness value evaluated by the fitness function to be optimized. The best position with the lowest fitness cost among all the particles in the swarm is set to P_{GBest}^i. Particles update their velocities and positions in order to track the optimal particle until a convergence criterion is achieved or a maximum of iterations are attained using the following equations:

$$V_{k+1}^i = wV_k^i + C_1 R_1 (P_{LBest}^i - X_k^i) + C_2 R_2 (P_{LBest}^i - X_k^i)$$

$$X_{k+1}^i = X_k^i + V_{k+1}^i$$

where R_1 and R_2 are random numbers in interval. A particle decides where to move next, considering its own experience, which is the memory of its best past position, and the experience of the most successful particle in the swarm. Acceleration coefficients, C_1 influences the cognitive behavior, which means how much the particle will follow its own best position while C_2 represents the social behavior, which means how much the particle will follow the best position of the swarm. w is the inertia weight factor.

3.3 The Proposed BFO-PSO Algorithm

In 2008, W. Korani proposed an improved BFO, namely BF-PSO. The BF-PSO combines both algorithms BFO and PSO. The aim is to make use of PSO ability to exchange social information and BF ability in finding a new solution by elimination and dispersal. In BFO, a unit length direction of tumble behavior is randomly generated. The random direction may lead to delay in reaching the global solution. For BF-PSO the global best position and the best position of each bacterium will decide the direction. During the chemotaxis loop, the update of the tumble direction is determined by:

$$\phi(j + 1) = V\phi(j) + C_1 R_1 (P_{Lbest} - P_{current}) + C_2 R_2 (P_{Gbest} - P_{current})$$

where P_{LBest} is the best position of each bacteria and P_{GBest} is the global best bacterial.

4 Experiment

The proposed method was implemented in MATLAB R2014a and executed on a core i3 processor, 3.20 GHz, 2 GB RAM computer.

4.1   Classical Data Set

To test the validity of this method, a standard data set, shown in Fig. 3a, was used. The data set which consisted of 2000 spots, distributing in two concentric circles separable in a 2-D feature space. It's hard to classify this data set with traditional methods because there were many noisy points between two classes. For instance, when we run the FCM algorithm directly, the result did not reflect

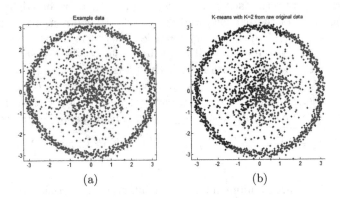

Fig. 3. (a) The original data set; (b) The cluster using FCM

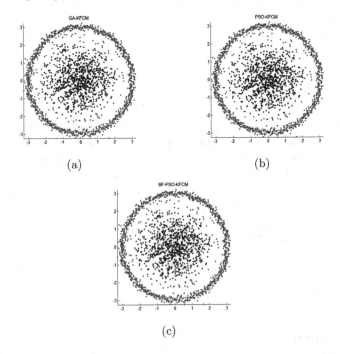

Fig. 4. (a) The cluster using GA+DM; (b) The cluster using PSO+DM; (c) The cluster using BFO+PSO+DM

the natural geometry of the data distribution. As shown in Fig. 3b, the data set was cut to two pieces briefly without showing any geometry in formation of the former graph.

As a comparison, the set was classified into two concentric circle by using diffusion maps, shown in Fig. 4. Some meaningful clusters respecting the intrinsic geometry of the data set were obtained. Genetic algorithm (GA) and PSO algorithm were used to test the better performance of hybrid BF-PSO algorithm. Compared to diffusion maps optimized by GA (Fig. 4a) or PSO (Fig. 4b) only, diffusion maps combined with BFO-PSO algorithm (Fig. 4c) obtained smaller object function representing better classify quality. Each algorithm process run 5 times to classify the standard data set, and results of object function were shown in Table 1. The new algorithm not only calculated well and had a good ability to deal with local extreme and global search capability, but also there were no any requests for the initial cluster centers and the entering order.

Table 1. The object function of based on different optimization algorithm

Time no	1	2	3	4	5
GA Diffusion maps	750.7954	750.7954	720.8364	756.2210	769.7340
PSO Diffusion maps	730.9793	657.6692	630.3283	623.0062	748.9318
BFO+PSO Diffusion maps	630.1426	615.1135	620.3785	616.0514	625.8664

4.2 Flight Data Set

To get reliable flight data we did the experiment in flight simulator. There were 5 crews of experienced pilots executed 2 different missions which were Manual departure and Standard instrument departure (SID). Each mission was carried out at two simulator modes, static and dynamic modes.

7 essential flight parameters, such as airspeed, pressure altitude, pitch angle, roll angle, rate of climb, vertical speed and angle of attack were chosen to calculate and study. The sample time of flight data was set to 30 Hz because of the limitation of simulator.

In our work, we extracted 5 features of each flight parameter: mean value, standard deviation, wavelet entropy, wavelet energy entropy and wavelet high/low frequency energy ratio.

Then use the proposed hybrid algorithm to classify features of flight data. Set parameters of the algorithm as follows: clustering categories as 2; diffusion dimension as 5; $S_b = 10$, $P = 10$, $N_c = 3$, $N_s = 4$, $N_r e = 2$, $N_e d = 2$, $P_e d = 0.25$, $C_1 = C_2 = 2$; $r = 150$.

The clustering results were shown in Fig. 5:

The proposed method was carried out 5 times using flight data, and the results were shown in Table 2. Manual departure was better than standard instrument departure by comparing their correct rates of clustering.

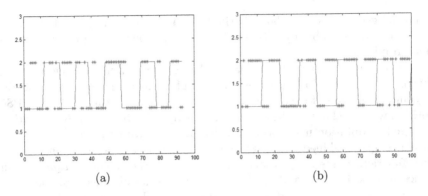

(a)   (b)

Fig. 5. (a) The cluster result at Manual departure task; (b) The cluster result at standard instrument departure task

Table 2. The failure rate of mode cluster at different task

Time no	1	2	3	4	5
Manual departure	37.63	39.78	40.86	37.63	39.78
Standard instrument departure	52.73	52.73	47.27	46.36	47.27

Two different simulator modes were easier to classify at the Manual departure task. The misclassification reached to about 37.63 % lowest, while the other one was only 45.45 %. This difference reflects the influence of the simulator movement, because the sensing path of pilot changed when vestibular system transmitted information for higher brain function showing in Fig. 1.

It illustrated that the performance at Manual departure was influenced by pilot's movement sensation. Compared to that at standard instrument departure which based on auto departure procedures, simulator movement has little impression on pilot sensory system.

5   Conclusion

This paper proposed a new hybrid algorithm to reduce high feature-dimension and recognize nonlinear flight data from different simulator modes. Hybrid diffusion maps and KFMC method could classify complicated data set and reflect the connectivity of the points within it. The proposed method was used to cluster the standard data set. The results indicated that the proposed method was robust to noise and had better performance compared to traditional ones. Then the flight data which was obtained from simulator was classified by this method. The cluster stated that the control performance of pilots was more sensible to the simulator movement at Manual departure task. It proved that the method was valuable to analysis whether the pilot performances had relationship with certain human sensing path.

References

1. Allerton, D.: Principles of Flight Simulation. Wiley, UK (2009)
2. Torrence, C., Compo, G.P.: A practical guide to wavelet analysis. Bull. Am. Meteorol. Soc. **79**(1), 61–78 (1998)
3. Coifman, R.R., Lafon, S., Lee, A.B., Maggioni, M., Nadler, B., Warner, F., Zucker, S.W.: Geometric diffusions as a tool for harmonic analysis and structure definition of data: diffusion maps. Proc. Nat. Acad. Sci. U.S.A. **102**(21), 7426–7431 (2005)
4. Jaakkola, M.S.T., Szummer, M.: Partially labeled classification with markov random walks. Adv. Neural Inform. Proc. Syst. (NIPS) **14**, 945–952 (2002)
5. Nadler, B., Lafon, S., Coifman, R.R., Kevrekidis, I.G.: Diffusion maps, spectral clustering and reaction coordinates of dynamical systems. Appl. Comput. Harmonic Anal. **21**(1), 113–127 (2006)
6. Kim, D.-W., Lee, K.Y., Lee, D., Lee, K.H.: Evaluation of the performance of clustering algorithms in kernel-induced feature space. Pattern Recogn. **38**(4), 607–611 (2005)
7. Graves, D., Pedrycz, W.: Performance of kernel-based fuzzy clustering. Electron. Lett. **43**(25), 1445–1446 (2007)
8. Graves, D., Pedrycz, W.: Kernel-based fuzzy clustering and fuzzy clustering: a comparative experimental study. Fuzzy Sets Syst. **161**(4), 522–543 (2010)
9. Zhang, D.-Q., Chen, S.-C.: A novel kernelized fuzzy c-means algorithm with application in medical image segmentation. Artif. Intell. Med. **32**(1), 37–50 (2004)
10. Maulik, U., Bandyopadhyay, S.: Genetic algorithm-based clustering technique. Pattern Recogn. **33**(9), 1455–1465 (2000)
11. Premalatha, K., Natarajan, A.: A new approach for data clustering based on pso with local search. Comput. Inform. Sci. **1**(4), p. 139 (2008)
12. Wan, M., Li, L., Xiao, J., Wang, C., Yang, Y.: Data clustering using bacterial foraging optimization. J. Intell. Inf. Syst. **38**(2), 321–341 (2012)
13. Selim, S.Z., Alsultan, K.: A simulated annealing algorithm for the clustering problem. Pattern Recognit. **24**(10), 1003–1008 (1991)

A Bi-level Optimization Approach to Get an Optimal Combination of Cost Functions for Pilot's Arm Movement: The Case of Helicopter's Flying Aid Functions with Haptic Feedback

Sami Cheffi[✉], Thomas Rakotomamonjy, Laurent Binet, Philippe Bidaud, and Jean Christophe Sarrazin

ONERA, Salon de Provence, France
sami.cheffi@onera.fr

Abstract. Force cueing and active control technology hold great opportunities in the next generation of helicopters. The overall goal would be to reduce the pilot workload and increase the situational awareness In this paper we present an approach to help in designing such forces through the understanding of human motor control and the relation that could be established with piloting an aircraft precisely pilot's arm movement. This method is based on the comprehension of the optimality criteria (cost functions and their weightings) within inverse optimal control combined with Fitt's experiment using an active side stick.

Keywords: Cost functions · Inverse optimal control · Pilot's arm movement · Fitt's law

1 Introduction

Helicopters, as a complex flying machine, have been the subject of great evolution since several decades; consequently, controlling such a machine has become a very costly task and requires a continuous attention. Arriving to the Fly by Wire commanding systems the workload of the pilot has been significantly increased and the idea of using haptic feedback started to be a very interesting solution to reduce such a workload and increase the situational awareness [1, 6].

As we know, in such a context, haptic feedback is using kinesthetic sense to find a new way to transmit some messages to the pilot that should be understood immediately. That's why forces that have to be implemented on side-sticks should be intuitive as much as possible.

The term intuitive here, has been the subject of many questions relative to the meaning of such a description of the force, and the manner it should be.

We propose in this paper an approach to have some answers to these questions through the understanding of human motor control and the relation that could be established with pilot's arm movement. This approach is based on optimal control theory

© Springer International Publishing Switzerland 2015
V.G. Duffy (Ed.): DHM 2015, Part II, LNCS 9185, pp. 248–257, 2015.
DOI: 10.1007/978-3-319-21070-4_25

combined with Fitt's task [2]. According to the optimal control theory natural movements are optimal after a learning phase. This optimality could be expressed by the optimization of a combination of cost functions that the central nervous system choose to coordinate many more degrees of freedom than necessary to accomplish a specific task [3].

According to Fitt's task, the performance of the movement is related to the task's difficulty and could be expressed through empirical values [2]. Within this approach, the performance of the movement could be expressed through the weightings of every cost function that should be in agreement with experimental data, and the way how it can vary with the difficulty of the task should give us new interpretations of the movement especially in the case of manipulating an active side stick.

Through these interpretations we should be able to design a force feedback that could help the pilot instinctively or may at least give a way to evaluate such forces.

The remainder of this paper is split into three sections, in the first one we introduce the notions used in this study like haptic feedbacks, optimal control and Fitt's task. The second one deals with the presentation of the basic ideas behind this research and the introduction of the method proposed. In the last section we discuss the results, concluding with its consequences on the future work.

2   State of the Art

2.1   Haptic Feedbacks

The control of a machine equipped with automated systems has been a very important field of research for many years especially when "human" have to keep his role in the loop as a commander so, he has to understand the communication present with such systems [4].

In our context, and as a powerful approach, haptic feedbacks were proposed, providing new channel of sensory transmission with the perception of contact forces implemented on control devises [5].

The interpretation of those forces require the use of muscles, tendons and articulations through multiple physiological receptors, combined with the role of the nervous system to understand the proprioceptive sensory information in the purpose of constructing a new representation of the body and muscle activity [4] and adapt a new strategy of motor control that respond and deal with the new information.

Several issues were highlighted when haptic feedbacks proved that it could be very useful on helicopters, as external aids able to maintain the pilot in the loop [7, 8, 21] especially when his mission has become a complex task that require a total coordination between him and the automated command systems. The main issue, is the ability of the pilot to interact with those feedbacks and for that many studies and approaches have suggested different ways to design such forces, like we can mention here as an example the direct haptic aid which consist of producing kinesthetic sensations that suggest the right direction to the pilot, also the indirect haptic aid which use the aspect of human in counteracting external forces implemented on the control device [8].

2.2 Optimal Control

Recent research on designing forces for active side-sticks, in the context of haptic feedbacks were based on the dynamics of visual errors [8], and to the best of our knowledge, there is not an understanding of the movement itself that is adopted to specify which force can suit and help the pilot in his manipulation.

Studies on human movement differs from discipline to another; there are theories that try to find principles behind human motion or just describe the observed one [3].

Being classified in the last category, optimal control theory confirm that human motor control is an optimal strategy in the coordination of different degrees of freedom of the body with respect of some criteria. In order to accomplish a motion, the musculoskeletal system offers a kinematic, dynamic and actuation redundancy with the use of many degrees of freedom than necessary. According to this theory, CNS selects the optimal criteria for the motor control through one or a combination of cost functions [3, 9–11].

Pointing tasks for human arm movement have been the subject of an intense research in this field and numerous plausible cost functions have been identified in the literature. Flash and Hogan proposed to minimize a kinematic criterion, the cartesian jerk [12] defined as the sum of the square of the third derivative of cartesian coordinates, for an arm movement in the horizontal plane only. The minimum torque change cost function which corresponds to the sum of arm joint torques first derivatives, was proposed by [13, 14]. The study used an arm model, studying plane movements. Many other criteria were identified like the geodesic model which suggests that the CNS select the shortest path in configuration space of Riemannian manifold with respect to the kinetic energy metric [15], energetic models which propose cost functions related to the minimization of work of torques [16] and neural models, designed to optimize the amount of motor neurons activity during multi-joints movement [17].

In order to find more optimal information about trajectories and with the progress of computational optimization and new algorithms coming from humanoid robotics field, combination of cost functions or hybrid cost function was introduced through the work of [18] where it was proposed to combine the hand force change and torque change criteria to determine the optimal trajectory of human arm movements in crank rotation tasks. Furthermore a combination of the absolute work of torques and the integrated squared joint acceleration was found as a hybrid cost function that fit the best the trajectory of an arm reaching a vertical bar [10].

The most important details in those hybrid cost functions is the weight associated to each criterion that seems to be like an indication of the participation's degree which the CNS is using while controlling the movement.

Based on recent research [3, 10, 11, 19, 20], an inverse optimal control technique is adopted to find such composite cost functions through the resolution of a bi-level optimization problem.

This technique is summarized within the following explanation:

The Global Cost Function

$$C(\alpha) = \sum_{i=1}^{n} \alpha_i C_i$$

With n is the number of criterion chosen C_i are the cost functions plausible for representing the optimality of the movement, and α_i are the weighting associated to each cost function (Figs. 1 and 2).

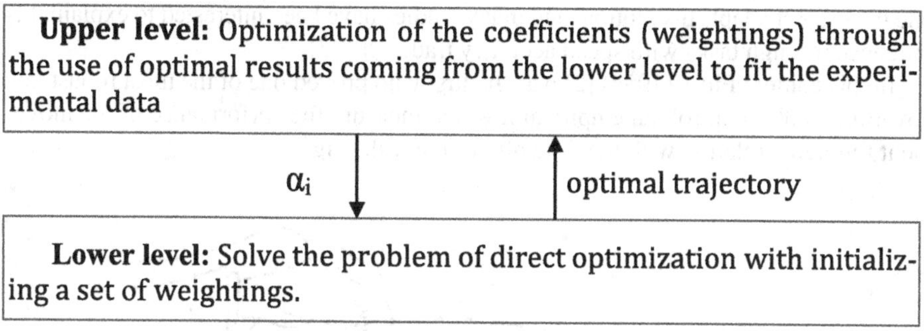

Upper level: Optimization of the coefficients (weightings) through the use of optimal results coming from the lower level to fit the experimental data

α_i ↓   ↑ optimal trajectory

Lower level: Solve the problem of direct optimization with initializing a set of weightings.

Fig. 1. Concept of the bi-level optimal control

Position(t)

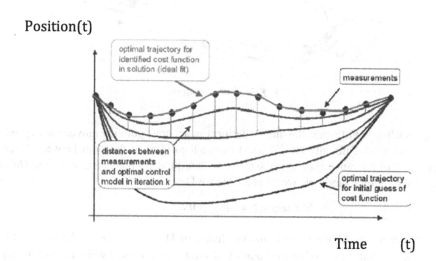

optimal trajectory for identified cost function in solution (ideal fit)

measurements

distances between measurements and optimal control model in iteration k

optimal trajectory for initial guess of cost function

Time   (t)

Fig. 2. Description of the goal of the bi-level optimal control: identification of cost function that fit the best experimental data [11]

Several methods were proposed to solve both levels depending on the arm model used and experimental conditions (task, limit of the movement…).

2.3 Fitt's Task

The control of the movement is a task that requires the integration of much information from environment and our neuro-musculoskeletal system, and the integration of such information determines the way how we control the movement. This process has been intensively studied from many experimental paradigms and discipline like biomechanics, cognitive science, and neuroscience.

Seen as both dynamical systems coupled, the actor and his environment interact with each other through forces provided by the user and sensory information structured by the environment [22]. Within the influence of physical constraint (forces) and sensorial one the subject adapts his motion, and many studies have been interested to explain this influence through tasks with speed accuracy trade-off [23].

In this context Fitt's (1954) [2] was the first who proved one of the most robust law governing motor control; an empirical law that measure the performance of the movement through a relation with the difficulty of the task (Fig. 3).

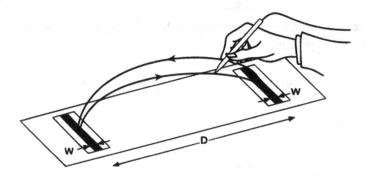

Fig. 3. Fitt's paradigm

According to Fitt's law, the time to perform an accurate pointing movement depends on the index of Difficulty (ID) defined as the logarithm of the ratio between target distance and tolerance (i.e. target size). This law predicts the movement time (MT) required to point a target of size W at a distance D:

$$MT = a + b * \log_2 (2D/W)$$

The term $\log_2 (2D/W)$ represents the Index of Difficulty (ID) of the task and is expressed in "bits" measuring the quantity of information treated while accomplishing the task. The higher the value of ID, the more difficult the task is.

Realizing Fitt's paradigm consists in pointing targets as fast and as accurately as possible. It could be used as a methodological tool in order to evaluate the performance in the use of the input devices [22].

3   Contribution of the Article

The contribution of this paper is twofold: first we present the approach of bi-level optimal control as a tool to describe pilot arm movement manipulating an active side stick. An approach that could help to understand the underlying optimization criteria of pilot's motor control with a dynamical arm model and several cost functions which are plausible to describe the movement.

The second contribution is related to the integration of Fitt's law with the realization of a pointing task in a simulation environment. Within this simulation, the performance of the pilot and many other indexes describing the movement like the variability (it gives an idea about accuracy i.e. the space of the target reached by user) are measured while manipulating the same side stick.

Combining these two contributions, two different descriptive vision of the motor control in a pointing task using an active side stick are unified in one framework in order to find new ideas in evaluating and specifying haptic feedbacks.

To do so, in the present study, we propose a method based on experimental setup using an active side stick as a control device for Fitt's task in a simulation environment [22].

4   Method

4.1   Participants

Participants are 10 right-handed volunteers. Having no previous history of upper extremity musculoskeletal disorders and all reported normal or corrected to normal vision.

All participants were experienced computer users (we are not going to use pilot participants for the moment) but none of the subjects had prior experience with the interface used in this task.

4.2   Tasks

The participants had to manipulate a pointer in a computer screen using only the roll angular displacement of an active side stick (WITTENSTEIN). The position of the pointer will move horizontally following the position (measured in degrees) of the side-stick.

The participants are required to reach as quickly as possible two targets, having the same dimension, separated with a known distance, and situated in the horizontal plane.

The trial consist of trying to reach those targets as quickly and as accurate as possible with doing 50 cycle. One cycle is defined as attaining both targets one time starting from the middle position. The trial is considered successful if the rate of missed targets (overshoot or undershoot) is strictly inferior to 15 % and the participants have to perform the same trial again if the minimum performance level required was not attained.

4.3 Experimental Design

Each condition was characterized by a quantified Index of Difficulty (ID). $ID = \log_2 (2D/W)$, the distance D (Fig. 4) is maintained constant and five widths W are used. The different values of the W parameter rendered a total of five experimental conditions with ID ranging from 3 to 7 bits with a 1 bit increment. The experimental phase was constituted by 8 trials for each of the different ID conditions. The order of the conditions was randomized to avoid any learning effect.

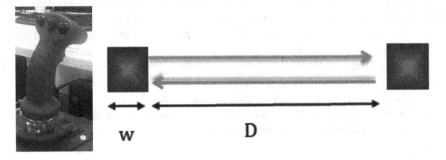

Fig. 4. Simulated Fitt's task & active side-stick

4.4 Experimental Setup

In order to applicate the bi-level optimal control, experimental data are needed and for that a specific setup was used to record the participant's motor activity from the 3D displacements of the upper limb segments and the electromyographic activities (EMG) in the effector space, with the position of the side-stick and the effort (forces) applied on it.

The 3D postures of the upper limb segments are recorded by four cameras optoelectronic (Flex 13 optitrack Motion System), at a 120 Hz frequency. Reflective markers are attached to specific places in the upper limb like the acromion for the shoulder and the lateral epicondyle for the forearm [24]. Following anatomical landmarks, joint angles could be reconstructed. EMG surface applied on group of Deltoid muscles pronator teres,

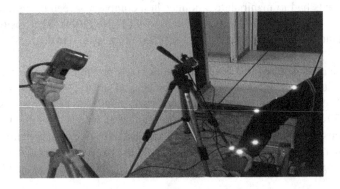

Fig. 5. System of motion capture

and brachioradialis muscles are recorded at 1980 Hz using a BIOPAC MP150 system with Ag/Ag-Cl bipolar surface electrodes (Skintact model FS 501, Innsbruck, Austria). Electrodes placement and locations were suggested by the SENIAM recommendations [25] (Fig. 5).

4.5 Data Collected

Through the experimental setup, data related to the kinematic of the upper limb segments EMG activity of the group muscles, the dynamic of the side stick (i.e.: it give an idea about the dynamic of end effector of the upper limb) are recorded by synchronizing the simulation of Fitt's task, the optitrack motion capture system and the BIOPAC MP150 system.

5 Human Arm Model

The use of an arm model is very crucial for the application of the bi-level optimal control problem as the purpose for the upper level is to find the best configuration of the arm (joint angles) that minimize a specific criteria. The use of such a musculoskeletal model even could enlighten us about some missing data that we could not reach by the experiment. That's why the work will be with XDE software which contains a big platform of several biomechanics models of the hole body seems to be a good solution to accelerate the research and avoid mistakes [26].

6 Discussion

For such a movement that was not yet explored, many cost functions were found from the literature that could be plausible to reproduce the optimal states of the motion. Based on pointing tasks essentially kinematic (jerk, acceleration, velocity, joint angles), dynamic (joint torques) energetic (work of torques) and neural models will be studied for our movement.

Finding all data needed for our arm motion using an active side stick in a Fitt's task (through the method proposed and the human arm model) and applicate the bi-level optimal control could lead us to a characterization of a task (could be simulated to piloting an aircraft in a slalom spot) within the variation of each cost function's coefficient.

The use of Fitt's task and the bi-level optimal control in this study lead to an evaluation of the performance of the motion through the variation of the weightings of each criterion (plausible to describe the movement) with the difficulty of the task.

7 Conclusion

In this study, we combine two different approaches to describe human motor control in order to give a better way to understand this complex task that the CNS seems doing daily.

Specifically, we are interested in pilot motor control in his arm movement manipulating the side-stick. The description of the method that we give in this paper could have an impact through the study of the influence of task's difficulties and haptic feedbacks on the performance of the movement and the variation of cost function's coefficient. That impact could help to design haptic forces in order to give a best way to assist the pilot's motion.

References

1. Mühlratzer, J., Konrad, G.: Active Stick Controllers for Fly-by-Wire Helicopters–Operational Requirements and Technical Design Parameters
2. Fitt's, P.M.: The information capacity of the human motor system in controlling the amplitude of movement. J. Exp. Psychol. **47**, 381–391 (1954)
3. Albrecht, S.: Modeling and Numerical Solution of Inverse Optimal Control Problems for the Analysis of Human Motions. Technische UniversitätMünchen (2013). http://mediatum. ub.tum.de/node?id=1136934
4. Sahnoun, M.: Conception et Simulation D'une Commande À Retour D'effort Pour Fauteuil, Roulant Électrique. Metz (2007). http://www.theses.fr/2007METZ039S
5. Casiez, G.: Contribution à l'étude des interfaces haptiques Le DigiHaptic: un périphérique haptique de bureau à degrés de liberté séparés. Lille (2004). http://www.lifl.fr/~casiez/ publications/TheseCasiez.pdf
6. Endsley, M.R.: Toward a theory of situation awareness in dynamic systems. Hum. Factors J. Hum. Factors Ergon. Soc. **37**(1), 32–64 (1995)
7. Wickens, C.D., Mavor, A.S., Parasuraman, R., McGee, J.P.: The Future of Air Traffic Control: Human Operators and Automation, pp. 1–336. The National Academies Press, Washington, D.C. (1998)
8. Olivari, Mario, Nieuwenhuizen, Frank M., Bülthoff, Heinrich H., Pollini, Lorenzo: Pilot adaptation to different classes of haptic aids in tracking tasks. J. Guidance Control Dyn. **37**(6), 1741–1753 (2014). doi:10.2514/1.G000534
9. Albrecht, S., Leibold, M., Ulbrich, M.: A bilevel optimization approach to obtain optimal cost functions for human arm movements. Numer. Algebra Control Optim. **2**(1), 105–127 (2012)
10. Berret, B., Chiovetto, E., Nori, F., Pozzo, T.: Evidence for composite cost functions in arm movement planning: an inverse optimal control approach. PLoS Comput. Biol. **7**(10), e1002183-1(18) (2011)
11. Mombaur, K., Truong, A., Laumond, J.P.: From human to humanoid locomotion - an inverse optimal control approach. Auton. Robot. **28**, 369–383 (2009)
12. Flash, T., Hogan, N.: The coordination of arm movements: an experimentally confirmed mathematical model. J. Neurosci. **5**, 1688–1703 (1985)
13. Uno, Y., Kawato, M., Suzuki, R.: Formation and control of optimal trajectory in human multijoint arm movement. Biol. Cybern. **61**(2), 89–101 (1989)
14. Wada, Y., Kaneko, Y., Nakano, E., Osu, R., Kawato, M.: Quantitative examinations for multi joint arm trajectory planning–using a robust calculation algorithm of the minimum commanded torque change trajectory. Neural Netw. **14**, 381–393 (2001)
15. Biess, A., Liebermann, D.G., Flash, T.: A computational model for redundant human threedimensional pointing movements: integration of independent spatial and temporal motor plans simplies movement dynamics. Neuroscience **27**(48), 13045–13064 (2007)

16. Berret, B., Darlot, C., Jean, F., Pozzo, T., Papaxanthis, C., et al.: The inactivation principle: mathematical solutions minimizing the absolute work and biological implications for the planning of arm movements. PLoS Comput. Biol. **4**, e1000194 (2008)
17. Guigon, E., Baraduc, P., Desmurget, M.: Computational motor control: redundancy and invariance. J. Neurophysiol. **97**, 331–347 (2007)
18. Ohta, K., Svinin, M.M., Luo, Z., Hosoe, S., Laboissiere, R.: Optimal trajectory formation of constrained human arm reaching movements. Biol. Cybern. **91**(1), 23–36 (2004)
19. Sylla, N., Bonnet, V., Venture, G., Armande, N., Fraisse, P.: Human arm optimal motion analysis in industrial screwing task. In: 2014 5th IEEE RAS EMBS International Conference on Biomedical Robotics and Biomechatronics, pp. 964–969 (2014). doi:10.1109/BIOROB.2014.6913905
20. Ulbrich, Michael, Leibold, Marion, Albrecht, Sebastian: A bilevel optimization approach to obtain optimal cost functions for human arm movements. Numer. Algebra Control Optim. **2**(1), 105–127 (2012). doi:10.3934/naco.2012.2.105
21. Hosman, R.J.A.W., Benard, B.: Active and passive side stick controllers in manual aircraft control, pp. 527–529 (1990). doi:10.1109/ICSMC.1990.142165
22. Loeches de La Fuente, H.: Étude multi-niveaux du contrôle d'un périphérique d'interaction de type joystick. Marseille (2014). http://www.theses.fr/s117852
23. Bootsma, R.J., Boulard, M., Fernandez, L., Mottet, D.: Informational constraints in human precision aiming. Neurosci. Lett. **333**(2), 141–145 (2002)
24. Wu, G., Van der Helm, F.C.T., Veeger, H., Makhsous, M., Van Roy, P., Anglin, C., McQuade, K.: ISB recommendation on definitions of joint coordinate systems of various joints for the reporting of human joint motion–Part II: shoulder, elbow, wrist and hand. J. Biomech. **38**(5), 981–992 (2005)
25. Hermens, H.J., Freriks, B., Disselhorst-Klug, C., Rau, G.: Developmentof recommendations for SEMG sensors and sensor placement procedures. J. Electromyogr. Kinesiol. **10**(5), 361–374 (2000)
26. http://www.kalisteo.fr/lsi/aucune/a-propos-de-xde

Development of a 3D Finite Element Model of the Chinese 50th Male for the Analysis of Automotive Impact

Hui-min Hu[1], Li Ding[2(✉)], Xianxue Li[2], Chaoyi Zhao[1], and Yan Yin[1]

[1] China National Institute of Standardization, Beijing, China
{huhm,zhaochy,yiny}@cnis.gov.cn
[2] Key Laboratory for Biomechanics and Mechanobiology
of Ministry of Education, School of Biological Science and Medical Engineering,
Beihang University, Beijing, China
{Ding1971316,li36101120}@buaa.edu.cn

Abstract. Occupant thoracic and abdominal injury during automotive crashes accounts for the biggest portion of all automotive injuries which is about 45 percent. So it's important to improve the vehicle's protective performance which leads to the high demand for crash test dummy. At present, crash test dummies are used in automotive impact in order to design and assess new vehicle safety performance. Hybird III I is widely used in the world and it's same in China. However Hybird III doesn't meet the Chinese anthropology which the Hybird III is bigger than Chinese. So it's in urgent need to establish the crash test dummy for Chinese. In this study, a finite element dummy with thorax and abdomen which is consistent with the 50th percentile Chinese male in order to predict the mechanism response of Chinese occupant during automotive impact and improve the impact automotive safety specifically for Chinese is developed.

Keywords: Finite element · Chest · Abdomen · Impact · Automobile

1 Introduction

Car has been essential for many people because of its convenience, however the problem of vehicle safety such as crash impacts is becoming more and more notable. In China, there were more than 100 thousands of people died because of traffic accidents which accounts 20 % of all the deaths derived from traffic accidents in the world [1]. According to the US National Accident Sampling System data which showed the damage parts of the body during the crash accidents, the head injuries accounted for 35.3 %, the chest injuries accounted for 26.7 %, the abdominal injuries accounted for 18.2 %, the lower limb injuries accounted for 4.6 % and then the upper limb and facial injuries [2]. From the above survey, we can know that the head, chest and abdomen are the most vulnerable parts to get injured during automobile crash accidents.

During the automobile crash accidents, the crash situations can be classified into frontal impact, side impact, rear impact and roll accident. Based on the survey, the frontal impact accounts for 57 %, and the side impact accounts for 27 % [3]. To improve the vehicle safety in the event of impacts, China has implemented the car

© Springer International Publishing Switzerland 2015
V.G. Duffy (Ed.): DHM 2015, Part II, LNCS 9185, pp. 258–265, 2015.
DOI: 10.1007/978-3-319-21070-4_26

design rules for occupant protection in frontal impact in 2003 and for the side impact in 2007 which the car manufacturers have to satisfy with the rules. In order to alleviate the cost and limitations of the automotive safety research through experiment, researchers have pursued the development of finite element models and the finite element modelling technology has been enabled with the advent of high-speed computing environment.

Understanding the mechanism behind the injuries during automotive impact is an important step in improving the impact crash safety of vehicles. Finite element modelling can represent the human body with accurate geometric or material properties and can simulate various complex situations [4–9].

The purpose of this study is to establish a finite element dummy with thorax and abdomen which is consistent with the 50th percentile Chinese male in order to predict the mechanism response of Chinese occupant during automotive impact and improve the impact automotive safety specifically for Chinese.

2 Methods and Model Description

2.1 Modeling Procedure

The finite element model consists of spine, ribs, heart, lungs and relative soft tissue. The spine, organs and soft tissue are established through three different approach. The geometry models of thorax and abdomen were finished in Solidworks of which the data was based on China national standard of human dimensions. The models of spine and ribs were developed in previous studies which were also based on the 50th percentile male dimensions. The organs like heart, lungs were established in Mimics from MRI data of a 50th percentile Chinese male. After the geometry model above were finished, the Hypermesh was used to mesh them into finite element model and then the finite element models were imported into Abaqus to analyze. The following will introduce each part in detail.

2.2 Finite Element Model of the Thorax and Abdomen

The geometry of the thorax and abdomen are based on China's National Standard GB 10000-88. The age group is 26–35 years old and all the samples are male. The 50 percentile data is used. The waist measurement, waist depth, waist width, chest measurement, chest width, chest depth, across shoulder width, neck width are used to develop the geometry model in Solidworks. The data is shown in Table 1. Firstly, the cross section curves of different parts, such as waist, chest, shoulder, are defined in Solidworks, and then they are lofted to form the 3D solid model just as shown in Fig. 1.

Then the thorax and abdomen model was meshed using Hypermesh and the finite element model contains 32338 nodes, 31244 elements which are mixed with C3D8R and C3D6. The finite element model of the thorax and abdomen is shown in Fig. 2.

Table 1. Measurement used in developing thorax and abdomen

Items	Waist measurement	Waist depth	Waist width	Chest measurement
Size (mm)	734	180	264	869
Items	Chest depth	Chest width	Shoulder width	Neck width
Size (mm)	212	281	376	120

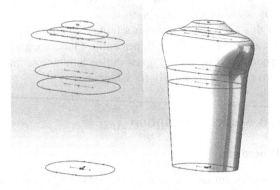

Fig. 1. Cross section curves and 3D solid model

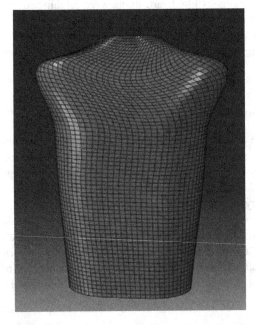

Fig. 2. Finite model of the thorax and abdomen

2.3   Finite Element Model of the Spine

The thoraco-lumbar spine has been developed in detail as shown in Fig. 3. The geometry of spine is based on the tomography data which was modeled in our previous study and now is scaled to represent the 50th percentile Chinese male spine. The spine contains 12 thoracic and 5 lumbar which is connected by 17 disks. The vertebral bodies and disks are all simulated using solid elements, however with different moduli. The whole spine element model contains 147655 nodes and 605943 elements which the type is C3D4.

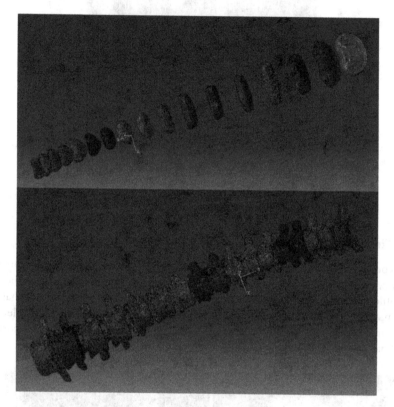

Fig. 3. Finite model of the spine

2.4   Finite Model of the Ribs

The ribs and sternum were modeled as shown in Fig. 4. The geometry of ribs and sternum is also based on the tomography data and process them to construct the 3D model with the most accuracy by Mimics software. Then the 3D model is scaled to represent the 50th percentile Chinese male ribs and sternum. To simplify the calculation, the ribs and sternum are modeled as one model except for the 11th and 12th ribs which ignores the ligaments and synchondrosis.

The geometry model then is processed and edited in Hypermesh software and meshed with trihedron. They are simulated using solid elements and share the same moduli. The whole model contains 154019 nodes and 480241 elements which mainly using C3D4 type.

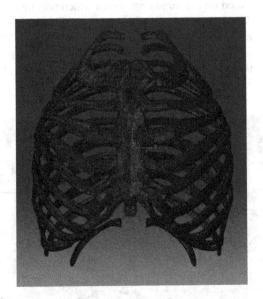

Fig. 4. Finite model of the ribs

2.5   Finite Element Model of the Heart and Lungs

The geometry of heart and lungs derives from previous study and is now modified in Hypermesh. Then they are meshed and scaled in Hypermesh to represent the 50th percentile male heart and lungs. They are simulated using solid elements and share the same material. The heart finite element model contains 3286 nodes and 15287 elements which are mixed with C3D8R and C3D4. The lungs finite element model contains 15660 nodes and 71266 elements which are all C3D4 (Fig. 5).

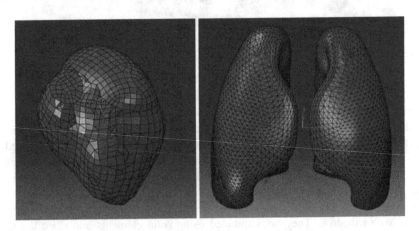

Fig. 5. Finite model of the heart and lungs

2.6   The Assembly Model

Since the different parts of the model are modeled in different coordinate systems, we should reassembly the models into one coordinate system. This work is done in the Abaqus Assembly module by rotation and translation. The assembled whole model is shown in Fig. 6.

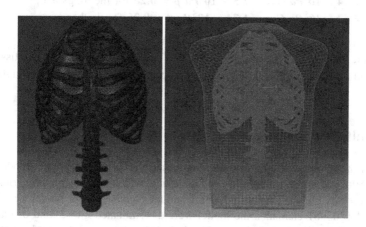

Fig. 6. The skeletal model with organs and the whole assembled model

All the anatomical components in the model are deformable and there is no rigid body. The articular joints between the ribs and the vertebrae, the facet joints between vertebrae, the joints between bones and outer soft tissue are defined by tied constraints. The interactions of the internal organs such as heart and lungs with outer soft tissue or bones are defined by contact interfaces.

3   Material Modeling

Since the thorax and abdomen consists of many different organs and each organ presents individual mechanical properties which makes it very complex to model, we simplified the whole model into two materials.

The constitutive laws for all the tissues in this model are either considered as linear elastic or linear viscoelastic. In this study, we refer the material settings in Ruan's paper [2, 10, 11]. Hard tissues, such as spine, ribs were modelled with liner elastic solid elements characterized by the stress-strain law:

$$\sigma = E\varepsilon \tag{1}$$

with,

$E = 4.2 \times 10^6$ Pa for spine and ribs.

Where E is the elastic modulus. The Poisson's ratio is set as 0.3.

Soft tissues, such as heart, lungs and other soft tissue were modelled with linear viscoelastic material characterized by:

$$Gt = G_\infty + (G_0 - G_\infty)e^{-\beta t} \tag{2}$$

with,

$G_0 = 2.24 \times 10^4 Pa, G_\infty = 7.5 \times 10^3 Pa, \beta = 0.25$ for the lungs and,

$G_0 = 4.42 \times 10^5 Pa, G_\infty = 1.74 \times 10^5 Pa, \beta = 0.25$ for the heart.

Where, G_0 and G_∞ are short-term and long-term shear moduli, which govern the viscoelastic response. β is the decay factor. The density of the model tissue was maintained at 1000 kg/m^3 to generate appropriate mass distribution throughout the model.

4   Results and Discussion

Based on the above work, finally, we established the 3D finite element model of the Chinese 50th percentile male thorax and abdomen, which consists of spine, ribs, heart, lungs and relative fresh. The mesh division and the elements of the model were 352958 nodes and 1203981 elements, the model were discriminated into 2 kind of material.

The results from this study suggested that the numerical finite element model established herein with intact structure and precise elements could be used as a powerful tool for biomechanics analysis and impact automotive safety research.

However, this finite element model was not been validated through the comparison of model predicted force-times and force-deflections with the experimental data from previous research. And also the large numbers of nodes and elements in order to simulate each detailed anatomical component will take much time to finish the calculation. The model built in this study has been simplified in material property, it may not represent the real mechanical response of human body. For real world occupant simulations, the model needs more improvement. And the large numbers of nodes and elements also need to be optimized.

Acknowledgements. Supported by the Fundamental Research Funds from Central Finance of China (282014Y-3353) and National Key Technology R&D Program (2014BAK01B05) and National Natural Science Foundation of China (51175021)

References

1. Xiao, K.: Traffic accident injuries in China (2006)
2. Ruan, J., et al.: Prediction and analysis of human thoracic impact responses and injuries in cadaver impacts using a full human body finite element model. Stapp Car Crash J. **47**, 299–321 (2003)
3. Li, F., Li, C.: Analysis on Application of Vehicle Side Impact Dummy (2007)

4. Deng, X., et al.: Finite element analysis of occupant head injuries: parametric effects of the side curtain airbag deployment interaction with a dummy head in a side impact crash. Aocid. Anal. Prev. **55**, 232–241 (2013)

5. Gursel, K.T., Nane, S.N.: Non-linear finite element analyses of automobiles and their elements in crashes. Int. J. Crashworthiness **15**(6), 667–692 (2010)

6. Li, Z., et al.: Development, validation, and application of a parametric pediatric head finite element model for impact simulations. Ann. Biomed. Eng. **39**(12), 2984–2997 (2011)

7. Li, Z., et al.: Rib fractures under anterior–posterior dynamic loads: experimental and finite-element study. J. Biomech. **43**(2), 228–234 (2010)

8. Majumder, S., Roychowdhury, A., Pal, S.: Simulation of hip fracture in sideways fall using a 3D finite element model of pelvis–femur–soft tissue complex with simplified representation of whole body. Med. Eng. Phys. **29**(10), 1167–1178 (2007)

9. Moes, N.C.C.M., Horváth, I.: Using finite element models of the human body for shape optimization of seats: optimization material properties. In: Proceedings of the International Design Conference, Dubrovnik, Yugoslavia (2002)

10. Ruan, J.S., et al.: Biomechanical analysis of human abdominal impact responses and injuries through finite element simulations of a full human body model. Stapp Car Crash J. **49**, 343–366 (2005)

11. Ruan, J.S., et al.: Impact response and biomechanical analysis of the knee-thigh-hip complex in frontal impacts with a full human body finite element model. Stapp Car Crash J. **52**, 505–526 (2008)

Biomechanical Analysis of Human Thorax and Abdomen During Automotive Impact

Hui-min Hu[1], Li Ding[2(✉)], Xianxue Li[2], Chaoyi Zhao[1], and Yan Yin[1]

[1] China National Institute of Standardization, Beijing, China
{huhm,zhaochy,yiny}@cnis.gov.cn
[2] Key Laboratory for Biomechanics and Mechanobiology of Ministry of Education, School of Biological Science and Medical Engineering, Beihang University, Beijing, China
{Ding1971316,li36101120}@buaa.edu.cn

Abstract. Injuries incurred to occupant during automotive frontal crashes range from every part of the human body, and especially for the thorax and abdomen. It's indeed to learn more about the impact biomechanical mechanism of human body in order to improve the impact safety of vehicles to protect the occupant. In this study, a previously developed finite model of Chinese 50th percentile male thorax and abdomen is used to study the biomechanical response under frontal impact. The stress-time, strain-time characteristics are analyzed. Quantitative results such deflection curve are obtained and indicate that the 6.7 m/s frontal impact leads to large deflection and stress which will damage the ribs, lungs and other organs. Since the experimental study with human cadavers is difficult to proceed, this finite element model based on the anthropometric data from Chinese 50th percentile male can be used to analyze the biomechanical response during automotive impact in order to improve the automotive impact safety.

Keywords: Biomechanical response · Automobile · Impact · Finite element

1 Introduction

The impact safety is one of the most important aspects during the automobile production process and it is mainly assessed by the human body injury [1]. So it's important to learn more about the biomechanical response of the human body during automotive impact in order to improve the automotive impact safety. Automotive accident analysis shows that thorax and abdomen are the most vulnerable parts which lead to death because the organs in these two parts are very important and vulnerable.

There are three approaches to study the biomechanical response of human body: (1) biological model: human cadaver or animal experiment. Mertz et al. [2, 3] have exposed the thoracic and abdominal regions of animals to frontal and lateral impacts of deploying airbags. The results showed that the same severity of injury could be produced for each impact direction for the same loading condition. However, since the animal have big difference from real human body, the experiment data is not satisfactory. Human cadaver

© Springer International Publishing Switzerland 2015
V.G. Duffy (Ed.): DHM 2015, Part II, LNCS 9185, pp. 266–273, 2015.
DOI: 10.1007/978-3-319-21070-4_27

is ideal experimental object, however human cadaver is rare and vary with age and gender which make it hard to do large-scale experiment. (2) mechanical model: researchers developed the crash test dummy to simulate the real human body. The crash test dummy simulates the human parts with springs, dampers and other mental parts [4–8]. By testing the flection and kinematic data, the impact biomechanical response is described. In China, Hybrid III is used in frontal impact experiment and EuroSID is used in lateral impact experiment. In the experiment of automotive impact, the crash test dummy is used to get the value of parameters such as force, acceleration and displacement and based on these basic parameters the HPC (head performance indictor), ThPC (chest performance indictor), FPC (thigh performance indictor) are calculated to indicate the automotive impact safety. Since HPC, ThPC and FPC are relative with the anthropological data, and those two kinds of dummies are based on the anthropological data from American and European, there are some differences with the Chinese people which will influence the results. (3) numerical model: the biomechanical response of human body or dummy can be modeled by either rigid-body dynamics or finite element methods. The finite element model can represent the flexibility and material behavior of the human body in detail and accurately but at a significantly higher computational cost. However, with the development of high-speed computing method, the finite element modeming technology has been used to predict the biomechanical response during automotive impact [7].

In this study, a previously developed finite element model of thorax and abdomen base on the Chinese male 50th percentile data is used to do some simulation on the automotive frontal and side impact in order to analyze the biomechanical response of the human body to improve the automotive impact safety.

2 Methods

2.1 Finite Model and Material

The finite element model of thorax and abdomen developed previously is used in this study. Figure 1 shows a view of the model that was based on the 50th Chinese percentile male dimensions which consists of spine, ribs, heart, lungs and relative soft tissue.

The whole finite element model contains 285801 nodes and 956984 elements. The model were discriminated into 2 kind of material. The constitutive laws for all the tissues in this model are either considered as linear elastic or linear viscoelastic. Hard tissues, such as spine, ribs were modelled with liner elastic solid elements characterized by the stress-strain law:

$$\sigma = E\varepsilon, \tag{1}$$

with $E = 4.2 \times 10^6$ Pa for spine and ribs. Where E is the elastic moduli.

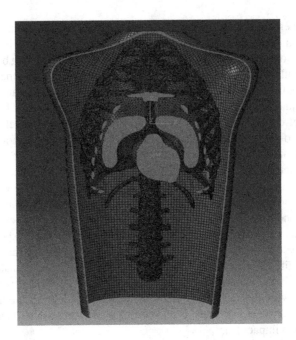

Fig. 1. Sectional view of the thorax and abdomen model

Soft tissues, such as heart, lungs and fresh were modelled with linear viscoelastic material characterized by:

$$G\,(t) = G_\infty + (G_0 - G_\infty)e^{-\beta t}, \tag{2}$$

with $G_0 = 230\,kPa$, $G_\infty = 436\,kPa$, $\beta = 0.635$. Where, G_0 and G_∞ are short-term and long-term shear moduli, which govern the viscoelastic response. β is the decay factor.

The skin was modelled with elastic material, which the Young's moduli is 31.5 MPa and the Poisson's ratio is 0.45.

Contact interfaces are defined between impactor and skin, skin and ribs, ribs and lungs, spine and skin. Tied constrains are defined between the vertebrae and disks.

2.2 Impact Conditions

The impact simulation was conducted by ABAQUS software and a dynamic explicit method was used, the step time was 50 ms. Since the model was used to simulate frontal blunt impact response. The blunt used for the frontal impact simulation was modelled as rigid cylinders just as Fig. 2 shows.

The blunt was given an initial velocity of 6.7 m/s and was set to generate a mass of 23.4 kg during frontal impact simulation. The blunt was meshed using solid elements.

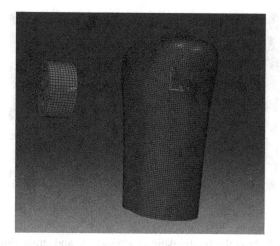

Fig. 2. Frontal and lateral impact

3 Results and Discussion

3.1 Impactor

Figure 3 shows the velocity of the impactor during the impact. From the results, we can see that the initial velocity is 6.70 m/s, the collision occurs at about 0.0275 s and declines because of the interaction between impactor and the human model.

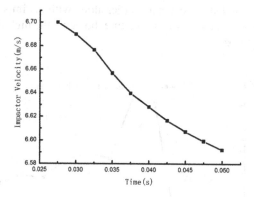

Fig. 3. Velocity of the impactor during impact

3.2 Skin

Figure 4 shows the map of displacement and stress after frontal impact. The impact area has the biggest deflection and decreases outwards. The stress concentration area occurs outside the impact area where large curvature occurs such as shoulders.

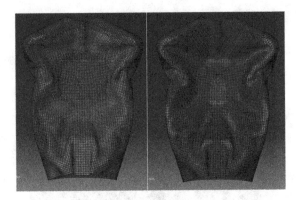

Fig. 4. Displacement and stress of skin

Figures 5 and 6 show the relationship of stress-time and strain-time during frontal impact. In about 0.01 s, the stress and strain increase to the maximum which are $7 \times [\![10]\!]^{\wedge}5$ Pa for stress and $2 \times [\![10]\!]^{\wedge}(-2)$ for strain. Then the stress and strain decrease to the half maximum slightly at 0.05 s. From the results we can conclude that the best time to reduce the injures during impact is the first 0.01 s so that we can improve automobile's impact safety at that time.

3.3   Ribs and Lungs

Figure 7 shows the stress and deflection characteristics of ribs under the 6.7 m/s frontal speed. The deflection and stress becomes larger along with the impact. Since the bone was set as elastic material, there was no fracture, however the high deflection rate will indicate the injury of ribs.

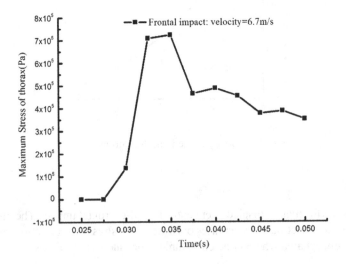

Fig. 5. Maximum stress of skin

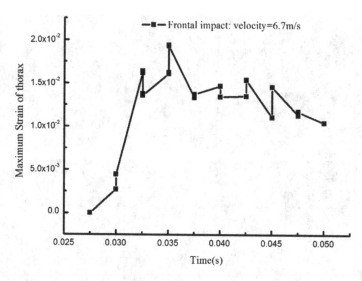

Fig. 6. Maximum strain of skin

Figure 8 shows the deflection of the lungs during the frontal impact. The deflection starts at about 0.035 s when the ribs deforms to contact the lungs. The deformation of lungs is based on ribs' deformation. From the results, the lungs have a large deformation about 10 cm at 0.050 s which will significantly damage the soft tissue of lungs.

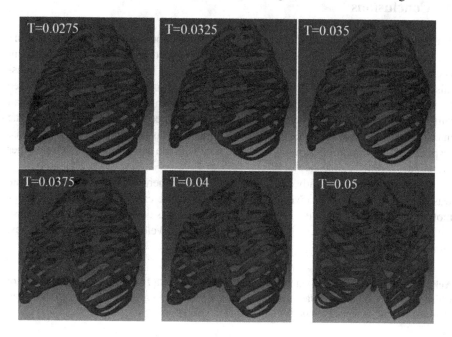

Fig. 7. Biomechanical response of ribs to frontal impact

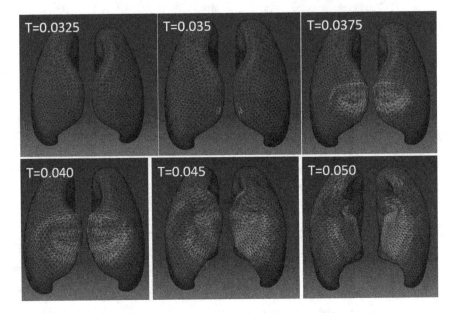

Fig. 8. Biomechanical response of lungs to frontal impact

4   Conclusions

The different injury types during impact appear to be dependent on the rate of loading because the soft tissues' viscoelastic property. Low speed impact's injury mechanism is compression of the organs and high speed impact will injure the occupant by transmission of a pressure wave. From the results of frontal impact simulation, we can see that the stress-time curve begins with a primary inertial impact peak because the human part at the impact site is quickly accelerated to the speed of the impact blunt. The maximum compression appears after the force plateau has begun to decline. The force response of the simulation shows good agreement with the experimental data from other literatures.

The results from this study can be used to analyze where and how the human tissue was affected during automotive frontal impact. Then we can try to improve the automotive impact safety targeted. Since the finite model was developed based on Chinese anthropology, it will play an important role in the development Chinese crash test dummy.

Acknowledgements. Supported by the Fundamental Research Funds from Central Finance of China (282014Y-3353) and National Key Technology R & D Program (2014BAK01B05) and National Natural Science Foundation of China (51175021)

References

1. Ruan, J., et al.: Prediction and analysis of human thoracic impact responses and injuries in cadaver impacts using a full human body finite element model. Stapp Car Crash J. **47**, 299–321 (2003)
2. Mertz, H., et al.: Response of animals exposed to deployment of various passenger inflatable restraint system concepts for a variety of collision severities and animal positions. In: Ninth Experimental Safety Vehicle Conference, Kyoto, Japan, pp. 352–368 (1982)
3. Mertz, H., Weber, D.A.: Interpretations of the impact responses of a 3-year-old child dummy relative to child injury potential. In: Ninth Experimental Safety Vehicle Conference, Kyoto, Japan, pp. 368–376 (1982)
4. Beheshti, H., Lankarani, H.M., Gopalan, S.: A hybrid multibody model for aircraft occupant/ seat cushion crashworthiness investigation. In: 5th International Conference on Multibody Systems, Nonlinear Dynamics, and Control (2005)
5. Haslegrave, C.M.: Dummies for crash testing motor cars. Appl. Ergon. **5**(3), 153–160 (1974)
6. Mullins, J.: The human crash test dummy. N. Sci. **194**(2602), 50–51 (2007)
7. Noureddine, A., Eskandarian, A., Digges, K.: Computer modeling and validation of a hybrid III dummy for crashworthiness simulation. Math. Comput. Model. **35**(7–8), 885–893 (2002)
8. Pearlman, M.D., Viano, D.: Automobile crash simulation with the first pregnant crash test dummy. Am. J. Obstet. Gynecol. **175**(4, Part 1), 977–981 (1996)

Toward a Model for Effective Human-Automation Interaction: The Mediated Agency

Kevin Le Goff[1,2], Arnaud Rey[2], and Bruno Berberian[1(✉)]

[1] Systems Control and Flight Dynamics Department, ONERA, Salon de Provence, France
Bruno.Berberian@onera.fr
[2] Laboratoire de Psychologie Cognitive, CNRS and Aix-Marseille Université, Marseille, France
legoff.kev@gmail.com

Abstract. In our increasingly technological world, automation largely improved some aspects of our life. Nonetheless, automation can also have negative consequences. Indeed, operators seem often helpless to takeover an automated system in case of failure. This "out-of-the-loop" problem occurs when operator is unable to understand the intentions and to predict the outcome of actions of the system, causing a decrease of control. The following article illustrates how the psychological approach of agency can help (1) to better understand this OOTL performance problem and (2) to propose design principles to improve human machine interaction in case of system automation.

1 Introduction

In our increasingly technological world, the influence of automation is perceived in each aspect of everyday life. At work or at home, human beings are accustomed to interact with sophisticated computer systems designed to assist them in their activities. Automation certainly makes some aspects of life easier: by allowing people with disabilities to be able to move and communicate; faster: with the generalization of computerized devices and the increase of productivity; and safer: the accident rate in aviation or high-risk industry has dropped down thanks to the implementation of automated systems [1]. This is far from over, thus, no one would be surprised in future years to see a car without driver let her/him cross the road.

Automation is often a suitable solution for functions that humans cannot achieve safely or reliably. Previous studies demonstrated that high level of automation reduced human operator workload and increase the level of productivity [2]. Nonetheless, the interposition of automated systems between human operators and processes transforms the nature of human work. As a matter of fact, the role of the human actors tends to evolve from direct control to supervision. This change is far from trivial and creates new burdens and complexities for the individuals and teams of practitioners responsible for operating, troubleshooting and managing high-consequence systems.

© Springer International Publishing Switzerland 2015
V.G. Duffy (Ed.): DHM 2015, Part II, LNCS 9185, pp. 274–283, 2015.
DOI: 10.1007/978-3-319-21070-4_28

2   Automation and OOL Performance Problem

When new automation is introduced into a system, or when there is an increase in the autonomy of automated systems, developers often assume that adding "automation" is a simple substitution of a machine activity for human activity (substitution myth, see [3]). Empirical data on the relationship between people and technology suggest that this is not the case and that traditional automation has many negative outcomes and safety consequences associated with it stemming from the human out-of-the-loop (OOL) performance problem [4, 5].

The OOL performance problem has been attributed to a number of underlying factors, including human vigilance decrements [6, 7], complacency [8, 9] and loss of operator situation awareness (SA) [10, 11]. Cognitive engineering literature has discussed at length the origins of vigilance decrements (e.g., low signal rates, lack of operator sensitivity to signals), complacency (e.g., over trust in highly reliable computer control) and the decrease in SA (use of more passive rather than active processing and the differences in the type of feedback provided) in automated system supervision and has established associations between these human information processing shortcomings and performance problems.

As a major consequence, the OOL performance problem leaves operators of automated systems handicapped in their ability to take over manual operations in the case of automation failure. Particularly, the OOL performance problem causes a set of difficulties including a longer latency to determine what has failed, to decide if an intervention is necessary and to find the adequate course of action [6]. The three following incidents from aviation, nuclear plant and finance domains illustrate such difficulties.

- Situation 1: Aviation
  The first example concerns Flight 447 from Air France. On May 31, 2009, the Airbus A330 took off from Rio de Janeiro bound to Paris. Four hours after the departure and due to weather conditions, ice crystals obstructed the Pitot probes. Hence, speed indications were incorrect and lead to a disconnection of the autopilot. Likely following this disconnection, the crew was unable to diagnose the situation and apply the appropriate procedure. Alternating appearances and disappearances of some indicators and alarms coupled with high stress probably prevented the crew to correctly evaluate the state of the system and act appropriately (for the official report, see [12]).
- Situation 2: Nuclear Power Plant
  The second example concerns the incident of the nuclear plant of Three Miles Island (Pennsylvania, USA), in 1979. A valve used to regulate the water inlet in the nuclear core was stuck open, although a light on the control interface indicated that the valve position was closed. However, this light did not indicate real position of the valve but instead that the closure order was given. Because of ambiguous information provided by the control interface, the operators were unable to correctly diagnose the problem for several hours [13]. During this period, a sequence of different failures and inappropriate actions lead to a partial meltdown of the nuclear core. Hopefully, the releases of radiations were not important enough to cause health and environmental damages. A major nuclear disaster was avoided.

- Situation 3: Stock Market

  In a completely different domain, we can mention one of the costliest computer bug. Knight Capital is a firm specialized in high frequency trading (automated technic used to buy and sell stocks in fractions of a second). On August 1, 2012, the firm tested a new version of its trading algorithm. However, due to a bug, the algorithm started pushing erratic trades. Because supervisors were not up to date of the system behavior, it took a long hour to understand that the problem came from the algorithm and coasted to Knight Capital about 400 million dollars [14].

Although these previous cases are from different domains, they highlight that when the automatic equipment fails, supervisors seem dramatically helpless for diagnosing the situation and determining the appropriate solution because they are not aware of the system state prior to the failure. Numerous experimental results confirm such difficulties. For example, Endsley and Kiris [4] provided evidence that performance during failure mode following a fully automated period were significantly degraded, as compared to a failure mode following a fully manual control. Merat and Jamson [15] reported similar conclusions. In a driving simulation task, they demonstrated that drivers' responses to critical events were slower in the automatic driving condition than in the manual condition. Because automation is not powerful enough to handle all abnormalities, this difficulty in takeover is a central problem in automation design. Moreover, with the development of autonomous cars, which should come onto our roads in a few years, everyone (not only expert operators) could be concerned by such difficulties, and the issue becomes universal.

These difficulties in takeover situations have been identified for a long time [1, 16] and different solutions have been proposed by the human factors society. Some of them consist in training human operator to produce efficient behavior in case of system failure. However, recent dramatic events indicate that such training does not ensure efficient takeover for trained situations, whereas the apparition of unexpected failure are not considered by such approach. Other solutions propose to manipulate the level of system automation, sharing the authority between the automation and the human operator (for example MABA-MABA methods, adaptive function allocation). Such approach rests on the hypothesis that new technologies can be introduced as a simple substitution of machines for people - preserving the basic system while improving it on some output measures. Unfortunately, such assumption corresponds to a vague and bleak reflection of the real impact of automation: automation technology transforms human practice and forces people to adapt their skills and routines [17].

If these traditional approaches have the virtue to partially decrease the negative consequences of automation technology, clear solutions are still missing to overcome these takeover difficulties [18, 19]. We argue that the key for designers is to focus on how automation technology transforms the human operator activity and what are the mechanisms of control involved in a supervisory task. We assume that the response to these questions remains a crucial challenge for successful design of new automated systems. In this paper, we propose a theoretical framework to explain this transformation.

3 OOL Performance Problem and System Predictability

As assumed by Norman [1], the lack of system predictability is certainly a central point in the comprehension of the OOL phenomenon and the associated takeover difficulties. With the advent in technology, current man-made complex systems tend to develop cascades and runaway chains of automatic reactions that decrease, even eliminate predictability and cause outsized events [20]. This is what we will call *system opacity*: the difficulty for a human operator to see the arrow from system intention to actual state and to predict the sequence of events that will occur.

However, such opacity is far from being a fatality. As pointed by Norman [1], the problem with automation is more its inappropriate design and application than over automation per se. Particularly, the lack of continual feedback and interaction appears as the central problem. Throughout the last years, computational and experimental evidences have proved the central place of feedback regarding the mechanisms that govern the control of our actions [21–25]. When people perform actions, feedback is essential for the appropriate monitoring of those actions. However, adequate feedback to the human operator is most of the time absent in case of system automation. Without appropriate feedback about the state of the system, people may not know if the actions are being performed properly or if problems are occurring. As a result, when an automatic equipment fails, people are not able to detect symptoms of troubles early enough to overcome them.

Interestingly, system engineers are blind to the paradox that we have never had more data than we have now, yet have less predictability than ever. To overcome such opacity, they have to propose adequate feedback about the state of the system. However, how to design a predictable system remains a difficult problem. A possible approach is to focus on how humans understand and control their own actions. Indeed, we can assume that operators interpret the intentions and the outcomes' actions of a system with their own "cognitive toolkit". Thus, understanding how this "cognitive toolkit" works could be relevant to propose design principles for potentially controllable systems.

4 Science of Agency as a Relevant Framework

When we act, we usually have a clear feeling that we control our own action and can thus produce effects in the external environment. This feeling has been described as "the sense of agency" [26], and is recognized as an important part of normal and human consciousness. Most people can readily sort many events in the world into those they have authored and those they have not. This observation suggests that each person has a system for authorship processing [27], a set of mental processes that monitors indications of authorship to judge whether an event, action, or thought should be ascribed to self as a causal agent [28]. Laboratory studies have attempted to shed more light on this mechanism and empirical data in recent psychology [29, 30], psychopathology [31, 32] and neuroscience [33, 34] have been accumulated. Interestingly, a variety of sources of information (e.g., one's own thoughts, interoceptive sensations, external feedback, etc.) could be involved in the authorship processing. Several indicators have been already proposed, including body and environment orientation cues [35], direct bodily feedback [36, 37], direct bodily feedforward [38, 39], visual and other indirect sensory feedback [40], social cues [41], agent goal information [42] and own behavior relevant thought [43–45]. Although, the mental processes contributing to the sense of agency are not fully understood at this time, the different approaches propose that we derive a sense of being the agent for our own actions by a cognitive mechanism that computes the discrepancies between the predicted consequences of our own actions' actual consequences of these actions, similarly to action control models [22, 24, 43]. Thus, predictability appears as a key notion regarding the mechanism of agency and researchers demonstrated that efferent signals, re-afferent signals, higher order knowledge and beliefs influence it.

Interestingly, Pacherie [46] argued that the different mechanisms underlying sense of agency for individual actions are similar to those underlying sense of agency one experiences when engaged in joint action. That is, the sense of agency in joint action is based on the same principle of congruence between predicted and actual outcomes. Sebanz, Bekkering and Knoblich [47] defined a joint action as "any form of social interaction whereby two or more individuals coordinate their actions in space and time to bring about change in the environment". Moreover, one of the criterions needed for the accomplishment of a joint action is the ability to predict other's actions and their outcomes. Predicting other's actions required areas involved in the human self-action control system [48]. This capability of prediction is crucial to achieve an efficient coordination in a joint action [49–51]. Vesper et al. [51] demonstrated that participants involved in a joint task were more predictable by reducing the temporal variability in order to facilitate the coordination.

If we consider that the predictability in human-system interactions and in human-human interactions operates in the same way, we can assume that the system opacity could dramatically change our experience of agency. This hypothesis receives an echo from the claim of Baron when he said:

"Perhaps the major human factors concern of pilots in regard to introduction of automation is that, in some circumstances, operations with such aids may leave the critical question, who is in control now, the human or the machine?" [52].

Recent empirical data have confirmed such degradation of our experience of agency in presence of automation [53]. Particularly, by manipulating the level of automation in an aircraft supervision task, we have demonstrated a decrease in agency (for both implicit and explicit measures) concomitant to the increase in automation. Consequently, we assume that a way to design a more controllable interface is to consider supervision as a joint action between a human operator and an artificial co-agent following the same principles as a biological co-agent. This proposition echoes that of Norman [1] when he assumed that *what is needed is continual feedback about the state of the system, in a normal natural way, much in the manner that human participants in a joint problem-solving activity will discuss the issues among themselves.* The use of the theoretical background of agency will make it easier to achieve this objective. This is why we argue, in this paper, for a mediated agency: an approach to HMI interactions that takes into account how the information provided by an automated system influences how an operator feels in control.

5   Agency Offers Tools and Measures

As previously assumed, system opacity is certainly a major cause of OOL performance problems. To overcome such system opacity, interactions designers could use the tools and measures, provided by the framework of agency (and by extension, the one of joint agency). Examples of such tools can be derived from the theory of apparent mental causation of Daniel Wegner [43]. His theory provided clues to determine the nature, the form and the timing of an appropriate feedback. Particularly, Wegner proposed that when a thought occurs prior to an action it is consistent with the action and the action has no plausible alternative cause, then we experience the feeling of consciously willing the action. This is what he called, priority, consistency and exclusivity principles. System engineers could use these principles to shape adequate feedbacks in order to make the automation more predictable. We already know that this capability of prediction is crucial to achieve an efficient coordination in a joint action [49–51]. Recently Berberian and colleagues provided evidence that these principles could be used to design Human-machine interfaces capable of compensating the negative effects of latency on action control [54]. We assumed that automated systems following such principles would make the operators more "agent", and then they would not be affected by the OOL performance problem. Thus, they would be faster and more reliable to take over an automated system in case of failure.

Another contribution from this framework to the human-machine domain is provided by the use of measures of agency. Although quantifying the degree of agency remains difficult, several measures have been proposed. Interestingly, we can distinguish two different kinds of measures (Explicit *vs.* Implicit) referring potentially to two separable agency processing systems [26, 55]. The explicit level refers to the "Judgment of agency", that is, the capability to attribute agency to oneself or another. This judgment is influenced by beliefs and external cues [56]. One can use classic declarative methods, such as surveys and self-reports to evaluate this aspect of agency. The implicit level refers to the "Feeling of agency", a low-level feeling of being an agent, mainly based on sensory-motor cues. Implicit markers of agency have been proposed by Haggard and colleagues, namely the intentional binding effect (IB). In a key study, they noticed that human intentional actions produce systematic changes in time perception. In particular, the interval between a voluntary action and an outcome is perceived as shorter than the interval between a physically similar involuntary movement and the same outcome event [57]. This phenomenon has been widely reported (for a review, see [58]). Although our understanding of the underlying mechanisms is not clear, IB may provide an implicit window into human agency. For the last decade, a lot of studies about agency were published, some used a method or another and some used both but still in simple and easy to control paradigms (for example, a visual signal appeared and the participant had to push a button). Regarding the applicability of these methods to design processes, future work will have to determine the efficiency of such methods in more complex situations encountered in the human-system interaction field. Berberian et al. [53] used both measures to evaluate the variation of agency depending on the level of automatism in an aircraft supervision task with different autopilot settings. They provided evidences that intentional binding measures are sensitive to graded variations in control associated with automation and was related to explicit judgments. This study demonstrates that IB could be used in a richer and more complex paradigm. These measures should therefore be combined to develop a framework for evaluating the OOL performance problem. Hence, ergonomists should bear in mind the different elements of the human sense of agency, and the different ways of measuring it, in order to correctly evaluate if an interface is sufficiently acceptable and controllable.

6 Conclusion

We have seen that, despite all the benefits of automation, there are still issues to be corrected (loss of control, less efficient monitoring…). This clearly establishes that some problems in human-machine interaction stem from a decreased predictability, due to an increase of complexity. However, designing relevant feedback and system-operator communication is clearly the key to avoiding these problems, but this remains a challenge. We proposed that using principles, tools and measures from the science of agency should lead to the introduction of a new methodology. "Being an agent" is a notion largely studied in neurosciences, psychology and philosophy. It would be also relevant, for the human-machine domain, to use a framework taking into account the difference between self-generated actions and those generated by other sources. This is why we argue for a mediated agency framework: an approach to HMI interactions that takes into account how the information provided by an automated system influence how an operator feels in control. We suggest that the science of agency in the field of human-machine interaction may be fruitful to elaborate concrete recommendations to design automatics system supervised by operators "in the loop" abating the negative consequence of OOL problem while maintaining the performance in the normal range. Measuring (explicitly or implicitly) the feeling of control may be important in evaluating different automated devices, and may also be relevant for evaluating operator's performances in supervisory tasks. In the end, a better understanding of how the sense of agency evolved in the case of interactions between humans and automated system would certainly refine the different models of agency and, more generally, models of control.

References

1. Norman, D.A.: The 'Problem' with automation: inappropriate feedback and interaction, not 'Over-Automation'. Philos. Trans. R. Soc. Lond. **327**, 585–593 (1990)
2. Kaber, D., Onal, E., Endsley, M.: Design of automation for telerobots and the effect on performance, operator situation awareness and subjective workload. Hum. Factors Ergon. Manuf. **10**, 409–430 (2000)
3. Woods, D.D., Tinapple, D.: W3: watching human factors watch people at work. Presidential Address, 43rd Annual Meeting of the Human Factors and Ergonomics Society (1999)
4. Endsley, M.R., Kiris, E.O.: The out-of-the-loop performance problem and level of control in automation. Hum. Factors J. Hum. Factors Ergon. Soc. **37**(2), 381–394 (1995)
5. Kaber, D.B., Endsley, M.R.: Out-of-the-loop performance problems and the use of intermediate levels of automation for improved control system functioning and safety. Process Saf. Prog. **16**(3), 126–131 (1997)

6. Billings, C.E.: Human-Centered Aircraft Automation: A Concept and Guidelines (NASA Tech. Memo. 103885). Moffet Field, CA: NASA-Ames Research Center (1991)
7. Wiener, E.L.: Cockpit automation. In: Wiener, E.L., Nagel, D.C. (eds.) Human Factors in Aviation, pp. 433–459. Academic Press, San Diego (1988)
8. Parasuraman, R., Molloy, R., Singh, I.L.: Performance consequences of automation induced complacency. Int. J. Aviat. Psychol. **3**, 1–23 (1993)
9. Singh, I.L., Molloy, R., Parasuraman, R.: Automation-induced monitoring inefficiency: role of display location. Int. J. Hum. Comput. Stud. **46**(1), 17–30 (1997)
10. Carmody, M.A., Gluckman, J.P.: Task specific effects of automation and automation failure on performance, workload and situational awareness. In: Jensen R.S., Neumeister, D. (eds.) Proceedings of the 7th International Symposium on Aviation Psychology, pp. 167–171. Department of Aviation, Ohio State University, Columbus (1993)
11. Endsley, M.R.: Automation and situation awareness. In: Parasuraman, R., Mouloua, M. (eds.) Automation and Human Performance: Theory and Applications, pp. 163–181. Lawrence Erlbaum, Mahwah (1996)
12. B.E.A.: Final Report on the accident of the flight AF 447 Rio de Janeiro-Paris (2012). http://www.bea.aero/fr/enquetes/vol.af.447/rapport.final.fr.php
13. Norman, D.A.: The Psychology of Everyday Things. Basic Books, New York (1988)
14. Jones, C.M.: What do we know about high-frequency trading? Columbia Business School Research Paper No. 13–11 (2013)
15. Merat, N., Jamson, A.H.: How do drivers behave in a highly automated car. In: Proceedings of the 5th International Driving Symposium on Human Factors in Driver Assessment, Training and Vehicle Design, pp. 514–521 (2009)
16. Bainbridge, L.: Ironies of automation. Automatica **19**(6), 775–779 (1983)
17. Dekker, S.W., Woods, D.D.: MABA-MABA or abracadabra? progress on human–automation co-ordination. Cogn. Technol. Work **4**(4), 240–244 (2002)
18. Baxter, G., Rooksby, J., Wang, Y., Khajeh-Hosseini, A.: The ironies of automation: still going strong at 30? In: Proceedings of the 30th European Conference on Cognitive Ergonomics, pp. 65–71. ACM, New York (2012)
19. Norman, D.A.: Living with Complexity. MIT Press, Cambridge (2010)
20. Taleb, N.N.: Antifragile: Things that Gain From Disorder. Random House Incorporated, New York (2012)
21. Kawato, M.: Internal models for motor control and trajectory planning. Curr. Opin. Neurobiol. **9**(6), 718–727 (1999)
22. Wolpert, D.M.: Computational approaches to motor control. Trends Cogn. Sci. **1**(6), 209–216 (1997)
23. Wolpert, D.M., Ghahramani, Z., Jordan, M.I.: An internal model for sensorimotor integration. Science **269**(5232), 1880–1882 (1995)
24. Blakemore, S.J., Wolpert, D.M., Frith, C.D.: Abnormalities in the awareness of action. Trends Cogn. Sci. **6**(6), 237–242 (2002)
25. Frith, C.D., Blakemore, S.J., Wolpert, D.M.: Explaining the symptoms of schizophrenia: abnormalities in the awareness of action. Brain Res. Rev. **31**(2), 357–363 (2000)
26. Gallagher, S.: Philosophical concepts of the self: implications for cognitive sciences. Trends Cogn. Sci. **4**, 14–21 (2000)
27. Wegner, D.M., Sparrow, B.: Authorship processing. In: Gazzaniga, M.S. (ed.) The New Cognitive Neurosciences, 3rd edn. MIT Press, Cambridge (2004)
28. Wegner, D.M., Sparrow, B., Winerman, L.: Vicarious agency: experiencing control over the movements of others. J. Pers. Soc. Psychol. **86**(6), 838 (2004)

29. Aarts, H., Custers, R., Wegner, D.M.: On the inference of personal authorship: enhancing experienced agency by priming effect information. Conscious. Cogn. **14**(3), 439–458 (2005)
30. Moore, J.W., Wegner, D.M., Haggard, P.: Modulating the sense of agency with external cues. Conscious. Cogn. **18**(4), 1056–1064 (2009)
31. Franck, N., Farrer, C., Georgieff, N., Marie-Cardine, M., Daléry, J., d'Amato, T., Jeannerod, M.: Defective recognition of one's own actions in patients with schizophrenia. Am. J. Psychiatry **158**(3), 454–459 (2001)
32. Farrer, C., Franck, N., Georgieff, N., Frith, C.D., Decety, J., Jeannerod, M.: Modulating the experience of agency: a positron emission tomography study. Neuroimage **18**(2), 324–333 (2003)
33. Tsakiris, M., Haggard, P.: The rubber hand illusion revisited: visuotactile integration and self-attribution. J. Exp. Psychol. Hum. Percept. Perform. **31**(1), 80 (2005)
34. Vallacher, R.R., Wegner, D.M.: A Theory of Action Identification. Psychology Press, New work (2014)
35. Gandevia, S.C., Burke, D.: Does the nervous system depend on kinesthetic information to control natural limb movements? Behav. Brain Sci. **15**(04), 614–632 (1992)
36. Georgieff, N., Jeannerod, M.: Beyond consciousness of external reality: a "who" system for consciousness of action and self-consciousness. Conscious. Cogn. **7**(3), 465–477 (1998)
37. Blakemore, S.J., Frith, C.D.: Self-awareness and action. Curr. Opin. Neurobiol. **13**, 219–224 (2003)
38. Blakemore, S.J., Frith, C.D., Wolpert, D.M.: Spatio-temporal prediction modulates the perception of self-produced stimuli. J. Cogn. Neurosci. **11**(5), 551–559 (1999)
39. Daprati, E., Franck, N., Georgieff, N., Proust, J., Pacherie, E., Dalery, J., Jeannerod, M.: Looking for the agent: an investigation into consciousness of action and self-consciousness in schizophrenic patients. Cognition **65**(1), 71–86 (1997)
40. Milgram, S.: Obedience to Authority. Harper & Row, New York (1974)
41. Langer, E., Roth, J.: Heads I win, tails it's chance. J. Pers. Soc. Psychol. **32**(6), 951–955 (1975)
42. Wegner, D.M.: The Illusion of Conscious Will. MIT Press, Cambridge (2002)
43. Wegner, D.M.: The mind's best trick: how we experience conscious will. Trends Cogn. Sci. **7**, 65–69 (2003)
44. Wegner, D.M., Wheatley, T.: Apparent mental causation: sources of the experience of will. Am. Psychol. **54**(7), 480–492 (1999)
45. Pacherie, E.: The phenomenology of joint action: self-agency vs. joint-agency. In: Seemann, A. (ed.) Joint Attention: New Developments, pp. 343–389. MIT Press, Cambridge (2012)
46. Sebanz, N., Bekkering, H., Knoblich, G.: Joint action: bodies and minds moving together. Trends Cogn. Sci. **10**(2), 70–76 (2006)
47. Sebanz, N., Frith, C.: Beyond simulation? Neural mechanisms for predicting the actions of others. Nat. Neurosci. **7**(1), 5–6 (2004)
48. Verfaillie, K., Daems, A.: Representing and anticipating human actions in vision. Vis. Cogn. **9**(1–2), 217–232 (2002)
49. Kilner, J.M., Vargas, C., Duval, S., Blakemore, S.-J., Sirigu, A.: Motor activation prior to observation of a predicted movement. Nat. Neurosci. **7**(12), 1299–1301 (2004)
50. Vesper, C., van der Wel, R.P., Knoblich, G., Sebanz, N.: Making oneself predictable: reduced temporal variability facilitates joint action coordination. Exp. Brain Res. **211**(3–4), 517–530 (2011)
51. Baron, S.: Pilot control. In: Wiener, E.L., Nagel, D.C. (eds.) Human Factors in Aviation, pp. 347–386. Academic Press, San Diego (1988)

52. Berberian, B., Sarrazin, J.C., Le Blaye, P., Haggard, P.: Automation technology and sense of control: a window on human agency. PLoS ONE **7**(3), 34075 (2012)
53. Berberian, B., Le Blaye, P., Schulte, C., Kinani, N., Sim, P.R.: Data transmission latency and sense of control. In: Harris, D. (ed.) EPCE 2013, Part I. LNCS, vol. 8019, pp. 3–12. Springer, Heidelberg (2013)
54. Synofzik, M., Vosgerau, G., Newen, A.: Beyond the comparator model: a multifactorial two-step account of agency. Conscious. Cogn. **17**(1), 219–239 (2008)
55. Moore, J.W., Middleton, D., Haggard, P., Fletcher, P.C.: Exploring implicit and explicit aspects of sense of agency. Conscious. Cogn. **21**(4), 1748–1753 (2012)
56. Haggard, P., Aschersleben, G., Gehrke, J., Prinz, W.: Action, binding, and awareness. In: Prinz, W., Hommel, B. (eds.) Common Mechanisms in Perception and Action, vol. 19, pp. 266–285. Oxford University Press, Oxford (2002)
57. Haggard, P., Clark, S., Kalogeras, J.: Voluntary action and conscious awareness. Nat. Neurosci. **5**(4), 382–385 (2002)
58. Moore, J.W., Obhi, S.S.: Intentional binding and the sense of agency: a review. Conscious. Cogn. **21**(1), 546–561 (2012)

Semantically Integrated Human Factors Engineering

Sebastien Mamessier[1,2]([⊠]), Daniel Dreyer[1,2], and Matthias Oberhauser[1,2]

[1] Airbus Group Innovations, Ottobrunn, Germany
[2] Creative Concept and Design Center, Ottobrunn, Germany
sebastien.mamessier@gatech.edu

Abstract. This work presents a modern approach to Human Factors Engineering enabling integrated simulation and human evaluation of early prototypes of flight deck systems in a immersive environment. The presented approach introduces pragmatic considerations regarding cognitive engineering frameworks such as Cognitive Work Analysis and Hierarchical Analysis for practical use with computational system simulations, laying down the foundation for efficient, quantitative Human Factors analysis in early product design phases. This principle is further demonstrated through a decentralized implementation leveraging the advantages of semantically connecting an immersive Virtual Reality environment with system simulations and semi-automated human factor analysis modules.

Keywords: Human factors · Cognitive engineering · Virtual reality · Semantics

1 Introduction

Human Factors and Ergonomics (HFE) has proven to bring significant value in improving performance and ease of use of complex systems. However it still suffers from a lack of adoption among industrial decision makers [3]. Recent efforts in Human System Integration (HSI) attempt to fill the gap between HFE methods and industrial processes to foster the use of human-centered methods [2,11]. Moreover, Human Factors considerations must be accounted for in early design phases to be able to influence design of subsystems in due date [7]. Along this goal, the iVISION project aims to use semantic technologies and virtual reality environments to assist engineers with Human Factors methods in early phases of cockpit and flight systems design process to avoid high re-design costs and unsatisfying performance-safety compromises.

A holistic Human Factors analysis of a complex socio-technical system like a modern flight deck requires the consideration of many variables such as the physical interface, flight systems and its underlying logic as well as procedures, role allocation and their impact on system performance and safety. Therefore, one needs a fully integrated simulation and evaluation architecture able to help

V.G. Duffy (Ed.): DHM 2015, Part II, LNCS 9185, pp. 284–294, 2015.
DOI: 10.1007/978-3-319-21070-4_29

conduct HFE analysis early in the design process. Current design processes suffer from various flaws among which we can identify:

1. The range of Human Factors methods used in industry is often limited to ad-hoc choices based on available knowledge, time and resources.
2. The coding and analysis of Human-In-The-Loop (HITL) experiments is tenuous and time-consuming.
3. Early user studies are either conducted on individual subsystems or incomplete and semi-functional systems whereas most issues originate from interaction between humans and subsystems and subsystems themselves.

This work presents an ecological simulation and design evaluation framework, combining benefits from Virtual Environments and Semantic Technology for a pragmatic use of Human Factors methods in early phases of complex socio-technical systems design.

1.1 Objectives

The overall objective of this work is to develop a modular, extensible, immersive, semi-automated evaluation system for Human Factors analysis of novel flight deck equipment, displays and concepts. This paper firstly introduces a high-level ontology for the description of complex socio-technical systems as well as pragmatics as guidelines for practical use. Secondly, a highly versatile simulation and Human-In-The-Loop framework architecture is introduced implementing these guidelines. Finally, a case-study implementation shows the advantages and capabilities of such an approach in the field of civil aviation and early flight deck design.

2 Background

The framework presented in this work finds its underlying concepts in Cognitive Engineering (CE) with a focus on ecological design (ED). This section reviews some key CE concepts and puts this work in perspective of the iVISION project.

2.1 Cognitive Engineering and Ecological Design

The question of modeling complex socio-technical systems has been studied extensively, ranging from safety-critical technical systems like control rooms of nuclear power plants to systems with a greater social impact such as stock markets, military command and control systems [16]. Hollnagel and Woods along with Rasmussen and Vicente were among the first researchers to include cognition in the system engineering process rather than treating the human factor as a linear information processor. Ecological design brings cognition outside of linear laboratory experiments as the entire work environment is argued to influence human action and performance.

A man-machine system must be viewed as a cognitive system that presents more variability and adaptability than a simple mechanical system. It produces intelligent action and its behavior is goal oriented, data and concept-driven [5]. Therefore HFE experts need to develop holistic models of such systems and gather data obtained in realistic work environments.

A multi-level functional representation of such systems is given by Rasmussen et al.: the Abstraction Hierarchy (AH) from which Ecological Interface Design (EID) suggests a direct implementation. AH is a multi-level stratified representation of a work domain allowing to cope with its complexity and supporting goal-directed problem solving [16]. A more behavioral representation is proposed by Hierarchical Task Analysis (HTA) which is comprised of a decomposition of system goals into subgoals and potentially cognitive tasks [1].

2.2 Shared Representations in Human Factors

Few authors make the effort of discussing interoperability between theoretical frameworks within Cognitive Engineering. Lind produced a remarkable ontological study of the concepts involved in Rasmussen and Vicente's Abstraction Hierarchy [9]. Ontological uncertainties exist in the concept of functions, the cardinality of mean-ends and whole-parts relations. Lind mentions the conceptual variability of the word *function* but does not attempt to treat the problem as it would require a thorough analysis of a *whole cluster of related concepts: goal, objective, function, disposition, action*. However, Jenkins et al. showed that when treated correctly, both methods can be complimentary and would benefit from formal communication means between frameworks [6]. Joint use is recommended however it is not made clear how to reconcile conceptual and ontological differences. Miller and Vicente illustrate ontological differences of HTA and Work Domain Analysis by applying both to the design of an interface for the DURESS II system [12].

2.3 The iVISION Project

Part of this work was conducted within the frame of the EU funded project: iVISION which aims at bringing together capabilities from three distinct scientific areas: Human Factors, Virtual Reality and Web Semantics. The overarching goal of iVISION is to allow Human Factors experts to benefit from immersive environments and semantic technologies to support cockpit design. On the human factors side, iVISION mostly focuses on methods derived from Hierarchical Task Analysis such as Critical Path Analysis (CPA) and Systematic Human Error Reduction and Prediction Approach (SHERPA).

3   High-Level Cognitive Engineering Ontology

This section describes the high-level ontology aligning Abstraction Hierarchy (AH) and Hierarchical Task Analysis (HTA) as both models are complimentary and prevail in the cognitive engineering community. Semantic relations are also defined with the *domain ontology* $\mathcal{S}$: an unstructured set of state variables describing the system and its environment, an example of which is shown later on in this article in Fig. 3.

Rasmussen and Vicente's abstraction hierarchy (AH) layers have been used with many different interpretations of its building blocks. Indeed, Vicente explains that the number of AH layers and their interpretation is open to variations [16], depending of the system under scrutiny and the type of analysis. We intend to lay down some AH pragmatics to ease practical ecological design and joint-use with task-oriented analysis paradigms such as HTA.

3.1 Abstraction Hierarchy Pragmatics

The following pragmatic considerations were derived from a literature review including Hajdukiewicz and Vicente theoretical note [4] and Vicente's article about Ecological Interface design progress and challenges [15]. They cover the five generic mean-ends related levels of the Abstraction Hierarchy.

Functional Purpose. Overall event-independent purpose of the system.
Example: *Fly passengers from A to B.*

Abstract Functions. Abstract system features relevant to measure achievement of overarching goal. Each item can be further described by a set of metrics integrating measurable system states.
Examples: *Passenger comfort, Fuel usage, Safe flight, Respect of regulations.*
Semantic binding: $f : S' \subset \mathcal{S} \to \mathbb{R}$.

Generalized Functions. Designate the functions controlling roughly independent sets of system states. Usually, achievement of each item requires a specific set of skills or technologies.
Examples: *Navigation, Steering, Communication, System management, Crew management.*
Semantic binding: `Set of states to control:` $S' \subset \mathcal{S}$.

Physical Functions. Describe the *families* of equipment used to control states mentioned in the *generalized functions*. Generic equipment might be described by necessary additional states.
Examples: *Manual control, Autopilot, FMS, Thrust control, Fuel pumps, Stall warning.*
Semantic binding: `Controlled states:` $S' \subset \mathcal{S}$, `Internal states:` $S'' \subset \mathcal{S}$, `Input events:` E.

Physical Forms. Physical instances of device families, displays for a specific design, including location and interfaces.
Examples: *Flight control unit interface, throttle design, side stick (3D shapes), fuel management display.*

Semantic binding: 3D Geometry , Feedback mapping, Interaction mapping, where a *feedback mapping* represents a modification of the 3D geometry, textures, based on system states and an *interaction mapping* describes the emission of events based on user interaction inputs.

Such pragmatics allows engineers to semantically bind an abstraction hierarchy to a domain ontology S.

3.2   HTA Pragmatics

The ontological alignment between Hierarchical Task Analysis and Work Domain Analysis was inspired by Hajdukiewicz and Vicente [4]. It is based on the definition of a task as a goal-directed operation that aims at changing a set of input state values to new output state values. Consequently, the connecting pieces between HTA and AH are the system states acted on for the former and described in the latter.

Therefore we can describe a *task* with a set of state variables - subset of S -, their initial and desired final values. This way, high-level tasks such as Landing the plane can be described in terms of changes in altitude, speed, gear position and physical tasks such as Press Autopilot 1 Engage button in terms of punctual changes in the cockpit element states. Cognitive tasks can also be interpreted in terms of changes in mental states. A formal, semantically bound description of HTA cognitive tasks and *plans* as originally introduced by Annett [1] will be treated as part of future work.

We aim to create and use semantically connected HTAs in the two following flavors.

Descriptive HTA. A *descriptive* HTA produces a task model from observations of operators in their work environment. It usually conducted by Human Factors experts in a paper-based fashion. Variability in operator behavior can be captured by conducting several HTAs and blending the results into more complicated *plans*.

Normative HTA. HTA models can also be *normative* as they describe the tasks to be performed by an operator to reach a certain goal. Interpreted as such, an HTA model can serve as an expert knowledge base for training purpose or to implement a human agent model for simulation purpose.

4   System Architecture

This section technically describes a computer architecture that enables ecological system design and evaluation by implementing the theoretical framework introduced in the previous section. We propose an extensible system architecture supported by semantic technologies and Virtual Reality. The purpose of such a system is to suppress technical integration challenges often hindering engineers from conducting early full-scale Human Factors analysis. It also allows engineers to provide decision-makers with quantitative human-related metrics early enough to influence design decisions.

Several components are semantically connected through the system, as shown in Fig. 1:

1. The work domain provides the unstructured domain ontology S and simulates system dynamics (ex: flight model + cockpit logic).
2. The virtual reality engine: handles VR rendering, head and finger tracking and collision detection.
3. The interaction interpreter: responsible for translation between VR events and the work domain.
4. The Human Factors module organizes the work domain using semantically aligned Human Factors methods that provide the engineer with modeling and analysis tools.

We chose to display the cockpit geometry and embedded systems to the operator in an immersive virtual reality (VR) environment similar to the one described in [10]. The pilot interacts with the virtual environment using a Head-Mounted-Display and accurate finger-tracking with collision detection as well as a physical stick, rudders and throttle. User inputs are then translated into the work domain ontology.

4.1   Decentralized Co-simulation

Extensibility is enforced by a decentralized network architecture assuring a constant entry cost for any additional subsystem or analysis tool. Every component is free to advertise or listen to *topics*, vehicles for state values, as shown in Fig. 1. We used the Robot Operating System (ROS) communication framework [14] to enforce this decentralized architecture.

4.2   Interaction Templates

An important task is to enforce meaningful communication between flight-related modules and the VR environment. A broadly adopted architecture for that type of problem is the Model View Controller (MVC) design pattern illustrated in Fig. 2.

MVC Design Pattern. The view is the cockpit geometry as shown in the VR environment, comprising the displays, outside visuals, button and lever states. The controller implements the user VR interactions such as touching objects, displays with virtually tracked fingers for instance. The model here is mostly the state of the work domain, continuously updated through the flight simulation. In practice, the MVC *update* and *manipulate* operations are to be procedurally implemented in one of the grey boxes (model, view or controller) with specific behavior for each element of the view, controller and model as shown in Fig. 2.

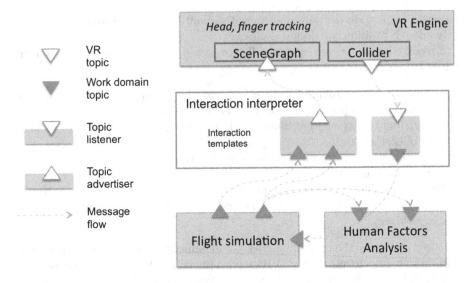

Fig. 1. Diagram of the decentralized system architecture.

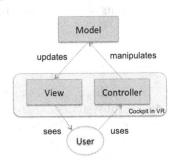

Fig. 2. Model-View-Controller design pattern

Interaction Templates. MVC works well in most software involving user inter-action since the model and the user interface are constants of the design problem. The implementation therefore reflects the specifics of the wanted behavior. In our framework, model, view and controller are the object of analysis and therefore are variables rather than constants. One needs to abstract further out the MVC design pattern to operationally accommodate different flight models, cockpit geometries and interaction modes. Moreover, in order to be formally analyzed, a cockpit behavior cannot be hardcoded and is therefore represented declaratively using interaction templates. Interaction templates are comprised of both a com-putational primitive that implements generic *update/manipulate* operations as well as placeholders for elements from the Model, View or Controller involved in the interaction. Examples of interaction templates are: *push-button with feedback led, touch-screen display, lever with discrete positions, stick, dimmer, etc.*

5   Case Study

We used the above-mentioned high-level ontology and architectural guidelines to implement a novel virtual reality flight simulation environment. The first step is to create an extensive work domain analysis of flight deck operations.

5.1   Aviation Domain Ontology

Numerical simulation of the flight parameters and flight deck systems require the storage and maintenance of *state variables*. Only states actually observable or controllable from a flight deck design point of view have been taken into account. For instance, sensor internal states and dynamics are ignored as sensor values are purely simulated. The dynamics of the subsystems were integrated to the runtime environment using X-Plane 10.

System and Environment States. An roughly structured flight deck work domain has been compiled as a set of categorized state variables, mostly inspired from *XPlane datarefs* [8], as shown in Fig. 3. There are dozens of different commercial airliners on the current market. It seems unreasonable to use a single model to describe their behavior. However it can be argued that many state variables can be shared across different aircraft and reuse of existing state variables should be promoted to ease comparative studies and interoperability with tools from other disciplines.

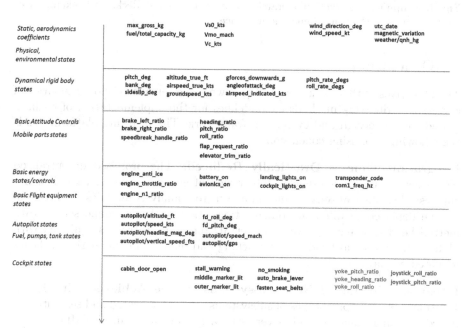

Fig. 3. An example subset of flight deck domain state variables

HF Models. To support Human Factors analysis, system and environment state variables can be semantically linked to an abstraction hierarchy. Figure 4 shows an example of flight deck abstraction hierarchy semantically linked with state variables.

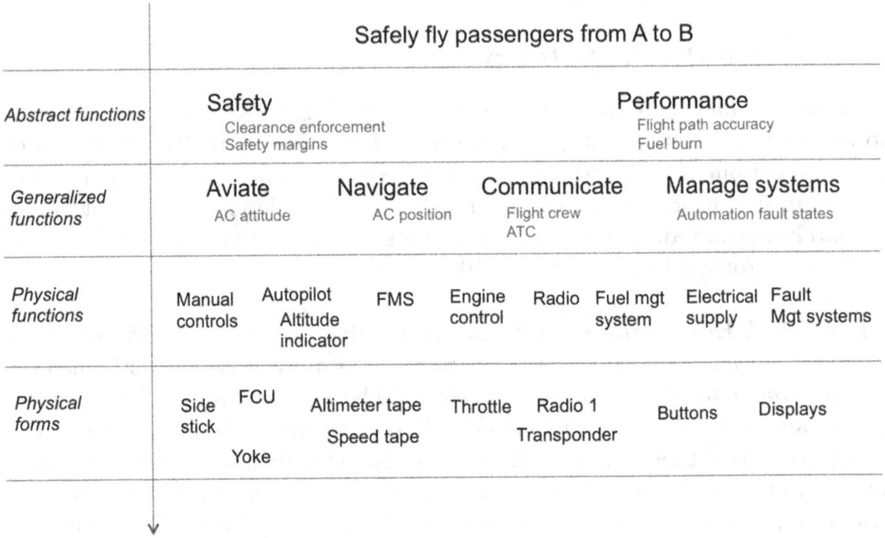

	Safely fly passengers from A to B			
Abstract functions	**Safety** Clearance enforcement Safety margins		**Performance** Flight path accuracy Fuel burn	
Generalized functions	**Aviate** AC attitude	**Navigate** AC position	**Communicate** Flight crew ATC	**Manage systems** Automation fault states
Physical functions	Manual controls Autopilot Altitude indicator FMS		Engine control Radio Fuel mgt system	Electrical supply Fault Mgt systems
Physical forms	Side stick FCU Yoke Altimeter tape Speed tape		Throttle Radio 1 Transponder	Buttons Displays

Fig. 4. Simplified abstraction hierarchy of a airliner flight deck, with examples of semantic links to the work domain state space.

6   Conclusion

The objectives of this work were to lay down some semantics and pragmatics of cognitive engineering methods as guidelines for the implementation of an integrated cockpit design and evaluation framework. The resulting platform yields the following promising conclusions.

Integration Time is Drastically Reduced. The proposed decentralized test bench enables much quicker integration of new subsystems, virtual reality engines, physiological sensors and human factors analysis modules. The system can be deployed in different configurations, ranging from mobile setups with inertial head tracking and web-browser 3D rendering to rooms equipped with high-accuracy optical head, finger tracking and high-fidelity rendering in head-mounted displays or VR caves.

Integrated Testing of New Subsystems can be Achieved with Early Prototypes. New prototypes of subsystems can be integrated and semantically linked to human factors models very easily. For instance, any HTML5 display prototype or Matlab flight control algorithm can interact with the full flight simulation and benefit from the same analysis capabilities.

Analysis of Human-In-The-Loop Experiments is Substantially Less Tenuous. Every interaction between the pilot and the cockpit is recorded and can be operationally replayed and analyzed offline, greatly simplifying the task of Human Factors experts. Therefore, a plurality of HFE methods can be operationalized. Pilot studies conducted with a preliminary version of this framework can be seen in [13].

The modularity of this tool is already leveraged through the adoption of new projects ranging from the evaluation of novel flight system management concepts to testing augmented reality head-worn displays for pilots. We believe new domains of applications and other Human Factors methods can easily benefit from this work.

7   Future Work

As mentioned in Sect. 3.2, HTAs can be used either in a descriptive or normative manner. Ongoing work is focusing of enabling robust semi-automated HTA generation from pilot experiments. Moreover, capturing expert knowledge into HTA models can also be used for agent modeling purposes or as a basis for intelligent support systems. It is also planned to enhance the existing system with eye-tracking pattern analysis and voice-detection features to allow for more extensive analysis including cognitive tasks.

Acknowledgements. This project has received funding from the European Union's Seventh Framework Programme for research, technological development and demonstration under grand agreement No. 605550.

References

1. Annett, J.: Hierarchical task analysis. In: Hollnagel, E. (ed.) Handbook of Cognitive Task Design, pp. 17–35. Lawrence Erlbaum Associates, Hillsdale (2003)
2. Booher, H.R.: Handbook of Human Systems Integration, vol. 23. Wiley, New York (2003)
3. Dul, J., Bruder, R., Buckle, P., Carayon, P., Falzon, P., Marras, W.S., Wilson, J.R., van der Doelen, B.: A strategy for human factors/ergonomics: developing the discipline and profession. Ergonomics 55(4), 377–395 (2012)
4. Hajdukiewicz, J.R., Vicente, K.J.: A theoretical note on the relationship between work domain analysis and task analysis. Theor. Issues Ergon. Sci. 5(6), 527–538 (2004)
5. Hollnagel, E., Woods, D.D.: Cognitive systems engineering: new wine in new bottles. Int. J. Man Mach. Stud. 18(6), 583–600 (1983)
6. Jenkins, D., Stanton, N., Walker, G., Salmon, P., Young, M.: Creating interoperability between the hierarchical task analysis and the cognitive work analysis tools. Report from the Human Factors Integration Defence Technology Centre, UK (2006)
7. Kelly, B.D.: Flight deck design and integration for commercial air transports. In: Harris, D. (ed.) Human Factors for Civil Flight Deck Design, pp. 3–31. Ashgate, Aldershot (2004)

8. Laminar Research: X-plane 10 datarefs (2014). www.xsquawkbox.net/xpsdk/docs/DataRefs.html

9. Lind, M.: Making sense of the abstraction hierarchy in the power plant domain. Cogn. Technol. Work **5**(2), 67–81 (2003)

10. Mamessier, S., Dreyer, D., Oberhauser, M.: Calibration of online situation awareness assessment systems using virtual reality. In: Duffy, V.G. (ed.) DHM 2014. LNCS, vol. 8529, pp. 124–135. Springer, Heidelberg (2014)

11. Mavor, A.S., Pew, R.W., et al.: Human-System Integration in the System Development Process: A New Look. National Academies Press, Washington (2007)

12. Miller, C.A., Vicente, K.J.: Comparison of display requirements generated via hierarchical task and abstraction-decomposition space analysis techniques. Int. J. Cogn. Ergon. **5**(3), 335–355 (2001)

13. Oberhauser, M., Dreyer, D., Mamessier, S., Conrad, T., Bandow, D., Hillebrand, A.: Bridging the gap between desktop research and full flight simulators for human factors research (accepted paper). In: Harris, D. (ed.) EPCE 2015. LNCS, vol. 9174. Springer, Heidelberg (2015)

14. Quigley, M., Faust, J., Foote, T., Leibs, J.: Ros: an open-source robot operating system. ICRA Workshop Open Source Softw. **3**, 5 (2009)

15. Vicente, K.J.: Ecological interface design: progress and challenges. Hum. Factors J. Hum. Factors Ergon. Soci. **44**(1), 62–78 (2002)

16. Vicente, K.: Cognitive Work Analysis: Toward Safe, Productive, and Healthy Computer-Based Work. Lawrence Erlbaum, Mahwa (1999)

Single-Variable Scenario Analysis of Vehicle-Pedestrian Potential Crash Based on Video Analysis Results of Large-Scale Naturalistic Driving Data

Renran Tian[1(✉)], Lingxi Li[1], Kai Yang[1], Feng Jiang[1], Yaobin Chen[1], and Rini Sherony[2]

[1] Transportation Active Safety Institute, Department of Electrical and Computer Engineering, Indiana University-Purdue University, Indianapolis, USA
{rtian,LL7,kaiyang,fejiang,ychen}@iupui.edu
[2] Collaborative Safety Research Center,
Toyota Motor Engineering and Manufacturing North America Inc.,
Erlanger, USA
rini.sherony@tema.toyota.com

Abstract. Vehicle-pedestrian crashes are big concerns in transportation safety, and it is important to study the vehicle-pedestrian crash scenarios in order to facilitate the development and evaluation of pedestrian crash mitigation systems. Many researchers have tried to investigate the pedestrian crash scenarios relying on crash databases or pedestrian behavior prediction models, both of which have some limitations like limited generalizability of the results, missing of important information, biased results. In this study, we propose to study the potential crash scenarios as one surrogate targets of the actual pedestrian crash scenarios. Extended from several previous studies, one single-variable scenario analysis is completed based on the video analysis results of one large-scale naturalistic driving data collection focusing on recording pedestrian behaviors in all kinds of situations. Through calculating potential conflict rates and applying chi-square tests for around 40 attributes from 12 scenario variables individually, this study has found out that number of pedestrians, pedestrian moving speed, pedestrian moving direction, vehicle moving direction, road type, road location, and existence of road separator/median are all important scenario variables for potential pedestrian-vehicle crashes.

Keywords: Naturalistic driving data collection · Pedestrian crash · Potential crash scenarios · Video analysis · Pedestrian behavior modeling

1 Introduction

Pedestrian safety is always a big concern in traffic safety, and pedestrian crashes are associated with a large number of injuries and fatalities every year. In the United States, the number for pedestrian fatalities has kept increasing in the past several years. In 2011, there are approximately 4,432 pedestrians killed which account for 14 percent of all traffic fatalities, and 69,000 pedestrian injured [1]. The fatality number has increased

© Springer International Publishing Switzerland 2015
V.G. Duffy (Ed.): DHM 2015, Part II, LNCS 9185, pp. 295–304, 2015.
DOI: 10.1007/978-3-319-21070-4_30

7 % to 4,743 in the following year of 2012 [2]. In order to alleviate the situation, more and more vehicle safety systems for pedestrian detection and pedestrian crash mitigation have been developed and installed in the modern vehicles to improve the effectiveness of vehicular active safety functions [3]. As summarized in the literature [4], it is important to understand pedestrian behaviors as well as the most common vehicle-pedestrian crash scenarios for developing and evaluating these pedestrian crash mitigation systems, and typically the researchers have been following three routes in studying the scenario variables: (1) relying on crash database, (2) constructing pedestrian behavior prediction models, or (3) relying on the large-scale naturalistic driving data collection.

Towards using the crash database, researchers have tried to use real crash data to aid the development of pedestrian detection systems [7], and to generate test scenarios and key variables for pedestrian mitigation system evaluation [8, 9]. As pointed out in [4], although using crash data can guarantee the generated crash scenarios representing real crash situations in various road types, these scenarios usually miss some important details and contain biased information. Towards the second route listed above, many published studies are focusing on systematically predicting pedestrian behaviors under different traffic conditions and modeling general vehicle-pedestrian crash scenarios [10–14]. These mathematical models are clearly good solutions to provide convenient and detailed pedestrian behavior information. However, researchers have also criticized that most of the current pedestrian behavior prediction models are focusing on specified traffic scenarios with limited capability to generalize the prediction results to overall road environment [4, 14].

To overcome the limitations of crash databases and pedestrian behavior prediction models, some efforts are made towards studying pedestrian-vehicle crashes using naturalistic driving data in the Transportation Active Safety Institute (TASI), Indiana University – Purdue University Indianapolis. Based on one large-scale naturalistic driving data collection focusing on pedestrian behaviors, researchers have tried to study single pedestrian behavior variable of walking step frequency [5], estimate the pedestrian/vehicle encountering risks in various traffic scenarios [4], and provide preliminary results of pedestrian behavior analysis as well as pedestrian-vehicle crash scenarios [6]. Based on the literature [15], it is reasonable in majority of cases to use near-miss events or potential conflict events for crash scenario construction. Thus, the authors have briefly discussed the potential conflict definitions, potential conflict cases achieving process, and the vehicle-pedestrian crash scenarios based on the potential conflict rates in different situations [6]. However, the discussions in [6] have some limitations:

- As one preliminary study, the dataset used for analysis is neither complete nor accurate;
- Several important factors are missing during the data analysis;
- There is no statistical analysis performed to test the significance of each factor.

Thus, in this study, we will extend the results described in [6] with using the whole dataset of the large-scale naturalistic driving data collection after reducing errors, including more variables in the analysis, and apply statistical analyses to test each factor.

2 TASI 110-Car Naturalistic Driving Study

From 2012 to 2013, the Transportation Active Safety Institute at the Indiana University – Purdue University Indianapolis has completed one large-scale naturalistic driving data collection focusing on understanding pedestrians' behavior during pre-crash and crash scenarios. A total of 110 cars with subject drivers were recruited around the city of Indianapolis starting from spring, 2012. Since the recruitments, every driver's driving data for the following one year were continuously recorded. The recorded data mainly include three parts that are synchronized during the whole data collection period:

1. Forward-view video data: relying on one video camera installed on the windshield of every data collection vehicle facing forward, high-definition video data were continuously recorded when the vehicle is moving representing the driver's view during all the time.
2. Vehicle GPS coordinates: relying on the GPS receiver installed in each vehicle, the longitude and latitude coordinates of the vehicle were recorded all the time when the subject was driving.
3. Vehicle acceleration data: relying on the accelerometer (g-sensor) installed in each vehicle, the vehicle accelerations in x-y-z directions were continuously retrieved and recorded at the rate of 10 Hz when the subject was driving.

After the one-year of data collection, a total of approximately 90 TBs of driving video data for over 1.44 million driving miles accumulatively across all the 110 subjects were recorded, with corresponding vehicle GPS coordinates and vehicle acceleration data also synchronized and recorded in the database. Upon the construction of the database, several steps of data analyses have been completed. Because the main purpose of the research focuses on pedestrian behaviors, one automatic pedestrian detection algorithm has been firstly applied on the collected video data to locate every scene with pedestrian(s). After manually checking all the pedestrian scenes detected automatically by the image-processing based algorithm to remove errors, no-interest scenes, and duplicated cases, short video clips were created towards each confirmed pedestrian scene. Then manual video analysis has been applied to the video clips by a group of trained data reductionists using several programs to detect potential conflict cases, to study pedestrian and driver behaviors, and to assign different scenario variables.

For more detailed information about the data acquisition apparatus, the constructed database structure, and the video analysis results, please refers to the literatures [4–6]. For more detailed information about the image processing based automatic pedestrian detection, please also refer to the literatures [16, 17].

3 Methodology for Data Analysis

The main purpose of this study is to investigate the potential conflict scenarios between the vehicles and pedestrians in the naturalistic road environment. As described above, literatures have shown that the potential conflict cases can represent the situations of the real crashes very well [15], and thus the potential conflict scenarios found in this research can also be used as the surrogate scenarios for real vehicle-pedestrian accidents to some extents.

The definition of potential conflict in this study follows the literature [4]: potential conflict case refers to the case that "real crash between the vehicle and pedestrian(s) will occur if neither the driver nor the pedestrian(s) changes the moving speed/moving direction, or the trajectories of the vehicle and the pedestrian are adjacent to each other during the time period which results in the movement responses from the driver and/or the pedestrian(s) to avoid the contact, although the responses may not be necessary."

As part of the overall data analysis process, the above Fig. 1 shows the whole picture of the project, as well as the data analysis process of the current study, marked as single-variable scenario analysis in the yellow solid line. The parts with green dashed line in the chart show the previous work, and the parts with red dotted line show the future work. Starting from the collected naturalistic driving video data, multiple steps of data analyses have been performed to achieve the potential conflict and non-potential conflict cases with values for different scenario variables assigned to each of them via intensive video analysis. Two types of scenario analysis can be done towards these processed cases including:

- Single-variable analysis: each scenario variable is treated to be independent, and the effect of individual scenario variable on the potential conflict rates can be calculated.
- Multi-variable analysis: multiple scenario variables are studied together, and compressive potential conflict scenarios can be achieved based on the calculated potential conflict rates.

Both of these two types of scenario analyses rely on the calculation of potential conflict rates using the following formula (1). When applying the formula (1) for single-variable analysis, certain scenario refers to one particular value for one individual scenario variable; however when applying the formula for multi-variable analysis, certain scenario refers to the combined values for a group of scenario variables.

$$Potential\ Conflict\ Rate = \frac{Number\ of\ Potential\ Conflict\ Cases\ Under\ Certain\ Scenario}{Total\ Number\ of\ Cases\ Under\ Certain\ Scenario}$$

$$(1)$$

Due to the scope of this paper, only single-variable analysis will be discussed, and the multi-variable analysis as well as matching the potential crash scenarios into accident scenarios will be completed in the future works. The following Table 1 shows the 12 variables studied for the single-variable analysis in this work, with descriptions about the variable definitions and the corresponding attributes. These variables include mainly pedestrian-related variables, road-related variables, vehicle-related variables, and environment-related variables. For each of the variable, we will calculate the potential conflict rate for every attribute respectively, and then apply chi-square analysis to test the significances of the effects.

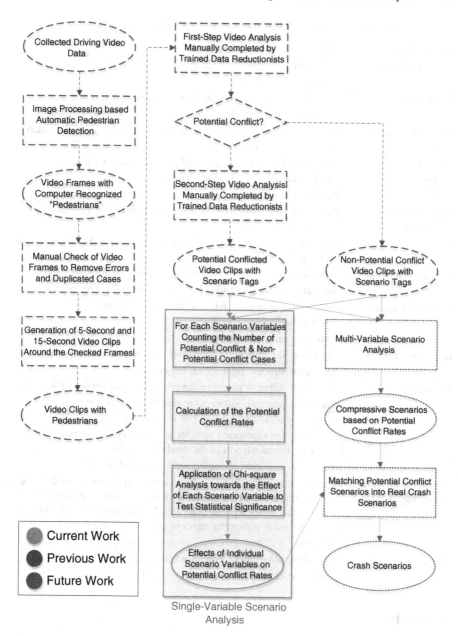

Fig. 1. Single-variable scenario analysis process as a part of the overall data analysis

Table 1. Scenario variables for the single-variable analysis

Variable name	Variable definition and attributes
Adult number	Definition: the number of adult pedestrians in the scene.
	Attributes: 0, 1, 2, >=3
Child number	Definition: the number of child pedestrians in the scene.
	Attributes: 0, 1, 2, >=3
Pedestrian walking speed	Definition: estimated pedestrian walking speed based on the video.
	Attributes: slow, normal, fast
Driving environment	Definition: brief categorization of the environment where the pedestrian-vehicle encounter happens.
	Attributes: rural, urban
Pedestrian moving direction	Definition: pedestrian moving trajectory during the pedestrian-vehicle encounter.
	Attributes: cross the road, with traffic (along the road), against traffic (along the road)
Pedestrian moving status	Definition: Movement status of the pedestrian before the event.
	Attributes: walking, standing, running, entering/exiting vehicle
Vehicle movement	Definition: moving behavior of the vehicle during the pedestrian-vehicle encounter
	Attributes: stop, straight, left turn, right turn, lane changing
Road alignment	Definition: the direction of the road that the vehicle is moving in.
	Attributes: straight, right curve, left curve
Road type	Definition: different places of the road where the encounter happens.
	Attributes: junction, intersection, mid-block cross walk
Road shoulder	Definition: shoulder is the part of a trafficway contiguous with the roadway for emergency use, for accommodation stopped vehicles, and for lateral support of the roadway structure.
	Attributes: with road shoulder, without road shoulder
Road median/separator	Definition: separator is the area of a trafficway between parallel roads separating travel in the same direction or separating a frontage road from other roads. Median is an area of a divided trafficway between parallel roads separating travel in opposite directions.
	Attributes: with road median/separator, without road median/separator
Driving condition	Definition: atmospheric conditions during the encounter.
	Attributes: clear, cloudy, rain, snow, backlight

4 Results

The above Fig. 2 shows the potential conflict rates calculated for all the attributes from the scenario variables, and the corresponding chi-square analysis results for each scenario variable individually. First of all, it looks like for both the number of adult pedestrians and the number of child pedestrians, their effects on potential conflict rate are significant. The charts show that with either more adult pedestrians or more child pedestrians, the chances to have potential conflict rates increase.

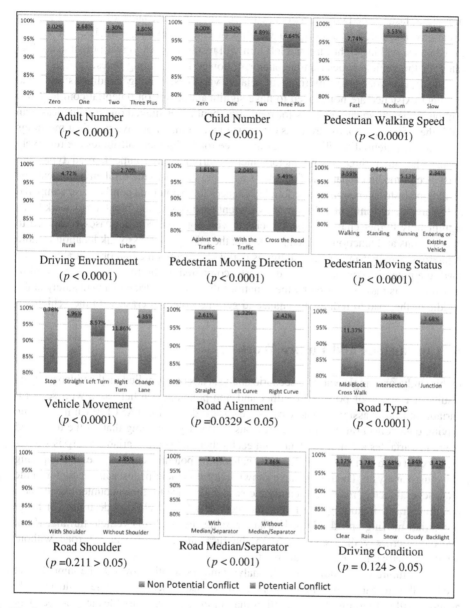

Fig. 2. Potential conflict rates and chi-square analysis results for different attributes from the 12 scenario variables individually.

Then for the pedestrian and vehicle behavior related variables, all of the pedestrian moving direction, pedestrian walking speed, pedestrian moving status, and vehicle movement are significant factors affecting the potential conflict rates. If looking into them separately, it looks like crossing the road is more dangerous to have potential conflict compared to walking along the road. Also when the pedestrian is running or moving in faster speed will be associated with much higher chance of potential conflict situations, compared to slow speed walking or entering/exiting vehicles. For vehicle movements, making right turn and left turn will result in much higher potential conflict rates for the vehicle-pedestrian encounter, followed by changing lanes.

Finally for road and environment related variables, driving conditions and road shoulder existence are not proved to have significant effects on potential conflict rates. Although the chi-square analysis for road alignment has achieved one p-value less than 0.05, the effects are not as strong as other factors, and may not have practical meanings since all the potential conflict rates for the three road alignment attributes are relatively small. The other three strong factors include driving environment, road type, and existence of median/separator. The results have shown that in the rural environment, the vehicle-pedestrian encounter has doubled chances to be potential conflict case compared to the urban environment. Also among different road types, mid-block cross walk has a significantly higher chance to be associated with potential conflict cases compared to intersections and junctions, which means that the mid-block cross walk location is more dangerous. Another interesting finding is that when there is median or separator for the road, the potential conflict chance decreases compared to the road without such infrastructure. This may be caused by the situations that the pedestrian can wait safely at the middle of the road to reduce the chance to get into potential crash with the vehicles.

5   Conclusions and Future Work

In this study, one single-variable scenario analysis has been applied on the video analysis results of a series of potential conflict and non-potential conflict cases with scenario variable attributes assigned. These cases are retrieved from the TASI 110-car naturalistic driving data collection through the previous works. By assuming that all the interested scenario variables are independent from each other, the single-variable analysis studies the effect of each variable individually by calculating potential conflict rates and applying chi-square analysis. The results have shown that for vehicle-pedestrian encounter in the road, several factors may significantly increase the chance for the encounter to become a potential crash, including: (1) larger numbers of adult or child pedestrian, (2) faster pedestrian moving speed, (3) pedestrian crossing the road, (4) vehicle turning, (5) at mid-block cross walk location, (6) in the rural area, and (7) at the road without separator/median in the mid of the road.

As for future work, multi-variable analysis may be applied towards the same dataset used in this research to achieve more comprehensive scenarios. The multi-variable analysis will not require the assumption that all the scenario variables are independent from each other, and will consider the combinations of different variables/attributes together as one scenario for the analysis. Also, the current results are only regards to potential crash scenarios between the vehicles and pedestrians in the road. It will be beneficial to match the scenarios with real crash scenarios to achieve more applicable results.

Acknowledgment. The authors would like to thank Toyota's Collaborative Safety Research Center for funding this project.

References

1. National Highway Traffic Safety Administration: Traffic safety factors – pedestrians (2011 Data). NHTSA report DOT HS 811 748 (2013)
2. National Highway Traffic Safety Administration: Traffic safety factors – pedestrians (2012 Data). NHTSA report DOT HS 811 999 (2014)
3. Gandhi, T., Trivedi, M.M.: Pedestrian protection systems: issues, survey, and challenges. IEEE Trans. Intell. Transp. Syst. **8**(3), 413–430 (2007)
4. Tian, R., Li, L., Yang, K., Chien, S., Chen, Y., Sherony, R.: Estimation of the vehicle-pedestrian encounter/conflict risk on the road based on TASI 110-car naturalistic driving data collection. In: IEEE Intelligent Vehicles Symposium, 8–11 June 2014, Dearborn, MI, pp. 623–629 (2014)
5. Tian, R., Du, E.Y., Yang, K., Jiang, P., Jiang, F., Chen, Y., Sherony, R., Takahashi, H.: Pilot study on pedestrian step frequency in naturalistic driving environment. In: IEEE Intelligent Vehicles Symposium (IV), 23–26 June 2013, Gold Coast, Australia (2013)
6. Du, E.Y., Yang, K., Jiang, F., Jiang, P., Tian, R., Luzetski, M., Chen, Y.: Pedestrian behavior analysis using 110-car naturalistic driving data in USA. In: 23rd International Technical Conference on the Enhanced Safety of Vehicles (ESV), 27–30 May 2013, Seoul, Korea (2013)
7. Kong, C., Nei, J., Yang, J.: A study on pedestrian detection models based on real accident data from IVAC database in Changsha of China. In: 2012 Third International Conference on Digital Manufacturing & Automation, July 2012, Guilin, China, pp. 136–139 (2012)
8. Good, D.H., Abrahams, R.L.: Vehicle speeds for pedestrian pre-crash system test scenarios based on US data. In: 2014 IEEE 17th International Conference on Intelligent Transportation Systems (ITSC), 8–11 October 2014, Qingdao, China (2014)
9. Coelingh, E., Eidehall, A., Bengtsson, M.: Collision warning with full auto brake and pedestrian detection – a practical example of automatic emergency braking. In: IEEE International Conference on Intelligent Transportation Systems, September 2010, Madeira Island, Portugal, pp. 155–160 (2010)
10. Wakim, C.F., Capperon, S., Oksman, J.: Design of pedestrian detection systems for the prediction of car-to-pedestrian accidents. In: IEEE International Conference on Intelligent Transportation Systems, October 2004, Washington, D.C., USA, pp. 696–701 (2004)
11. Flach, A., David, K.: A physical analysis of an accident scenario between cars and pedestrians. In: the IEEE 70th Vehicular Technology Conference, pp. 1–5, Anchorage, AK (2009)
12. Zhuang, X., Wu, C.: Modeling pedestrian crossing paths at unmarked roadways. IEEE Trans. Intell. Transp. Syst. **14**(3), 1438–1448 (2013)
13. Chen, Z., Ngai, D.C.K., Yung, N.H.C.: Pedestrian behavior prediction based on motion patterns for vehicle-to-pedestrian collision avoidance. In: IEEE International Conference on Intelligent Transportation Systems, October 2008, Beijing, China, pp. 316–321 (2008)
14. Papadimitriou, E., Yannis, G., Golias, J.: A critical assessment of pedestrian behavior models. Transp. Res. Part F Traffic Psychol. Behav. **12**(3), 242–255 (2009)
15. National Highway Traffic Safety Administration: Evaluating the relationship between near-crashes and crashes: can near-crashes serve as a surrogate safety metric for crashes? NHTSA report DOT HS 811 382 (2010)

16. Yang, K., Du, E.Y., Delp, E.J., Jiang, P., Chen, Y., Sherony, R., Takahashi, H.: A new approach of visual clutter analysis for pedestrian detection. In: 16th International IEEE Conference on Intelligent Transportation Systems, 6–9 October 2013, The Hague, The Netherlands (2013)
17. Yang, K., Du, E.Y., Delp, E.J., Jiang, P., Jiang, F., Chen, Y., Sherony, R., Takahashi, H.: An Extreme Learning Machine-based Pedestrian Detection Method. In: IEEE Intelligent Vehicles Symposium (IV), 23–26 June 213, Gold Coast, Australia (2013)

Driving-Behavior Monitoring Using an Unmanned Aircraft System (UAS)

Calvin Zheng, Andreina Breton, Wajeeh Iqbal, Ibaad Sadiq,
Elsayed Elsayed, and Kang Li[✉]

Rutgers University, Piscataway, NJ 08854, USA
kl419@rci.rutgers.edu

Abstract. Abnormal driving behaviors have been used as cues to identify Driving While Intoxicated (DWI) drivers and prevent DWI-related accidents. Currently law enforcement officials rely on visual observation for detecting such behaviors and identify potentially DWI drivers. This approach however, is subject to human error and limited to vehicles in a very small region. To overcome these limitations, we propose to use an Unmanned Aircraft System (UAS) for driving-behavior monitoring to prevent accidents and promote highway safety. A high-resolution optical camera on the UAS is used to capture the movement of vehicles on the road. The vehicle trajectories are tracked from the captured videos to identify the misbehaviors. This allows for a quicker response time from law enforcement. A risk model is also developed for analyzing the severity of misbehaviors while providing a basis to take appropriate action to reduce dangerous activity. We developed a UAS prototype to showcase the practicality and effectiveness of the proposed system. It was demonstrated that dangerous driving activity on highways can be effectively and timely detected and analyzed.

Keywords: Driving behavior monitoring · Unmanned aircraft system · Driving safety

1 Introduction

Abnormal driving behaviors can be used as cues to identify Driving While Intoxicated (DWI) drivers and prevent DWI-related accidents. These cues have been commonly used by law enforcement officials to identify potentially drunk drivers as summarized by the National Highway Traffic Safety Administration (NHTSA) in 2010 [1]. This approach however, is subject to human error and is theoretically limited to only observing a few vehicles at a time due to human mental processing limitations.

Recently, unmanned systems in the traffic monitoring, management, and control are starting to take center stage [2, 3]. They can be launched and deployed within a very short period time and offer bird's eye view over a large area with a relatively low cost. Exploratory UAS based systems are currently being developed and tested in the United States. For example, Ohio State University [2] utilizes UAS to fly over a freeway for observing flows, speeds, densities, off ramp weaving, and vehicle trajectories. At the

© Springer International Publishing Switzerland 2015
V.G. Duffy (Ed.): DHM 2015, Part II, LNCS 9185, pp. 305–312, 2015.
DOI: 10.1007/978-3-319-21070-4_31

University of Florida [4], UAS has been used for traffic monitoring applications. Image processing and speed calculation algorithms were used to identify vehicles and respective vehicle speeds. These projects suggested that UAS based monitoring systems have the potential for traffic and driving-behavior monitoring due to their mobility, large field of view, and capability of following vehicles [2]. However, the existing studies are limited in the overall focus of traffic monitoring. They focus on offline post processing analysis of traffic systems; lacking online image processing systems that detect and track vehicles for real time analysis. To overcome these limitations, this paper proposes a framework for utilization of Unmanned Aircraft System (UAS) technology for driving-behavior monitoring to prevent accidents and promote highway safety. The framework for the proposed application contains methodology for real time vehicle tracking using image processing, vehicle risk modeling through statistical analysis, prototype development, and testing. The real time tracking shows immediate autonomous detection of vehicles, thus allowing for a quicker response time from law enforcement and the risk modeling helps analyze the severity of misbehaviors while providing a basis to take appropriate action to reduce dangerous activity. A designed prototype as well as testing applications is highlighted to show the practicality and effectiveness of the proposed system. The proposed system allows for driving misbehaviors to be detected and analyzed simultaneously thus accounting for more dangerous driving activity on highways and ultimately making roadways safer.

2   System Design

Our framework for driving behavior monitoring and risk analysis using the Unmanned Aircraft System is shown in Fig. 1. First, users select roads for monitoring based on their experience. A flight plan is then generated and uploaded wirelessly to the UAS. The UAS system then automatically takes off and maneuvers according to the flight plan to hover and observe traffic. While hovering, live videos are transmitted wirelessly by the UAS to the ground station computer for near real-time processing. Based on the metrics calculated from the processing, the system identifies the observed behaviors and calculates driving-behavior related risks. In this study, we have developed a heavy duty multi-rotor drone system based on Pixhawk [5] and a vision-based risk analysis system to monitor traffic, identify driving-behavior, and calculate associated risks. The details of the process are discussed below.

2.1   Flight Path Planning

Our system allows the user to choose specific roads to conduct traffic observations for risk analyses. Once roads are selected, the road-path coordinates are uploaded to Mission Planner, which is an open source ground control software. Mission Planner then routes the flight plan into the PixHawk board. The Pixhawk controls the rotors on the UAV during flight for maneuvering along the pitch, yaw, and roll axes. After uploading the flight plan to the drone, the user can send the command to launch the UAV and execute the mission via the Mission Planner interface.

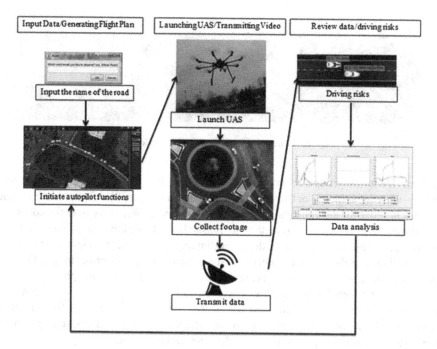

Fig. 1. The proposed framework for driving behavior monitoring

2.2 Driving Behavior Monitoring

Upon reaching the hover point, the UAS transmits video via an onboard video transmitter device. The ground station computer receives analog video via a video receiver, and converts it into a digital format that interfaces with the software for video processing algorithms to be applied and for subsequent key metrics to be calculated. The ultimate objective of calculating behavior risk is based on the observation and quantification of eight different possible driving behaviors.

To observe the eight potential misbehaviors, six key metrics must be identified and quantified. These key metrics consist of Vehicle ID, Speed, Forward Distance, Lane Change, Lane Change Time, and Acceleration. The calculation of these key metrics is therefore the first task of the computer vision algorithm to ultimately determine and quantify the misbehaviors.

The calculation of the six key metrics requires both the position of a vehicle relative to a lane line along with the identification and tracking of a vehicle across video frames. The first priority is to determine the locations of the lanes and lane lines in the video feed, and identify a vehicle identification tracking approach as shown in Fig. 2.

In order to identify these key metrics, the computer vision algorithm, developed and executed in MATLAB, must first detect and track vehicles as well as detect the lanes via user selection. Motion-Based Multiple Object Tracking algorithm by MathWorks, Inc. assists with the detection of vehicles. Essentially, background subtraction is used in which stationary pixels are identified as background and moving pixels are identified as foreground by the system. After separation of the foreground from the background, a blob

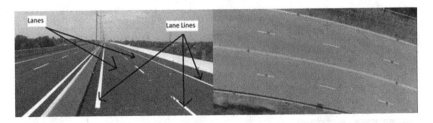

Fig. 2. Lanes and lane lines and land detection

analyzer identifies groups of connected pixels which likely correspond to moving objects –moving vehicles, in this case. Additionally, a Kalman filter is used to track the vehicles in order for the vehicles' key metrics to be stored effectively over the course of multiple frames. For lane detection, the user is asked to indicate how many lanes are being observed, and based on the answer, the algorithm requests the user to select two points on each lane line. The algorithm then checks to see if the user made any errors in selections by converting the initial frame to binary, and assessing if the user selected points on white portions of the image (because highway lane lines are mostly white). The algorithm then draws lines on the initial frame and stores the equations of the lines for reference throughout the algorithm processing. With vehicles detected and tracked and lanes identified, the algorithm proceeds to calculate the six key metrics.

2.3   Calculate Driving-Behavior Risk

Behavior decision making and risk quantification can be done by assessing the six key metrics identified for each vehicle in the software component of the system design. Each behavior has an associated risk value which is dependent on how severe the observed behavior is. Therefore, behavior identification is broken down into two categories: decision making and risk analysis. Decision making identifies the behavior being exhibited as normal or irregular, and risk analysis quantifies the severity of each behavior as well as combination of behaviors that may be observed.

To classify driving behaviors as irregular, classification thresholds were established through research. Previous traffic/driving studies and governmental surveys were studied to find the normal and extreme parameters of each key metric other than vehicle ID. Each metric value is collected for the time and distance the observed vehicle is in the view of the UAS.

In this driving behavior monitoring system, risk is defined as the probability of collision due to the different metric parameters that the observed vehicle is demonstrating. Different vehicle speeds, lane change patterns and forward distance maintaining behaviors yield different risk probabilities. These observable behaviors have associated risk values which correspond to four of the six key metrics: vehicle speed, number of lane changes, lane change time and forward distance. The overall risk is defined as weighted probability function of the four the individual risk values. The weights of each individual risk component are selected based on frequency and relevancy to collision risk. For example, tailgating and speeding behaviors are more commonly observed in traffic then weaving behavior therefore they have more weight on the overall risk. Using the weighted probability equation, a detailed and comprehensive collision risk score can be assigned to vehicles in observance. The total risk function is described as follows.

$$TotalRisk = \sum R_i w_i$$

$$\sum (w_i \ldots w_j) = 1$$

$$R_i = Risk_i$$

$$w_i = weight_i$$

Two statistical methods are used to calculate the four components of the total risk function. However in general, individual risks are calculated by comparing the observed metric values to values exhibited during normal driving behavior. This means that vehicles displaying normal driving behavior will exhibit metric values that are similar to the normal values with some small variation. For example, vehicles exhibiting normal speed behavior will have metric values that are comparable to the speed limit but not identical. Therefore the normal speed metric can be assumed to be normally distributed with a mean value, the speed limit, and a standard deviation. The same assumptions are made for the forward distance, lane change and lane change time normal behavior metrics.

Risk associated with the speed, number of lane changes, and lane change time also utilizes the distributions of the metric values but is calculated using a different set of equations. The risk associated with these metrics compares how different the observed metric values are to the normal values. If the observed metric distribution matches that of normal behavior, the associated risk is zero. However if the observed metric value distribution differs from the normal, risk is calculated using the Bhattacharyya bound and Bhattacharyya coefficient equations. The Bhattacharyya-bound, DB, and coefficient, Bc, equations are described below. The Bhattacharya coefficient Bc calculates the probability of overlap – thus the risk is calculated as 1-Bc.

$$D_B(1,2) = \frac{1}{4} \ln \left(\frac{1}{4} \left(\frac{\sigma_1^2}{\sigma_2^2} + \frac{\sigma_2^2}{\sigma_1^2} + 2 \right) \right) + \frac{1}{4} \left(\frac{(\mu_1 - \mu_2)^2}{\sigma_1^2 + \sigma_2^2} \right)$$

$$B_c = \frac{1}{e^{D_B}}$$

$$Risk = 1 - B_c$$

$$\mu_1, \mu_2 = MetricMeanValues$$

$$\sigma_1, \sigma_2 = MetricStdvValues$$

Both methods of risk calculation are used to calculate the four different risk values corresponding to the six key metrics each vehicle will display. Because certain vehicle behaviors can indicate high risk by themselves, the total risk function is utilized conditionally so that if one of the components of the function yields an extreme value, the overall risk is indicated as high in the user interface. Immediate action will be taken when high risk behaviors are observed. This can ultimately help identify more dangerous drivers that the current monitoring methods do not account for.

The mathematical quantification of collision risk and identification of irregular behaviors is interfaced into the computer vision system using Matlab computer software. Each vehicle behavior as well as the individual and overall risk scores is embedded as separate functions into the software of the overall system. To implement the risk functions, standard deviations and mean values for normal behaviors as well as misbehaviors need to be approximated. The approximations are inferred values based off of initial research. They have been tuned to give a reasonable and reliable risk quantification. Future testing and research can be conducted to find more accurate approximations for these values.

3   Validation

To demonstrate the code and designs created, physical hardware for a UAS and ground station were designed to test the system. There are many components to the UAS, all which need to work in order for the overall system to function. The basic hardware components include the frame, motors, batteries, RC controller, Pixhawk autopilot, power distribution board, gimbal, and camera. Figure 3 shows the basic structure of the overall hardware system.

The overall frame, along with the rotors, and landing gear is produced with carbon fiber material. This frame was chosen due to its high durable, lightweight characteristics. Along with a 16000 mAh Lipo battery, the UAS is able to sustain 20–40 min of flight, depending on weight and intensity of flight. The eight motors can produce a max thrust of 3.4 kg each, which allow the UAS to carry an additional 20 kg of weight on top of the current hardware it is equipped with. The UAS stands 2 ft. tall and is 4.5 ft. in diameter.

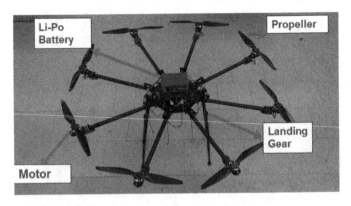

Fig. 3. Our heavy duty UAS prototype

The vision system attached to the belly of the UAS consists of a Tarot gimbal with a GoPro Hero3 camera. A gimbal is used to ensure the video is relatively stable for processing, and the Hero3 will provide good quality video. The video can be recorded using the micro SD card in the GoPro camera or it can be transmitted through the live video transmission: FlySight FPV monitor system. Coupled with a Hauppauge 610 USB-Live 2 Analog Video Digitizer and Video Capture Device, the UAS is able to send live video to a ground station control for immediate processing.

Testing the prototype by having it hover over highways presents many risks and is restricted by FAA and local law enforcement regulations. Therefore two different testing methods were used: remote control (RC) car behavior simulations, and controlled environment road tests.

Using RC cars instead of real cars to simulate the eight driving misbehaviors proved safer and still effective. Each RC car was 1/24 in scale of a real car. A test track with multiple lanes on a similar scale was also created to mimic the real environment as close as possible. All scales were taken into account to ensure calculations made were correct. Figure 4 below is a sample video capture of the RC track during a test run.

Speeds were scaled for realism. These tests were conducted indoors, with the overhead camera fixed, tested independently from the UAV unit.

To mitigate risks, controlled environments on university grounds were tested on at altitudes compliant with FAA regulation. The designed prototype was tested for flight routing, live video transmission as well as real time processing capabilities. The UAS footage was also recorded and tested in post-processing. Figure 5 shows two sets of test footages that were processed.

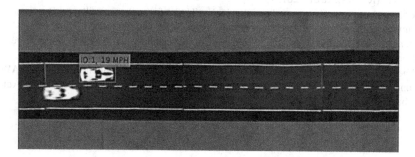

Fig. 4. Test track video capture

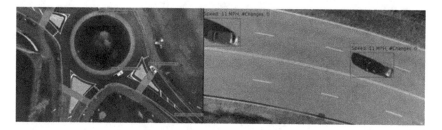

Fig. 5. Speed detection algorithms tested on real footage

4   Conclusion

This paper presents the first UAS-based system to autonomously monitor traffic, automatically identify multiple potentially dangerous driving behaviors and simultaneously calculate risk scores in real time. The work proposes a data-driven, objective approach to traffic law enforcement, and can be used to identify drivers with a high probability of DWI, or drivers that exhibit irregular and potentially dangerous behavior; both of which are potential dangers to surrounding drivers. Unmanned Aircraft Systems are a frontier for breakthrough applications, and this system is a unique attempt to utilize the advantages of a UAS-based system for traffic monitoring – namely, the ability to maneuver at any desired altitude to monitor multiple vehicles, the ability to follow a high-risk vehicle for further monitoring, and the ability to easily review and analyze data. The system proposed is a promising venture, and a gateway to further research in the area, with the hope of reducing traffic accidents and ultimately saving lives.

References

1. NHTSA, U.S: The Visual Detection of DWI Motorists. US Department of Transportation, Washington, DC (2012)
2. Kanistras, K., Martins, G., Rutherford, M.J., Valavanis, K.P.: A survey of unmanned aerial vehicles (UAVs) for traffic monitoring. In: International Conference on Unmanned Aircraft Systems (ICUAS), IEEE (2013)
3. Puri, A.: A survey of unmanned aerial vehicles (UAV) for traffic surveillance. Department of Computer Science and Engineering, University of South Florida (2005)
4. Zhang, L.-Y., Peng, Z.-R., Li, L., Wang, H.: Road boundary estimation to improve vehicle detection and tracking in UAV video. J. Cent. S. Univ. **21**(12), 4732–4741 (2014)
5. Meier, L., Tanskanen, P., Heng, L., Lee, G.H., Fraundorfer, F., Pollefeys, M.: PIXHAWK: a micro aerial vehicle design for autonomous flight using onboard computer vision. Auton. Rob. **33**(1–2), 21–39 (2012)

Human Modeling in Medicine and Surgery

A Mobile Application for the Stereoacuity Test

Silvia Bonfanti, Angelo Gargantini, and Andrea Vitali[✉]

Department of Economics and Technology Management,
Information Technology and Production, University of Bergamo (BG), Dalmine, Italy
{silvia.bonfanti,angelo.gargantini,andrea.vitali1}@unibg.it
http://3d4amb.unibg.it

Abstract. The research paper concerns the development of a new mobile application emulating measurements of stereoacuity using Google Cardboard. Stereoacuity test is based on binocular vision that is the skill of human beings and most animals to recreate depth sense in visual scene. Google Cardboard is a very low cost device permitting to recreate depth sense of images showed on the screen of a smartphone. Proposed solution exploits Google Cardboard to recreate and manage depth sense through our mobile application that has been developed for Android devices. First, we describe the research context as well as the aim of our research project. Then, we introduce the concept of stereopsis and technology used for emulating stereoacuity test. Finally, we portray preliminary tests made so far and achieved results are discussed.

1 Introduction

Having two eyes, as human beings and most animals, located at different lateral positions on the head allows binocular vision. It permits for two slightly different images to be created that provide a means of depth perception. Through high-level cognitive processing, the human brain uses binocular vision cues to determine depth in the visual scene. This particular brain skill is defined as *stereopsis*. Some pathologies, such as blindness in one eye and strabismus, cause a total or partial stereopsis absence. The examination of stereopsis ability can be evaluated by measuring stereoscopic acuity. Stereoscopic acuity, also named stereoacuity, is the smallest detectable depth difference that can be seen by someone with normal two eyes and brain functions.

Testing the total or partial loss of stereovision can lead to the detection of visual diseases like *amblyopia*. Amblyopia, otherwise known as 'lazy eye', is reduced visual acuity that results in poor or indistinct vision in one eye that is otherwise physically normal. This condition affects 2–3 % of the population, which equates to conservatively around 10 million people under the age of 8 years worldwide [10]. Children who are not successfully treated when still young (generally before the age of 7) will become amblyopic adults. The projected lifetime risk of vision loss for an individual with amblyopia is estimated around at least 1–2 % [8]. For these reasons, screening for amblyopia in early childhood is

This work is partially supported by GenData 2020, a MIUR PRIN project.

V.G. Duffy (Ed.): DHM 2015, Part II, LNCS 9185, pp. 315–326, 2015.
DOI: 10.1007/978-3-319-21070-4_32

done in many countries to ensure that affected children are detected and treated within the critical period. The main goal is to help children to achieve a level of vision in their amblyopic eye that would be useful should they lose vision in their non-amblyopic eye later in life.

However, classical stereoacuity tests suffer from many problems: they are rather costly and can be performed only be specialized personnel. Moreover, they have a low level of sensitivity (vision problems may go undetected) and low specificity (vision problems are falsely reported).

For these reasons, we have been working on developing an efficient and affordable test, using for instance personal computer and 3D systems as in [5–7,9]. The system we proposed in [7] is still rather demanding in terms of equipment: it requires a desktop PC and a 3D vision system. In this paper we present a system which is composed by a simple Cardboard that realizes the 3D vision and whose cost is negligible as well as an Android smartphone together with a simple app described in this work. The proposed solution promises to be simple to use, affordable and accurate.

Firstly, we present some background regarding the use of 3D technologies for the virtual reality and we explain how the Google Cardboard works. Then, we introduce the stereoscopic acuity and some classical tests normally used to measure it. Furthermore, we introduce the mobile application we have developed in order to perform the stereoacuity test. Finally, several preliminary results are presented and future works are discussed.

2 Scientific Background

In recent years, many researchers have been involved in research works to design IT solutions to make more realistic the experiences with a 3D virtual environment. The aim is to permit users to interact with virtual environments as done in the real world. To this end, a set of devices has been developed to emulate the most important human senses which are tact and eyesight. There are devices that permit tracking of hands/fingers, such as Leap Motion device, Duo3D and Intel Gesture Camera (Fig. 1). These devices allow interacting with 3D objects using hands/fingers gestures and thin objects held in the hand. These solutions can be used for medical applications such as design for lower limb prosthesis [3]. 3D systems have been developed to recreate depth sense on PC screen using LCD shutter glasses, such as NVIDIA® 3D Vision^{TM} system and Google Cardboard. 3D systems work in this way: they provide the two eyes with two different images of the same scene with a slightly offset viewing angles which correspond to the different viewpoints of our left and right eye. This vision produces an illusion of real depth of the scene and it is the basis of the *3D virtual reality*.

On computers and TVs, this effect is generally obtained by requiring the users to wear a special type of glasses. These are capable of separating the images display on the screen into two separate scenes for the left and right eye. The NVIDIA® 3D Vision^{TM} technology, which we used in another similar work [7], requires a standard personal computer with a NVIDIA graphic card

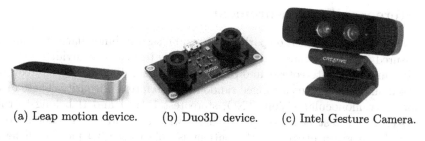

(a) Leap motion device.   (b) Duo3D device.   (c) Intel Gesture Camera.

Fig. 1. Devices to track hands/fingers.

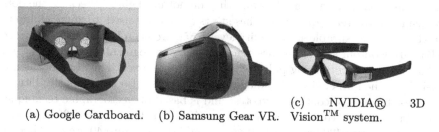

(a) Google Cardboard.   (b) Samsung Gear VR.   (c)   NVIDIA®   3D Vision™ system.

Fig. 2. 3D devices.

(also entry level NVIDIA graphic boards work) and a monitor 3D Vision ready with a refresh rate of 120 Mhz as well as a NVIDA 3D glasses. The monitor alternates images for the two eyes and the glasses are able to synchronize the display of the images shown by the monitor through the synchronized emitter to be connected either PC USB port or directly to the graphic board. The Google Cardboard (Fig. 2a) is a simple box with two lenses that used in combination with a smartphone, constitutes a simple yet powerful virtual reality viewer. The smartphone must be inserted in the box and the user looks inside in order to see the images displayed by the phone. It permits a stereo vision by sending two different images to the two eyes. It works with different smartphones and can be easily adapted to be used by children. The system proposed in this paper also works with other types of VR viewers (e.g., Samsung Gear VR).

In this research work, we pay attention to 3D technology, which allows to simply emulate stereo vision. 3D vision systems are used to study different eye diseases, such as amblyopia and measurement of stereoacuity [1,2,4]. Regarding the use of virtual reality, IBit and our reserach project, i.e. 3D4Amb, are two research groups who are exploiting NVidia 3D technology in order to treat amblyopia disease in young children. Moreover, 3D4Amb has started to develop a set of PC-desktop applications to emulate different visual tests that are usually performed by oculists and orthoptists, such as Lang test and stereoacuity test. In this paper, we present a new application to emulate stereo acuty test exploiting Google Cardboard to create depth sense through the use of an Android smartphone.

3 Stereoacuity Measurement

Stereoacuity is the smallest disparity that can be seen in binocular vision and it is measured in second of arc (arcsec). Stereoacuity tests can be divided into two groups: random dot stereotests and contour stereotests. Random dot stereotests are based on dots patterns arranged randomly with lateral disparity. These tests do not allow monocular vision. TNO, stereotest Lang I and II belong to this group. TNO is a test based on set of sheets with red and green random dots. Using red and green eyeglasses the patient is able to see 3D pictures if he is healthy. This test measures stereoacuity level from 2000 arcsec to 15 arcsec. Lang I and II are based on random dots and they do not need glasses because the dots are displaced to create disparity. These tests are mostly used in young children, but the lower measurable stereoacuity level is 550 arcsec in Lang I and 200 arcsec in Lang II. Contour stereotests are made up by two recognizable images, stagger, and shown to patients using polarized or anaglyph glasses. This category is not sensitive as the former since the images are recognized also monocularly. Titmus stereotest belongs to contour stereotest and is based on vectographic technique. This test measures three levels of stereoacuity: high level around 3600 arcsec, medium level from 400 arcsec to 100 arcsec and low level upto 40 arcsec. There is a test that is a joint of random dot stereotests and contour stereotests, i.e., randot test. It is composed by two tables, the first is based on contour stereotest but background is replaced with dots. This technique prevents the monocular vision. Using this first table the measurable stereoacuity level is from 400 arcsec to 20 arcsec. The second table is based on random dots and it measures stereoacuity from 500 arcsec to 250 arcsec. All these tests can generate a false negative because they have the following disadvantages:

- Shown images are always the same, so the patients can memorize them and give right answers even if they do not see the right image.
- Children can be helped by parents or doctors, so the test is not truthful.

In order to reduce the number of false negative, we have devised the following policies:

- the shape is randomly chosen every time;
- the user that delivers the test has no clue about which shape is currently displayed.

Recently, a new stereoacuity test has been developed, i.e., 3DSAT [7]. This test has been carried out using PC with 3D capabilities and NVIDIA® 3D Vision™ technology. It is based on randot test and monocular vision is absent. During these tests, the images always change without a logical order and only the patient can see them. This increases the results truthfulness because no one can help the patients.

4 Stereoacuity Test App

The application we present in this paper is called "StereoAcuity Test" and it is developed for Android devices. The smartphone screen is split in two parts. Each

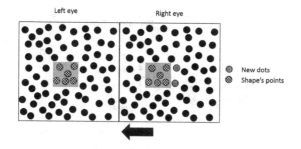

Fig. 3. Randot: principle of operation.

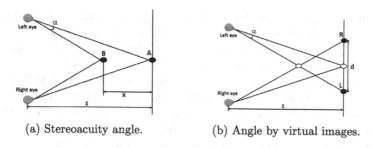

(a) Stereoacuity angle.   (b) Angle by virtual images.

Fig. 4. Howard-Dolman Stereoacuity angle and angle by virtual images

eye sees one set of dots: one for the left eye and one for the right eye. The left eye sees a random dot image, while the right one sees the same image except for the dots within the shape that must be guessed. The points inside the shape are horizontally shifted (leftward) by a desired number of pixel. The blank space to the right of the shape is replaced by other dots. Principle of operation is shown in Fig. 3.

4.1   Angle Measurement

Stereoscopic acuity, also named stereoacuity, is the smallest detectable depth difference that can be seen by someone with two eyes and normal brain functions. Its measure was introduced by Howard and Dolman who explained stereoacuity with a mathematical model as shown in Fig. 4a. The observer is shown a black peg (A in the figure) at a distance z. A second peg (B), in front of it, can be moved back and forth until it is just detectably nearer than the fixed one. Stereoacuity is this difference (x) between the two positions, converted into an angle of binocular disparity (α).

The same effect can be replicated by using a 3D virtual system (like the Cardboard) by creating two virtual points (R and L), each to be seen by one eye, translated by a distance d, as shown in Fig. 4b. The disparity distance d can be converted into the angle of disparity α in radiants by the following equation:

$$\alpha = \arctan \frac{d/2}{z}$$

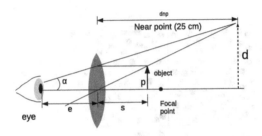

Fig. 5. Using a Cardboard.

To convert α into the usual unit of seconds of arc, a multiplicative constant is used. The use of angles permits to evaluate the perceived dimensions of objects according to distance of the observer from the same objects. The stereacuity of humans is excellent when its value is around 60 seconds of arc.

In our case, we have to take into account the presence of the Cardboard lens. The Cardboard is provided with a positive lens with a short focal length (large dioptric power) to enlarge the image on your retina, much like the corrective lens for hyperopia does. In this way the images displayed on the phone appear in focus although the phone is very close to the eyes. This positive lens is usually referred to as a magnifying glass or a simple magnifier. It forms an enlarged image that cna be see by the eye, typically taken as 0.25 m. Figure 5 illustrates how the Cardboard lenses work.

A simple magnifier is characterized by its magnification power, usually denoted as a number with a mult, like 2x. The magnification power is a measure of how much bigger the image appears with the magnifier than it does at the retina with the unaided eye. The calculation of the angle subtended by an object of height p shown on the screen at distance s from the lenses, is the following:

$$\alpha = \arctan\left(\frac{p}{s}d_{np}\frac{1}{2}\frac{1}{e + d_{np}}\right)$$

Given a disparity in terms of pixels, for which one can compute the dimension of the shown object p by considering the phone pixel density, the distance e of the eye from the lenses, the distance s of the phone from the lenses in the Cardboard, and the d_{np}, then the formula above permits to obtain the angle α.

Table 1 reports some configuration examples with selected smartphones and pixel disparities assuming a value for the eye distance of 5 mm. As shown in the table, the angle can vary from around 1500 to min 120/150 s of arc for the smartphones. The minimum angle is obtained by a disparity of 1 pixel. With higher pixel density screens, the test can reach smaller angles; for instance, with a new generation of screens capable of around 800 pixels per inch, the minimum angle will become around 78, which represents a typical excellent stereoacuity.

Table 1. Stereoacuity angle for smart-phones and disparity

SmartPhone	Screen size (")	pixels		ppi	1 pixel in mm	pixel disparity	angle (seconds)
		width	height				
Galaxy S5	5,1	1920	1080	431,9	0,059	1	156,5
						2	312,9
						5	782,3
						10	1564,6
LG G3	5,5	2560	1440	534,0	0,048	1	126,6
						2	253,1
						5	632,8
						10	1265,5
Meizu MX4 Pro	5,5	2560	1536	542,8	0,047	1	124,5
						2	249,0
						5	622,5
						10	1245,1
Samsung (planned, 2015)	5,1	3840	2160	863,9	0,029	1	78,2

4.2 How the Application Works

The activity proposed by the software is divided into two parts: training and test phases. They are accessible from the main screen of application shown in Fig. 6.

The **training** phase has been developed to make people understand how the test works and in which part of the screen they have to search the shape (Fig. 7a). The user has to force oneself to search the shape, but it is simplify since the figure has a different color compared to background. The patient can scroll shapes until he understands how use the application with Google Cardboard.

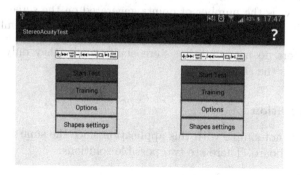

Fig. 6. Main screen

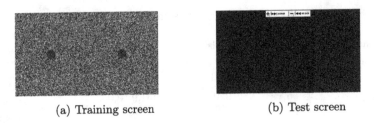

(a) Training screen   (b) Test screen

Fig. 7. Application screens

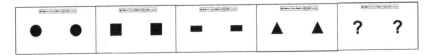

Fig. 8. Test answers.

After the training the user can start the **test**. The screen is split in two parts and it is overstuffed by points (Fig. 7b) inside which shapes are hidden.

The patient looks inside the Cardboard until he finds the 3D shape. After that, using the iteration devices, he chooses the shown image from a set of default forms (Fig. 8).

The user sees a different shape with a decreasing level of stereoacuity. Stereoacuity level depends on the number of pixels whose shape is horizontally shifted.The higher number of pixel, the higher the stereoacuity level and the stereoacuity angle are. He/she starts from the higher level and guesses the shape until he makes a mistake or guesses all levels. At this point of the test, he/she certifies a stereoacuity level and the stereoacuity angle.

Furthermore it is possible to change both difficulty of test and the shape settings from the main screen. The *"Shapes settings"* button allows users to set the figures dimensions. The bigger shapes are,the easier discover is them during the test. *"Select test level"* button contains options that entail level changing:

- Points dimension: is the dimension of the points generated on the screen. They are like 2 pixel per side as default.
- Points density: is the number of points generated on the screen to draw the shape and the background. Higher is this value greater is the number of points.

These parameters do not condition stereoacuity angle, they only increase the difficulty of guess the shapes.

4.3 User Iteration

User iteration is not simple with this application since the smartphone is inside the Google Cardboard. There are two possible solutions:

- Stereo headset buttons (Fig. 9a)
- Bluetooth stereo headset (Fig. 9b)

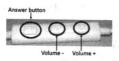

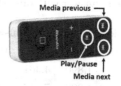

(a) Stereo headset.   (b) Bluetooth stereo headset.

Fig. 9. Instruments used by users.

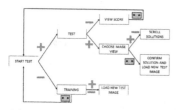 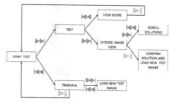

(a) Interaction cycle with stereo headset.

(b) Interaction cycle with bluetooth stereo headset.

Fig. 10. Interaction cycles using either normal or bluetooth stereo headset.

The stereo headset is composed by three buttons, i.e., plus (+) button, minus (−) button as well as answer button. The iteration diagram is shown in Fig. 10a. It is possible to choose test phase (using + button) or training phase (using − button) from the main screen. Inside the training phase, the patient can scroll all shapes using +/− buttons and return to main screen using answer button. During the test phase, the patient uses + button to enter in the choose answer procedure, he/she scrolls them using +/− buttons and confirms using answer button. During the test user can interrupt it pushing − button. At the end of the test the application displays the score and it is possible to close it using answer button.

It is possible also use a bluetooth stereo headset (Fig. 10b). These buttons substitute stereo headset buttons with the following relation:

- + button = media next button
- − button = media previous button
- answer button = play/pause button

5   Test Results

We performed some tests with the main aim of finding the best combination between points density and points dimension. Each test session is made up by seven levels and each level has different offset (number of leftward pixel). The user has to guess the shown shape. If the answer is right, then he carries on with the test until he reaches the first level, otherwise he finishes the test with

Table 2. Meantime to answer with different points dimension and points density $= 0.9$.

Points dimension	Meantime to answer [sec]					Meantime mean
	User 1	User 2	User 3	User 4	User 5	
1 pixel	1,890	4,461	4,066	6,018	3,597	4,006
2 pixel	1,896	7,717	2,905	2,793	2,697	3,602
3 pixel	2,059	14,496	2,714	3,113	3,174	5,111

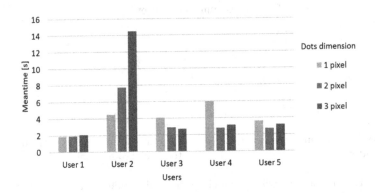

Fig. 11. Meantime to answer.

a certain certified level. We have carried out tests to five users (without visual diseases) with different point dimensions and different point densities. For each level we measured the time to guess and the mean of all values is reported in Table 2 (only for point density $= 0.9$ since the time to guess is lower). In the last column is computed the mean of all meantime for a certain point dimension. The lower value is obtained for point dimension equals to 2 pixel and this is set as default value in the application.

6   Future Works

At present, the iteration between user and application is made by stereo headset buttons or bluetooth stereo headset (see Sect. 4.3). Future work points to develop a twin application. The basic idea of this application is that the same application can be used by doctor and patient running on two different smartphones. Patient and doctor start the application on their smartphone and set the mode of operation. Doctor opens a listener port and waits until the patient smartphone sends a message. When the applications recognize each other the doctor can control the patient test without using stereo headset. At the end of the test, patient smartphone sends to the doctor test results and it saves all in a data base.

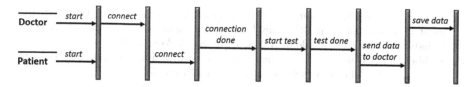

Fig. 12. Twin application.

7   Conclusions

We have presented an Android application calls "StereoAcuity Test" that emulates randot test using a smartphone and Google Cardboard. Our test procedure ensures the accuracy of the results because only the patient sees the smartphone screen. Stereoacuity angles are a bit higher than some standard test, but this is due to the pixel density of each smartphone. We have demonstrated if the pixel density increases, the stereoacuity angle decreases.

Future development will be done in order to control the test by another smartphone and thus, define additional test to collect other data.

References

1. Achtman, R.L., Green, C.S., Bavelier, D.: Video games as a tool to train visual skills. Restorative Neurol. Neurosci. **26**(4–5), 435–446 (2008)
2. Breyer, A., Jiang, X., Rütsche, A., Mojon, D.S.: A new 3D Monitor-Based random-dot stereotest for children. Invest. Ophthalmol. Vis. Sci. **47**(11), 4842 (2006)
3. Colombo, G., Facoetti, G., Rizzi, C., Vitali, A.: Socket virtual design based on low cost hand tracking and haptic devices. In Proceedings of the 12th ACM SIG-GRAPH International Conference on Virtual-Reality Continuum and Its Applications in Industry, VRCAI 2013, pp. 63–70. ACM, New York (2013)
4. de Bougrenet de la Tocnaye, J.L., Cochener, B., Ferragut, S., Iorgovan, D., Fattakhova, Y., Lamard, M.: Supervised stereo visual acuity. J. Disp. Technol. **8**(8), 472–478 (2012)
5. Facoetti, G., Gargantini, A., Vitali, A.: An environment for domestic supervised amblyopia treatment. In: Duffy, V.G. (ed.) DHM 2014. LNCS, vol. 8529, pp. 340–350. Springer, Heidelberg (2014)
6. Gargantini, A., Bana, M., Fabiani, F.: Using 3D for rebalancing the visual system of amblyopic children. In: 2011 International Conference on Virtual Rehabilitation (ICVR), pp. 1–7, June 2011
7. Gargantini, A., Facoetti, G., Vitali, A.: A random dot stereoacuity test based on 3d technology. In: Proceedings of the 8th International Conference on Pervasive Computing Technologies for Healthcare, PervasiveHealth 2014, pp. 358–361, ICST (Institute for Computer Sciences, Social-Informatics and Telecommunications Engineering), Brussels (2014)
8. Rahi, J.S., Logan, S., Timms, C., Russell-Eggitt, I., Taylor, D.: Risk, causes, and outcomes of visual impairment after loss of vision in the non-amblyopic eye: a population-based study. The Lancet **360**(9333), 597–602 (2002)

9. Vitali, A., Facoetti, G., Gargantini, A.: An environment for contrast-based treatment of amblyopia using 3D technology. In: International Conference on Virtual Rehabilitation 2013, Philadelphia, PA, USA, 26–29 August 2013
10. Webber, A.L., Wood, J.: Amblyopia: prevalence, natural history, functional effects and treatment. Clin. Exp. Optom. 88(6), 365–375 (2005)

Automatic Identification of Below-Knee Residuum Anatomical Zones

Giorgio Colombo[1], Giancarlo Facoetti[2(✉)], Caterina Rizzi[3],
and Andrea Vitali[3]

[1] Department of Mechanical Engineering, Polytechnic of Milan, Milan, Italy
giorgio.colombo@polimi.it
[2] BigFlo S.R.L. (BG), Dalmine, Italy
giancarlo.facoetti@bigflo.it
[3] Department of Management, Information and Production Engineering,
University of Bergamo (BG), Dalmine, Italy
{caterina.rizzi,andrea.vitalil}@unibg.it

Abstract. The research work presented in this paper is part of an innovative framework that deals with the design process of lower limb prostheses. The quality of the whole prosthesis depends on the comfort of the socket, which realizes the interface between the patient body and the mechanical parts. We developed a CAD system, named Socket Modelling Assistant that guides the user during the design of the socket, exploiting domain knowledge and design rules. In this work we present a preliminary study that describes the implementation of a software module able to automatically identify the critical areas of the residuum to adequately modify the socket model and reach the optimal shape. Once the critical areas have been identified, the Socket Modelling Assistant can apply proper geometry modifications, in order to create the load and off-load zones for a good pressure distribution over the residual limb.

Keywords: Lower limb prosthesis · Neural network · Prostheses socket · CAD

1 Introduction

This research work is part of a project whose aim is to develop an innovative design framework for lower limb prosthesis design [1]. In particular, we refer to the module, named Socket Modelling Assistant (SMA), that permits to replicate the traditional, handmade socket design process and embeds design rules and orthopedic technicians' knowledge.

One of the most important steps of socket design is the identification of critical zones that have to be modified to ensure the realization of a comfortable socket. In fact, due to the anatomical characteristic of the residuum, the appropriate pressure over specific areas is crucial to provide the right fit and prevent pain. We focused the attention on below knee residuum, which is characterized by the following critical zones (Fig. 1): patella, medial tibia, patella tendon, lateral femoral condyle, crest of the tibia, tibia terminal, head of the fibula, lateral tibia, popliteal depression and fibula end [2, 3].

© Springer International Publishing Switzerland 2015
V.G. Duffy (Ed.): DHM 2015, Part II, LNCS 9185, pp. 327–335, 2015.
DOI: 10.1007/978-3-319-21070-4_33

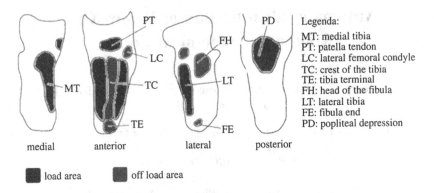

medial   anterior   lateral   posterior

Legenda:
MT: medial tibia
PT: patella tendon
LC: lateral femoral condyle
TC: crest of the tibia
TE: tibia terminal
FH: head of the fibula
LT: lateral tibia
FE: fibula end
PD: popliteal depression

load area   off load area

Fig. 1. Anatomical zones of below knee residuum

Therefore, our main goal has been to develop a module to be integrated within SMA that can identify automatically the mentioned areas. Once they are recognized, SMA can perform the corresponding deformations, in automatic way, in order to create the so-called load and off-load socket zones [1].

The implemented recognition algorithm exploits a supervised learning approach [4], in which a number of artificial neural networks have been trained for the recognition of a specific anatomical zone. In particular, we focused on the automatic recognition of the patella, the patella tendon and the tibia terminal.

2 Training Dataset

Artificial Neural Networks (ANN) are machine learning computational models inspired by the biological brain and are useful to approximate complex functions that depend on a large number of inputs [5].

In supervised learning, a given ANN is trained with a samples dataset consisting of a number of input data and their corresponding correct output (usually computed/labeled by human experts). After the training, the ANN is able to estimate the transfer function between input and output and to generalize its response.

In our specific case, the training dataset is composed by a set of 3D models of the residuum (STL files), on which prosthetists have labeled the anatomical zones. In particular, in order to carry out preliminary tests, experts marked the patella center, the patella tendon and the tibia terminal (Fig. 2).

One of the drawbacks of supervised learning is that it requires a good number of training data. This is an important issue because, due the nature of our context, it's quite challenging to get a sufficient amount of lower limb residuum models.

We used 5 models as seed shapes to generate new residuum models. Performing random scaling and skewing geometric operations on each seed have generated a new set of models. The generated models are synthetic but are useful to train a recognition system, because they respect the proportions and shapes of a real human limb.

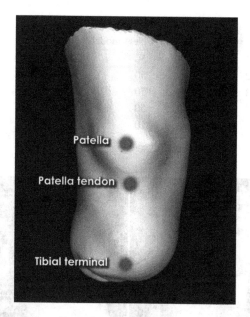

Fig. 2. Patella, patella tendon and tibia terminal labelled by experts

Generation of new synthetic data by performing geometric transformations on real data is a useful technique used, for example, in optical character recognition systems [8].

Models generated from the first 4 seeds have been used to train the neural network (with a proportion of 80 % for the training set, and 20 % for the validation set), while the models generated from the fifth seed have been used to test the performance of the networks on new cases. The models distribution for the training, validation and test dataset is represented in Table 1.

3 Features Extraction

In order to convert the 3D geometric data in an input suitable for a neural network, we created a grid of 20 × 25 points in correspondence of the frontal view. Then, we casted a ray, perpendicular to the grid (Z axis), from each of the grid points, computing its intersection on the residuum model surface (Fig. 3).

The distances between the grid points plane and the intersection points represent our features, thus the neural network input is represented by a matrix of 20 × 25 distances. Distances have been normalized in −1.0 /+ 1.0 range (Fig. 4).

In a given dataset sample, a correct output corresponds to each input. In this case, the output consists of the position of the marker that experts assigned during the manual labeling phase.

Specifically, the output is represented as X and Y coordinates on the grid, in correspondence of the centre of a given anatomical zone (assuming the Z axis perpendicular to the grid).

Table 1. Dataset creation

Seed	Scaling	Skewing	New models	Dataset
Seed 1	x, y, z	x, y, z	50	*Training set* 80 %
Seed 2	x, y, z	x, y, z	50	*Validation set* 20 %
Seed 3	x, y, z	x, y, z	50	
Seed 4	x, y, z	x, y, z	50	
Seed 5	x, y, z	x, y, z	10	Test set

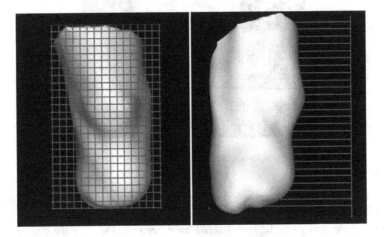

Fig. 3. Ray casting on 3d model surface

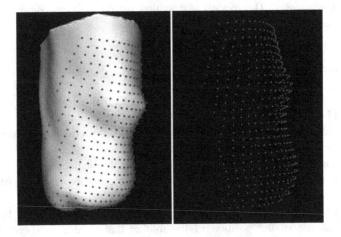

Fig. 4. Features extraction

4   Neural Network Architecture and Training

The neural network type used to recognize the anatomical zones is a feed-forward network [6] composed by three layers (Fig. 5). The input layer has 500 neurons (20 × 25 grid points), the hidden layer has 30 neurons and the output layer has 2 neurons, that represent the X and Y coordinates of the centre of the anatomical zone to be identified.

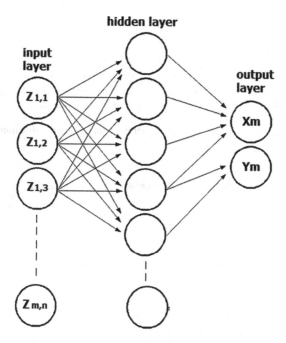

Fig. 5. Neural network architecture

The activation function of the hidden neurons is the sigmoid function, while the input and output neurons have a linear activation function. The network has been trained with the back propagation algorithm [6].

For each anatomical area to be identified (i.e., patella, patella tendon and tibia terminal), a specific neural network has been trained with the back propagation algorithm.

Since the size of the training dataset was small, to avoid over-fitting we adopted the early-stopping approach. We trained several networks, and stopped the training when the validation error started to increase [7]. Then we kept the network with the minimum validation error. Figures 6, 7, 8 show the training error and validation error during the training epochs, respectively for the patella, patella tendon and tibia terminal networks.

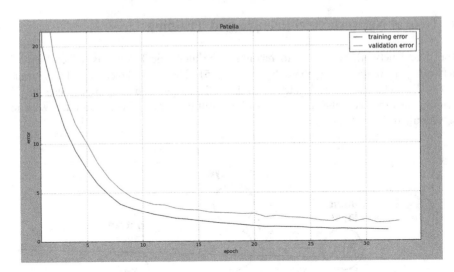

Fig. 6. Neural network for patella area recognition training and validation error graph

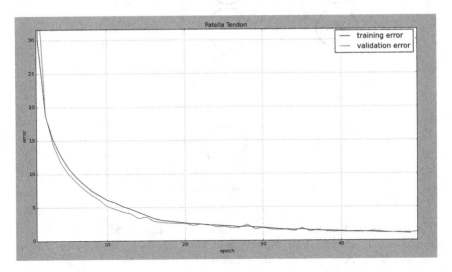

Fig. 7. Neural network for patella tendon area recognition training and validation error graph

5 Results

Once the neural networks have been trained, we tested their performance on models generated from the seed 5. The test error represents the distance between a given anatomical area marker position, estimated by the network, and the real marker position, labeled by human experts. Table 2 shows the test errors, that is a measure of the performance of the networks. The test dataset has been composed by 10 models labeled by human experts, and not used during the training.

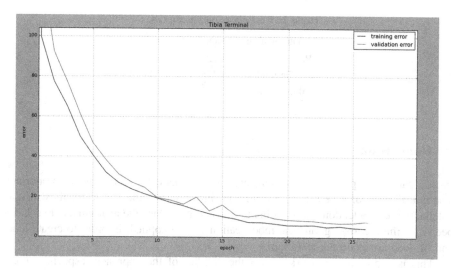

Fig. 8. Neural network for tibia terminal area recognition training and validation error graph

Figure 9 shows the markers positions of each anatomical area: red markers have been placed by humans experts, while green markers have been placed on the coordinates estimated by the neural networks. Considering the application field, the performances of the neural network are good, as stated by domain experts.

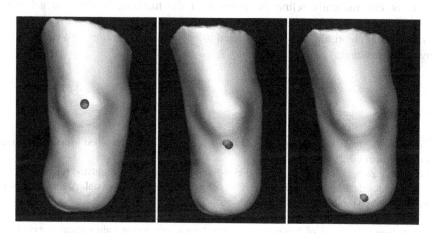

Fig. 9. Patella, patella tendon and tibia terminal predicted (green) and real (red) marker positions.

Table 2. Test errors on unseen cases

Anatomical area	Mean test error
Patella	3.127
Patella tendon	3.345
Tibia terminal	2.137

6 Conclusions

In this paper, we presented a system able to automatically recognize the important anatomical areas of a below-knee residuum. In particular, the system deals with the patella, the patella tendon and the tibia terminal zones. Once the anatomical areas have been identified, correct geometric modification can be applied, in order to create load and off-load zones on the residuum.

This is a preliminary work to test the validity of the approach, especially concerning the extraction of the learning features from the 3D model of the residual limb.

Results are promising, however we have planned to develop further the learning model, expanding the training dataset and adding new learning features. It could be worth to investigate the generation of new synthetic data by merging operation: creating a new residuum model by blending the geometries of two existing models.

Once the recognition system will be embedded into the Socket Modelling Assistant, new learning data can be acquired. During the design process, the system identifies and marks the anatomical areas position; the user can accept the automatic choice of the system, or can manually refine the position of the markers, in order to get more precision. This operation generates a new sample learning data, useful to train further the recognition algorithm. We have planned to apply the recognition algorithm also to above knee residuum.

References

1. Colombo, G., Facoetti, G., Rizzi, C.: A digital patient for computer-aided prosthesis design. Interface Focus 3(2), 20120082 (2013)
2. Lee, W.C., Zhang, M., Mak, A.F.: Regional differences in pain threshold and tolerance of the transtibial residual limb: including the effects of age and interface material. Arch. Phys. Med. Rehabil. **86**, 641–649 (2005)
3. Wu, C.L., Chang, C.H., Hsu, A.T., Lin, C.C., Chen, S.I., Chang, G.L.: A proposal for the pre-evaluation protocol of below-knee socket design: integration pain tolerance with finite element analysis. J. Chin. Inst. Eng. **26**, 853–860 (2003)
4. Haykin, S.: Neural Networks and Learning Machines – Pearson. Prentice Hall, Upper Saddle River (2008)
5. Bishop, C.M.: Pattern Recognition and Machine Learning - Information Science and Statistics. Springer, Heidelberg (2006)
6. Fine, L.T.: Feedforward Neural Network Methodology - Information Science and Statistics. Springer, Heidelber (1999)

7. Zhang, T., Yu, B.: Boosting with early stopping: convergence and consistency. Ann. Stat. **33** (4), 2005 (2013)
8. Coates, A., Carpenter, B., Case, C., Satheesh, S., Suresh, B., Wang, T., Wu, D.J., Ng, A.Y.: Text detection and character recognition in scene images with unsupervised feature learning. In: 12th International Conference on Document Analysis and Recognition, 440–445 (2013)

Visual Comparison of 3D Medical Image Segmentation Algorithms Based on Statistical Shape Models

Alexander Geurts, Georgios Sakas, Arjan Kuijper[✉], Meike Becker,
and Tatiana von Landesberger

TU Darmstadt, Darmstadt, Germany
arjan.kuijper@igd.fraunhofer.de

Abstract. 3D medical image segmentation is needed for diagnosis and treatment. As manual segmentation is very costly, automatic segmentation algorithms are needed. For finding best algorithms, several algorithms need to be evaluated on a set of organ instances. This is currently difficult due to dataset size and complexity.

In this paper, we present a novel method for comparison and evaluation of several algorithms that automatically segment 3D medical images. It combines algorithmic data analysis with interactive data visualization. A clustering algorithm identifies regions of common quality across the segmented data set for each algorithm. The comparison identifies best algorithms per region. Interactive views show the algorithm quality.

We applied our approach to a real-world cochlea dataset, which was segmented with several algorithms. Our approach allowed segmentation experts to compare algorithms on regional level and to identify best algorithms per region.

Keywords: Medical image segmentation · Visual comparison · Visual analytics · Segmentation evaluation

1 Introduction

In medicine, detection of organs and organic structures in 3D images is an important task during diagnosis and treatment. Manual segmentation is very expensive as it requires expertise and is very time consuming. Therefore, automatic segmentation algorithms are needed. The development of these algorithms is difficult due to image resolution, image noisiness and organ variation.

The development of segmentation algorithms requires a detailed evaluation of segmentation results and their comparison across various algorithms or algorithm variations. The evaluation of segmentation quality often takes a set of ground truth images (i.e., expert segmentations) and compares them to automatic segmentation results. Then the segmentation quality is compared across algorithms (see Fig. 1). It is important to identify where algorithms systematically fail and to identify best performing algorithms. This needs to be done on

© Springer International Publishing Switzerland 2015
V.G. Duffy (Ed.): DHM 2015, Part II, LNCS 9185, pp. 336–344, 2015.
DOI: 10.1007/978-3-319-21070-4_34

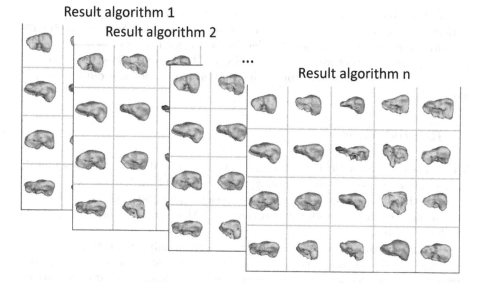

Fig. 1. Example problem: Need for comparing results of several algorithms, each segmenting multiple organ instances.

a local (per point or region) level, as some algorithms may perform better on one part of the organ (e.g., top) and at the same time fail in other region (e.g. bottom). In these cases, an expert needs to know in which part of the organ, which algorithm is better suitable and how well it performs.

Current algorithm evaluation and comparison methods support the algorithm assessment only in a limited way. Often one remains at a global evaluation, which means that for each mesh a score is created that evaluates the algorithmic segmentation. Since this only gives a rough overview of the quality, it does not allow to see whether the algorithms have problems in specific regions. In contrary, local evaluation methods require a detailed inspection of each individual result, without the possibility to compare the results algorithmically. A visual comparison is in this case limited to several instances due to screen size. Moreover, it is time consuming and subjective. So there is a need for new methods allowing for detailed comparison of segmentation quality for several algorithms.

In this paper, we present a novel method for comparison and evaluation of several 3D medical image segmentation algorithms. Our approach combines algorithmic data analysis with interactive data visualization. A specialized clustering algorithm identifies regions of common quality across data set for each algorithm. It thereby allows for comparison of segmentation algorithms on local level. The comparison identifies best algorithms per region. Interactive views show the algorithm quality on various levels of detail. We concentrate on algorithms based on statistical shape models. These algorithms are widely used owing to their robustness and good quality.

We applied our approach to a real-world cochlea dataset which was segmented with several algorithms. Our approach allowed segmentation experts to compare algorithms on regional level and to identify best algorithms per region.

The paper is structured as follows. Section 2 presents related work in this area. Section 3 details on our approach. Section 5 concludes and outlines future work.

2   Related Work

We review related publications. We first review standard 3D segmentation evaluation methods used by medical imaging experts. We then focus on visual analytics methods for the evaluation of SSM-based segmentations. As our focus is not on segmentation, we note that review of SSM based segmentation methods can be found in [9].

Currently, medical image segmentation experts mainly employ two evaluation methods: algorithmic and visual. Algorithmic evaluation relies on a set of global metrics [8]. The metrics include Average Surface Distance, Maximum Surface Distance or Dice Coefficient. The global measures provide only a coarse information on segmentation quality. They do not discriminate between two results which are badly segmented in different regions (e.g., top and bottom of an organ). Visual inspection concerns individual instances shown in 2D and 3D views such as ITK Snap (www.itksnap.org) or overlay the two meshes using transparency, color-coded local distances between vertices, e.g., [2,5,6,13]. These views are very detailed, but require manual inspection of all instances individually. They are not suitable for several algorithms with multiple instances.

Visual Analysis for evaluation of segmentation results and comparative visualization is the topic of several recent works reviewed in [7,11]. Some works analyze the effect of segmentation parameters on the result (e.g., [14]). They do not compare several instances for several algorithm results, which is in the focus of our work. Other works focus on shape variability analysis [3,10] without evaluating segmentation quality.

Cardness et al. [4] presented an interactive visualization system for analyzing segmentation quality. Local segmentation quality view is combined with the calculation of global segmentation quality metrics. This approach, however, does not enable quality comparison. Von Landesberger et al. [11] presented several methods for supporting creation and evaluation of medical image segmentation algorithms. They show the distribution of global quality values across the dataset and select instances with high or low quality values for detailed inspection. This visualization compares only global quality values, it does not allow for comparing local quality across the dataset. A recent publication [15] analyzes the progress of segmentation quality during the segmentation process. It analyzes segmentation quality for one organ in each segmentation iteration. This approach allows for analyzing and comparing local quality improvements, but is constrained to one sample. Quality comparison across samples or across algorithms is not possible.

3 Approach

We have developed an approach that consists of two types of visual evaluations supported by quality-based clustering (see Fig. 2):

- *Global Quality View*: The data are globally evaluated in a scatterplot matrix. It offers pairwise comparison of algorithm's quality pro instance. It is based on global quality criteria. It also allows to select instances for further regional analysis.
- *Quality-based Clustering*: Quality-based clustering identifies regions with systematic quality characteristics across the test dataset. Clusters are then further processed in order to determine algorithms with best output quality pro region.
- *Regional Quality View*: Regional view shows the clustering and algorithm quality results.

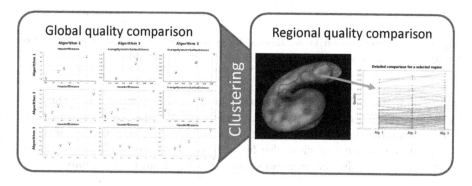

Fig. 2. Overview of our approach. First, global quality comparison in a scatterplot matrix is performed. It offers pairwise comparison of algorithm quality pro instance. Then clustering is performed to identify regions with systematic quality characteristics and to identify best algorithms pro region. The results are explored in regional view.

Global Quality View: This view allows the user to compare algorithms for each instance in a set (see Fig. 2). It provides first insights into an overall algorithm quality and enables their comparison across algorithms. The comparison employs common global segmentation quality measures, such as Hausdorff Distance and Average Surface distance [8].

Global Quality view shows a scatterplot matrix of algorithm comparisons (see Fig. 3). The scatterplots show pairwise comparisons of algorithms, where the points are segmentation instances (see Fig. 4). Upper right matrix shows comparison for average surface distance, lower left triangle shows results for Hausdorff distance. Diagonal shows result quality pro algorithm. In each scatterplot, each X-axis represents quality of one algorithm, and the Y axis shows the

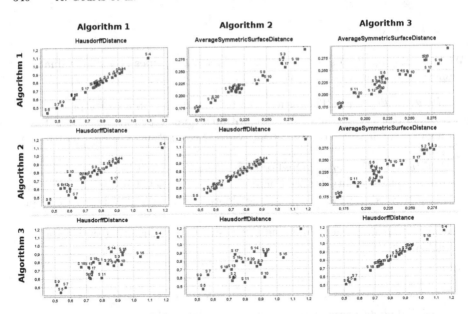

Fig. 3. Global comparison view allowing for a pairwise comparison of segmentation quality values across algorithms and organ instances in a dataset.

quality of another algorithm. The scatterplot allows the user to assess the quality of each segmentation (bottom left corner - good, upper right corner - bad). It also allows to analyze which algorithm is better for a particular instance.

The user can use this view also for selecting instances for further regional analysis. For example, the user can exclude outliers from further analysis.

Quality-based Clustering and identification of best algorithms: Landmarks of an organ are clustered according to their quality values so that regions with similar quality appear. We use a connectivity-extended hierarchical agglomerative clustering. After the regions are detected, we automatically identify which algorithms are best for each region. Suitable algorithms are those with low Average surface distance in a region. As several algorithms can lead to very good and similar results, we use a user-defined quality tolerance level for best algorithms. For example, all algorithms with values less than the best algorithm value + tolerance are deemed suitable for a particular region.

Regional Quality View: The regional quality comparison view allows the user to gain an insight into which algorithms are suitable for which region of an organ. It shows the results of a previous algorithmic analysis.

The regional comparison view shows the identified regions using a black border (see Fig. 5 left). Within each region, the best algorithm is indicated by a color. If several algorithms are suitable for a region, then they are displayed using weaving of colors within this region, as inspired by [12]. In this way, the

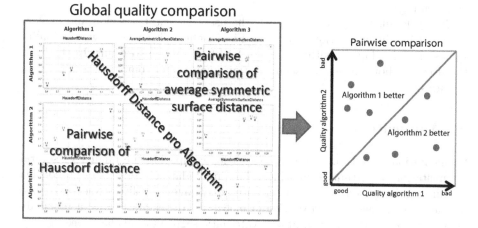

Fig. 4. Explanation of global comparison view. The scatterplots show pairwise comparisons of algorithms, where the points are segmentation instances. Upper right matrix shows comparison for average surface distance, lower left triangle shows results for Hausdorff distance. Diagonal shows result quality pro algorithm. In each scatterplot, each X-axis represents quality of one algorithm, and the Y axis shows the quality of another algorithm.

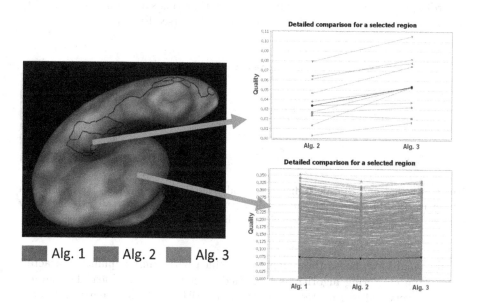

Fig. 5. Regional quality comparison

segmentation experts can see which algorithms perform best on the organ and in which region.

For a detailed quality assessment, the user can select a region and explore quality values in an additional view (see Fig. 5 right). This view shows the quality values of all landmarks within a region for all suitable algorithms. In this way, the user can both assess the segmentation quality and compare the algorithm qualities.

4   Application

Segmentation experts used our approach for comparing the quality of several segmentation algorithms for cochlea. The input dataset consists of 20 cochlea instances gained from a CT Scanner with an average intraslice voxel size of 0.18 and an average interslice voxel size of 0.38 mm. All instances have a manually created ground truth segmentation. Automatic segmentations have been generated using three variations of the SSM-based algorithm by Becker et al. [1].

Global view (see Fig. 3) shows that average distance is lower than 0.3 mm, thus the samples are very well segmented. All algorithms have broadly similar result quality. As the samples (i.e., points) are close to the diagonal in most scatterplots, there seem to be no large differences among algorithms. Looking at the individual samples shows that samples 5 and 9 (S5 and S9) have the best segmentation results. Interestingly, Sample 4 (S4) has extraordinary bad quality according to Hausdorff distance for all algorithms, but it has "normal" quality according to average distance. This indicates that this sample has good quality on average, but has some badly segmented regions (see Fig. 6).

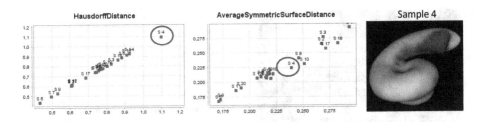

Fig. 6. Average and Hausdorff distance for all samples in the dataset. Sample 4 is an outlier in Hausdorff distance, but not in Average Distance. This is due to one badly segmented region (dark red) (Color figure online).

Regional view shows the regions on cochlea with similar quality characteristics. The clustering algorithms identified 21 regions on cochlea. The largest region is very well segmented by all three algorithms. It has a mean quality of 0.075 mm (see Fig. 5 bottom). The algorithm could also identify a very well segmented region in the middle of cochlea. However, solely the Algorithms 2 and 3 have been determined as the best in this region (see Fig. 5 top).

5   Conclusions and Future Work

We presented a new system for visual comparison of several segmentation algorithms on a dataset containing multiple 3D images. Our approach allows the user to analyze and visualize the quality of segmentation algorithms according to local quality.

We applied our approach to a cochlea dataset segmented with three versions of a SSM-based algorithm. Segmentation experts were able to assess the quality of algorithms on a dataset.

In the future, we would like to extend the scalability of our approach.

References

1. Becker, M., Kirschner, M., Sakas, G.: Segmentation of risk structures for otologic surgery using the probabilistic active shape model (PASM), **9036**, 903600–903600-7 (2014)
2. Busking, S., Botha, C.P., Ferrarini, L., Milles, J., Post, F.H.: Image-based rendering of intersecting surfaces for dynamic comparative visualization. Vis. Comput. **27**(5), 347–363 (2011)
3. Busking, S., Botha, C.P., Post, F.H.: Dynamic multi-view exploration of shape spaces. Comput. Graph. Forum **29**(3), 973–982 (2010)
4. Cárdenes, R., Bach, M., Chi, Y., Marras, I., de Luis, R., Anderson, M., Cashman, P., Bultelle, M.: Multimodal evaluation for medical image segmentation. In: Kropatsch, W.G., Kampel, M., Hanbury, A. (eds.) CAIP 2007. LNCS, vol. 4673, pp. 229–236. Springer, Heidelberg (2007)
5. Dick, C., Burgkart, R., Westermann, R.: Distance visualization for interactive 3d implant planning. IEEE Trans. Vis. Comput. Graph. **17**(12), 2173–2182 (2011)
6. Gerig, Guido, Jomier, Matthieu, Chakos, Miranda: Valmet: A New validation tool for assessing and improving 3D object segmentation. In: Niessen, Wiro J., Viergever, Max A. (eds.) MICCAI 2001. LNCS, vol. 2208, p. 516. Springer, Heidelberg (2001)
7. Gleicher, M., Albers, D., Walker, R., Jusufi, I., Hansen, C.D., Roberts, J.C.: Visual comparison for information visualization. Inf. Vis. **10**(4), 289–309 (2011)
8. Heimann, T., van Ginneken, B., Styner, M., et al.: Comparison and evaluation of methods for liver segmentation from CT datasets. IEEE Trans. Med. Imaging **28**, 1251–1265 (2009)
9. Heimann, T., Meinzer, H.P.: Statistical shape models for 3D medical image segmentation: A review. Med. Image Anal. **13**(4), 543–563 (2009)
10. Klemm, P., Lawonn, K., Rak, M., Preim, B., Toennies, K.D., Hegenscheid, K., Völzke, H., Oeltze, S.: Visualization and analysis of lumbar spine canal variability in cohort study data. In: Proceedings of the International Workshop on Vision, Modeling and Visualization, pp. 121–128 (2013)
11. von Landesberger, T., Bremm, S., Kirschner, M., Wesarg, S., Kuijper, A.: Visual analytics for model-based medical image segmentation: Opportunities and challenges. Expert Syst. Appl. **40**(12), 4934–4943 (2013)
12. Luboschik, M., Radloff, A., Schumann, H.: A new weaving technique for handling overlapping regions. In: Proceedings of the International Conference on Advanced Visual Interfaces, AVI 2010, pp. 25–32. ACM, New York (2010). http://doi.acm.org/10.1145/1842993.1842999

13. Schmidt, J., Preiner, R., Auzinger, T., Wimmer, M., Gröller, M.E., Bruckner, S.: Ymca - your mesh comparison application. In: IEEE VIS 2014. IEEE Computer Society, Nov 2014
14. Torsney-Weir, T., Saad, A., Moller, T., Hege, H.C., Weber, B., Verbavatz, J., Bergner, S.: Tuner: principled parameter finding for image segmentation algorithms using visual response surface exploration. IEEE Trans. Vis. Comput. Graph. **17**(12), 1892–1901 (2011)
15. von Landesberger, T., Andrienko, G., Andrienko, N., Bremm, S., Kirschner, M., Wesarg, S., Kuijper, A.: Opening up the black box of medical image segmentation with statistical shape models. Vis. Comput. **29**(9), 893–905 (2013). doi:10.1007/s00371-013-0852-y

Analyzing Requirements Using Environment Modelling

Dominique Méry[1] and Neeraj Kumar Singh[2]([✉])

[1] Université de Lorraine, LORIA, BP 239, Nancy, France
Dominique.Mery@loria.fr
[2] McMaster Centre for Software Certification,
McMaster University, Hamilton, Canada
singhn10@mcmaster.ca

Abstract. Analysing requirements is a major challenge in the area of safety-critical software, where requirements quality is an important issue to build a dependable critical system. Most of the time, any project fails due to lack of understanding of *user needs*, missing functional and non-functional system requirements, inadequate methods and tools, and inconsistent system specification. This often results from the poor quality of system requirements. Based on our experience and knowledge, an environment model has been recognized to be a promising approach to support requirements engineering to validate a system specification. It is crucial to get an approval and feedback in early stage of system development to ensure completeness and correctness of requirements specification. In this paper, we propose a method for analysing system requirements using a closed-loop modelling technique. A closed-loop model is an integration of system model and environment model, where both the system and environment models are formalized using formal techniques. Formal verification of the closed-loop model helps to identify missing system requirements or new emergent behaviours, which are not covered earlier during the requirements elicitation process. Moreover, an environment model assists in the construction, clarification, and validation of the given system requirements.

Keywords: Environment modelling · Closed-loop modelling · Analysing requirements · Verification

1 Introduction

Requirements engineering (RE) provides a framework for simplifying a complex system to get a better understanding of system requirements by using several formal and informal techniques. It plays an important role in early stage of system development to meet system qualities, success of the system, and reducing the cost of overall development. The prime causes of project failure are lack of understanding of system behaviour, missing functional and non-functional requirements, and inconsistent system requirements, which often lead to poor quality of requirements specification. Increasing complexities and system requirements require to

© Springer International Publishing Switzerland 2015
V.G. Duffy (Ed.): DHM 2015, Part II, LNCS 9185, pp. 345–357, 2015.
DOI: 10.1007/978-3-319-21070-4_35

pay more attention towards requirements engineering to omit a system failure [1]. *"what the system should do?"* is an initial goal of requirements engineering. Incompleteness, ambiguity, inconsistencies, and vagueness, are the most common problems encountered during the elicitation and specification of system requirements. However, the prime objective of any requirements engineering tool is to address these common problems [1].

To identify missing system requirements, inconsistency or new emergent behaviours in early stage of system development for developing a quality, safety, and dependable system, we need to look beyond the system itself, and into the working environment, including human interactions. Requirements traceability is a branch of the requirements management within the software development. Requirements traceability is concerned with documenting the life of requirements and to allow bi-directional traceability in the system requirements, and product produced like source codes and test cases. It enables users to identify the origin of each requirement and track every change, which was made to this requirement. Validation of requirements specification is an integral and essential part of requirements engineering. Validation is a process of checking, together with stakeholders, whether the requirements specification meets its stakeholders' intentions and expectations [2].

In this paper, we propose a method for analysing system requirements using environment modelling. The environment model and system model form a closed-loop system to trace missing requirements or new emergent behaviours. The closed-loop model is an integration of system model and environment model, where both the system and environment models are formalized using formal techniques. Formal verification of this closed-loop model helps to identify missing system requirements or new emergent behaviours, which are not covered earlier during the requirements elicitation process. This closed-loop modelling approach helps to get confidence in early stage of system development. This approach offers numerous benefits of the proposed approach as follows:

- Closed-loop modelling in early stage of system development;
- Identifying gaps or inconsistencies in system requirements;
- Strengthening the given system requirements;
- To support "what-if" analysis during formal reasoning;
- Traceability of missing behaviours that leave the system in undesired state;
- Automatic identification of an emergent behaviour;
- Validation of the system assumptions;
- Financial benefits that can allow to change the system requirements.

The remainder of this paper is organized as follows. Section 2 presents related work. Section 3 presents a short description of requirements engineering. Section 4 presents an overview of environment modelling. Section 5 presents a case study to model a closed-loop system for verifying system requirements. Section 6 discusses the environment modelling approach for analysing system requirements. Section 7 concludes the paper.

2   Related Work

Requirements analysis is an important step in the software development lifecycle that allows for eliciting, analysing, and recording the system requirements. The requirements should be unambiguous, satisfying completeness, formally verified, proper documented, and traceable. A list of errors related to software requirements is given in [3]. This paper also presents a detailed survey on different types of errors that are the root causes for failing the critical systems. The root causes are program faults, human errors, and process flaws. There are several methods are applicable for requirements analysis like prototyping and simulation. The exiting methodologies are not sufficient, and we are still striving for better methods for improving the requirements analysis process.

Prototype refers to an incomplete version of the system development that simulates a system partially when system requirements are indefinite and system behaviours are unclear [4]. Goguen et al. [5] have proposed a novel approach for constructing a prototype using formal specification, where this work advocates the use of an algebraic specification language for executing the given specification. A run-time technique for monitoring the system requirements for satisfaction purpose is presented in [6], where the system requirements are monitored for violations, and system behaviour is dynamically adapted a new behaviour. New introduced behaviour changes the system requirements that must meet the higher-level goals.

There are few approaches reported in the literature related to environment modelling. Kishi et al. [7] have proposed an environment modelling approach for an embedded system. A new language is proposed in [8] for modelling an environment and required behaviour to simulate an environment. The UML class diagram and sequence diagram are also used together for modelling and simulating an environment in [9]. Kreiner et al. [10] have presented a process to develop an environment model for simulation purpose, where this environment model can be used to simulate the automatic logistic systems.

An environment modelling is not limited for simulation purpose only. There are some works reported in the literatures that discuss testing based on an environment of a system. This type of environment modelling is applicable for rigorous testing of a given system. Auguston et al. [11] have discussed the development of environment behavioural models using Attributed Event Grammar for testing an embedded system. Heisel et al. [12] have proposed the use of a requirement model and an environment model using the UML state machines for testing. A testing approach for synchronous reactive software is presented in [13] using the temporal logic based on the environmental constraints.

3   Requirements Engineering

Requirements characterize a system related to functional and non-functional behaviours, system properties and safety constraints that must be satisfied by a developing system. The Institute of Electrical and Electronics Engineers (IEEE) defines a requirement as a condition or capability that must be met or possessed by a system or system components to satisfy the contract, standard, specification, or other formally imposed document [14]. Requirements engineering allows the use of systematic techniques for ensuring completeness, consistency and relevance of system requirements [15]. Requirements engineering has numerous phases for requirements elicitation, analysis, specification, verification, and management. The requirement elicitation is a process for identifying, reviewing, checking, and documenting a stakeholder needs for a given system. The requirements analysis is a process that allows to check a stakeholder needs and system constraints using formal and informal techniques. The requirements specification is a process for documenting a stakeholder needs and constraints unambiguously and precisely using formal or semi-formal techniques. The requirements verification allows to ensure completeness, correctness, understandable and consistent of system behaviour according to stakeholders. The requirements management uses for managing, coordinating, and documenting the system development life-cycle.

In requirements engineering the elicitation process is important to capture rationales and sources precisely in order to understand the requirements evolution and verification. Requirements analysis advocates desirable properties of the software development processes, and numerous problems are identified during the development process. It involves for finding variations and commonalities in the system development process. Moreover, it also allows feedback mechanism to provide essential information for reducing complexity by eliminating complex requirements by simple requirements. There are several techniques that are useful for improving the quality of requirements for dependable critical systems. In this paper, we propose a new technique for analysing requirements using environment modelling by developing a closed-loop model. A closed-loop model is an integration of system model and environment model, where both the system and environment models are specified using formal modelling language. This approach has potential benefits to trace missing requirements or new emergent behaviours. All these approaches, methods, techniques and tools proposed for analysing the requirements are useful as long as its adoption decision is present preferably during the early stages of the projects, and we need to understand how a decision on analysing requirements is made and which factors influence an adoption of the requirements engineering. Here, we present the conceptual treatment for analysing the system requirements using environment modelling for identifying peculiar requirements, which eventually provide us with a theoretical lens to examine this adoption in a systematic manner.

4   Environment Modelling

If environment models are to be used for safe dependable critical systems, they should not only be sufficiently detailed, but should also be easy to understand and modify as an environment and critical system evolve. To handle the complexity of a realistic system environment, a modelling language should have provision for modelling at several levels of abstraction. A modelling language should also have well-defined syntax and semantics for the tools to specify an environment model accurately that should be understandable by humans. A modelling language should also provide features for modelling real world concepts, real-time features, and other concepts, such as non-determinism, required by the components of an environment. Formal methods based modelling languages, such as Event-B, Z and VDM can be used to fulfill the required features for modelling an environment.

In this work, we are using the same notations to model an environment that are used for modelling the software systems. It is important to note that the methodology for environment modelling is significantly different from the system modelling. While modelling for an industrial case, we have abstracted the functional details of the environment components to an extent that hide the system complexities. For modelling an environment behaviour, non-determinism is widely used, which is not nearly as common when modelling an internal behaviour of a system.

For verifying and tracing the missing requirements or new emergent behaviours of a system based on its environment, the behaviour details of the environment are as important as its structural details. Structural details of a critical system environment are important to understand the overall composition of an environment using actuators and sensors, characteristics of various components, and their relationships. We select the Event-B modelling language to model these details using stepwise incremental refinement, where each refinement step is built by the *correct-by-construction* approach. The incremental refinement also adds the required safety properties to develop a safe and correct environment. The behavioural details of environment components are required to specify the dynamic aspects of an environment, for example, to determine the possible environment states, before and after its interactions whenever system is in effect, and to specify the possible interactions between the system and its environment.

In the following subsections, we discuss a modelling methodology for developing an environment model (the heart). Then the heart model will be used to develop a closed-loop model for a cardiac pacemaker. This closed-loop model of the pacemaker and heart can be used further for analysing system requirements and to identify missing requirements or new emergent behaviours.

4.1   Heart Model

The heart is a muscular organ that functions as the body's circulatory pump. It contains four chamber (see Fig. 1(a)), which contract and relax periodically. For contracting and relaxing, the heart requires an electrical stimulus that is generated by the sinus node. This electrical stimulus travels down through the conduction pathways. The electrical current flows progressively in the heart muscle using special conduction cells. To design an environment model of the heart, we select a set of landmark nodes (A, B, C, D, E, F, G, H) on the conduction network (see Fig. 1(b)), that controls the contraction and relaxing functionalities of the heart. Here, we describe only core idea for developing the heart model. Interested readers can find the modelling process in [16,17]. We introduce the necessary elements using formal notations to define the heart system as follows:

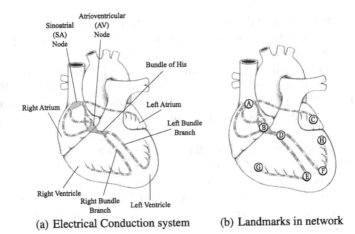

(a) Electrical Conduction system   (b) Landmarks in network

Fig. 1. The electrical conduction and landmarks of the heart system [16]

Definition 1 (The Heart System). *Given a set of nodes N, a transition (conduction) t is a pair (i, j), with i, j ∈ N. A transition is denoted by i ⤳ j. The heart system is a tuple HSys = (N, T, N_0, TW_{time}, CW_{speed}) where:*

- *N = { A, B, C, D, E, F, G, H } is a finite set of landmark nodes in the conduction pathways of the heart system;*
- *$T ⊆ N × N$ = { A ↦ B, A ↦ C, B ↦ D, D ↦ E, D ↦ F, E ↦ G, F ↦ H } is a set of transitions to represent electrical impulse propagation between two landmark nodes;*
- *N_0 = A is the initial landmark node (SA node);*
- *TW_{time} ∈ N→TIME is a weight function as time delay of each node, where TIME is a range of time delays;*
- *CW_{speed} ∈ T → SPEED is a weight function for the impulse propagation speed of each transition, where SPEED is a range of propagation speeds.*

Property 1 (Impulse Propagation Time). *In the heart system, the electrical impulse originates from the SA node (node A), travels through the entire conduction network and terminates at the atrial muscle fibres (node C) and at the ends of the Purkinje fibres in both sides of the ventricular chambers (node G and node H). The impulse propagation time delay differs for each landmark node. The impulse propagation time is represented as the total function TW_{time} ∈ N → $\mathbb{P}$(0..230). The impulse propagation time delay for each node is represented as: $TW_{time}(A)$ = 0..10, $TW_{time}(B)$ = 50..70, $TW_{time}(C)$ = 70..90, $TW_{time}(D)$ = 125..160, $TW_{time}(E)$ = 145..180, $TW_{time}(F)$ = 145..180, $TW_{time}(G)$ = 150..210 and $TW_{time}(h)$ = 150..230.*

Property 2 (Impulse Propagation Speed). *The impulse propagation speed also differs for each transition (i ⤳ j, where i, j ∈ N). The impulse propagation speed is represented as the total function CW_{speed} ∈ T → $\mathbb{P}$(5..400). The Impulse propagation speed for each transition is represented as: $CW_{speed}(A ↦ B)$ =*

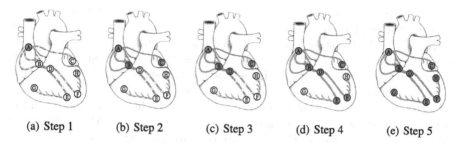

(a) Step 1   (b) Step 2   (c) Step 3   (d) Step 4   (e) Step 5

Fig. 2. Impulse propagation through landmark nodes [16]

$30..50$, $CW_{speed}(A \mapsto C) = 30..50$, $CW_{speed}(B \mapsto D) = 100..200$, $CW_{speed}(D \mapsto E) = 100..200$, $CW_{speed}(E \mapsto G) = 300..400$ and $CW_{speed}(F \mapsto H) = 300..400$.

The generated electrical stimulus from the sinus node propagates through the conduction network and selected landmark nodes (see Fig. 2). This electrical activity synchronizes the contraction of atria and ventricles. Changing conduction speed affects the natural rhythm and produces abnormalities. The abnormalities lead to various types of arrhythmias. The *bradycardia* is generated due to slow conduction speed, and the *tachycardia* is generated due to fast conduction speed. *Property* 1 and *Property* 2 describe a range of values for impulse propagation time delay for each landmark node and impulse propagation speed for each conduction path, respectively.

The heart blocking is an important term for describing a disorder of conduction of the impulse that stimulates heart muscle contraction. Disturbances in conduction may appear as slow conduction, intermittent conduction failure or complete conduction failure. These three kinds of conduction failure are also known as 1st, 2nd and 3rd degree blocks. We can show these different kinds of heart block throughout the conduction network using selected landmark nodes (see Fig. 3).

A set of spatially distributed cells forms a CA (Cellular Automata) model, which contains a uniform connection pattern among neighbouring cells and local computation laws. The CA is a discrete dynamic system corresponding to space and time that provides uniform properties for state transitions and intercon-

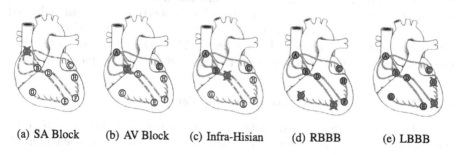

(a) SA Block   (b) AV Block   (c) Infra-Hisian   (d) RBBB   (e) LBBB

Fig. 3. Impairments in impulse propagation due to the heart blocks [16]

nection patterns. The cardiac muscle cells of the heart are presented in the following states: *Active, Passive* or *Refractory*. Initially, all cells are *Passive*, where each cell is discharged electrically and has no influence on its neighbouring cells. When an electrical impulse propagates, the cell becomes charged and eventually activated (*Active* state). The *Active* cell transmits an electrical impulse to its neighbour cells. The electrical impulse is propagated to all the cells in the heart muscle. After activation, the cell becomes discharged and enters in the *Refractory* state within which the cell cannot be reactivated. After a time, the cell changes its state to the *Passive* state to await the next impulse [17].

5   Case Studies

This section describes a closed-loop model of the cardiac pacemaker and heart, where the cardiac pacemaker responses according to functional behaviour of the heart [16,17]. The main objective of this closed-loop model is for finding inconsistencies, verifying essential safety properties, identifying an emergent behaviour, and strengthening the given system requirements. Due to limited space, we only provide a brief description of the closed-loop system development. A detailed formalization, including safety properties is available in [17,18].

5.1   Abstract Model

To define an abstract model of a closed-loop system, we develop a combined model of the cardiac pacemaker and heart, where the cardiac pacemaker actuates and senses according to the heart behaviour. The environment model of the heart behaves according to observations of an impulse propagation in the conduction network. For developing an abstract model, initially we capture the electrical features thorough defining a set of landmark nodes, impulse propagation times, impulse propagation paths, and impulse propagation speeds. The given parameters describe possible normal and abnormal behaviours of the heart. The cardiac pacemaker model contains sensors, actuators, and timing intervals. The timing intervals are upper rate limit, lower rate limit, and refectory periods for atria and ventricular chambers. The abstract model contains numerous events related to the heart and cardiac pacemaker models to describe the closed-loop model considering several interesting safety properties to establish a desired behaviour for satisfying the given system requirements. We introduce a clock, where time increases progressively by 1 (ms). This clock event controls the time line of pacing and sensing activities including heart impulse propagation.

5.2   Refinement 1: Threshold and Impulse Propagation

This refinement step introduces the impulse propagation that originates from the sinus node and travels down through the conduction network using the landmark nodes. The electrical impulse reaches at the Purkinje fibers of the ventricles. We describe the impulse propagation activities using a set of events, where electrical impulse passes through the several intermediate landmark nodes and finally sinks to the terminal nodes (C, G, H). The conduction model uses a clock counter to model a real-time system to satisfy the required temporal properties. A set of new events simulates a desired behaviour of the impulse propagation into the heart conduction network, where each new refined event formalizes impulse flow between two landmark nodes. The cardiac pacemaker model is enriched by introducing concrete behaviour of sensors for both the atrial and ventricular chambers, where sensors filter a desired sensing value through comparing with selected standard threshold values. The standard threshold value for atria is always lower than the ventricular chamber. The heart conduction behaviour is continue monitored by the cardiac pacemaker model to allow or inhibit to pace into the heart chamber to control a desired behaviour of the heart according to the standard threshold value under the required timing intervals.

5.3 Refinement 2: Hysteresis and Perturbation the Conduction

This refinement step introduces an abnormal behaviour by introducing the heart blocking activities, and *hysteresis* operating mode. The blocking behaviour specifies perturbation in the heart conduction network to realize an actual abnormal behaviour of the heart. A set of events is introduced using progressive refinement to simulate possible desired blocking behaviours. This blocking activities generate abnormalities into the electrical impulse propagation, which are destined through partition the landmark nodes in the conduction network. The cardiac pacemaker model introduces a new operating mode known as *hysteresis*, which prevents the constant pacing. This mode allows a patient to have his or her own underlying rhythm as much as possible. The *hysteresis* is a programmed feature whereby the pacemaker paces at a faster rate than the sensing rate. A list of events describes this feature for the cardiac pacemaker model.

5.4 Refinement 3: Rate Modulation and Cellular Model

This is the last refinement of the closed-loop system, where a cellular level description is added to the heart, and the rate modulation is added to the cardiac pacemaker. This refinement provides a simulation model that allows to describe the impulse propagation at the cellular level using cellular automata. An electrical impulse propagates at the cells level. A set of events is used to formalize a desired behaviour of the heart using cellular automata. The cardiac pacemaker model is enriched by describing a rate adapting pacing technique. The rate adapting pacing technique gives freedom to select automatically a desired pacing rate according to physiological needs. Automatic selection of a desired pacing rate helps to increase or decrease the pacing rate and assists a patient for controlling the heart rate according to daily activities. The rate modulation sensor is used to determine the maximum exertion performed by a patient. This increased pacing rate refers to the *sensor indicated rate*. Reducing the physical activities helps to progressively decrease the pacing rate down to the lower rate. A set of new refined events models increasing and decreasing pacing rates of the cardiac pacemaker.

5.5   Proof Statics

In this section, we briefly discuss how a closed-loop system modelling approach can be used to analyse system requirements for finding missing requirements. Table 1 expresses the proof statistics of the development of the closed-loop model of the cardiac pacemaker within the heart environment. These statistics measure the size of the model, the proof obligations (POs) generated and discharged by the Rodin prover and those that are interactively proved.

Table 1. Proof statistics

Model	Total number of POs	Automatic proof	Interactive proof
Closed-loop model of One-electrode pacemaker			
Abstract model	304	258 (85 %)	46 (15 %)
First refinement	1015	730 (72 %)	285 (28 %)
Second refinement	72	8 (11 %)	64 (89 %)
Third refinement	153	79 (52 %)	74 (48 %)
Closed-loop model of Two-electrode pacemaker			
Abstract model	291	244 (84 %)	47 (16 %)
First refinement	1039	766 (74 %)	273 (26 %)
Second refinement	53	2 (4 %)	51 (96 %)
Third refinement	122	60 (49 %)	62 (51 %)
Total	3049	2147 (70 %)	902 (30 %)

This closed-loop development results in 3049 (100 %) POs, in which 2147 (70 %) POs are proved automatically, and the remaining 902 (30 %) POs are proved interactively using the Rodin prover. The environment (heart) model is used together with the system (pacemaker) model for verification purpose, that generates automated oracles. These oracles are new proof obligations those are not appeared independently in the system (pacemaker) and environment (heart) models. These generated proof obligations are produced according to the expected system behaviour corresponding to the environment model. A set of new generated POs helps to discover new behaviours by checking formal proofs or undischarged POs. However this approach also helps to check validation of the given assumptions, and identification of new emergent behaviours in the cardiac pacemaker.

6   Analysing Requirements Based on Environment Models

In this section, we briefly discuss how our environment modelling approach is used to analyse system requirements for identifying missing system requirements or new emergent behaviours. The formal model of environment (heart) in Event-B describes the environmental properties in various refinement layers. The developed environment model is used together with the system (cardiac pacemaker) model for verification purpose, that generates automated oracles. These oracles are new proof obligations that do not appear independently in the system model and in the environment model. These generated POs are produced according to the expected system behaviour corresponding to the environment model. However, these generated POs also allow to have more precise actions corresponding to the given guards that should be strengthen to meet expected dynamic behaviours of the cardiac pacemaker, including timing constraints and pacing and sensing activities. Moreover, the closed-loop model can be used for various purposes during the system development, such as automated code generation and automated test case generation.

In this work, we have focused on formalizing the closed-loop system behaviour of a cardiac pacemaker using several incremental refinements. The goal of this closed-loop model is to provide the nondeterministic behaviour such that an environmental error state is reached during the formal verification, if any fault is present. In fact, to have effective heuristics we need to have precise knowledge of the error states. This information is easily added in the models using stereotypes. All the relevant states/transitions that lead to those error states can be exploited for the automatic derivation of a desired function.

In some relevant cases, it is possible to automatically derive very precise desired functions. This happens when time constraints need to be satisfied, for example a cardiac pacemaker must actuate at exact time interval. Modellers do not need to write these heuristics, they are in fact automatically derived from the given environment model. This is essential, because in general software modellers do not have access to such expertise to write proper desired functions for search algorithms. The results of this experiments show that our closed-loop modelling methodology can be used for a fully automated system verification that is effective in revealing new emergent behaviours, missing system requirements and inconsistencies in the given system. Although the system modelling and environment modelling can be designed in many ways using different strategies, the closed-loop modelling methodology and analysing requirements technique described here would still remain the same.

7 Conclusion

In this paper, we have discussed system requirements analysis using environment modelling. The integration of system model and environment model forms a closed-loop system to trace new emergent behaviours or missing requirements. For practical reason and to facilitate to handle a large complex system, we use the Event-B modelling language to support incremental refinement for modelling, structuring and defining the safety constraints. We have briefly discussed how an environment model is used to simulate required operating environment for a given system using formal logics. The main advantage of this environment model is to assist in the construction, clarification, and validation of the given system requirements.

We have modelled an environment model for the heart for investigating the expected behaviours of a cardiac pacemaker. Given that a cardiac pacemaker interacts with the heart exactly at this level (i.e., electrical impulses), this model is a very promising "environmental model" to be used in parallel with a pacemaker model to form a closed-loop system. This model therefore has an immediate use in "the grand challenges in formal methods" where an industrial pacemaker specification has been elected as a benchmark. The closed-loop modelling of the heart and cardiac pacemaker involves formalizing and reasoning about pacemaker behaviour under normal and abnormal heart conditions.

A set of requirements is given in the closed-loop model for modelling general and patient specific conditions. Based on these requirements, we have presented an interactive and physiologically relevant closed-loop model for verifying basic and complex operations of a cardiac pacemaker. The main benefits of this work are as follows:

- To support verification and validation activities;
- Identifying gaps or inconsistencies in system requirements;
- Strengthen the given system requirements;
- To support "What-if" analysis during formal reasoning;
- Closed-loop modelling in early stage of system development;
- Analysing requirements, reducing cost, and virtualization;
- Increase confidence level and decrease the failure risks;
- To satisfy V&V requirements for domain specific certification standards;
- Automatic identification of new emergent behaviours;
- Validation of the system assumptions.

The main objectives of our work are to promote the use of such kind of closed-loop modelling approach to bridge a gap between software engineers and stakeholders to build a quality system, and to discover all ambiguous information from the requirements. Moreover, this approach helps to verify the correctness of behaviour of a system according to stakeholder requirements. There are scientific and legal applications as well, where the formal model based closed-loop modelling approach has certain scenarios to glean more information or better understandings of a system and assist to improve the final given system.

Acknowledgement. This work was supported by grant ANR-13-INSE-0001 (The IMPEX Project http://impex.loria.fr) from the Agence Nationale de la Recherche (ANR).

References

1. Bubenko Jr., J.A.: Challenges in requirements engineering. In: Proceedings of the Second IEEE International Symposium on Requirements Engineering, pp. 160–162, March 1995
2. McDermid, J.: Software Engineer's Reference Book. CRC Press Inc, Boca Raton (1991)
3. Lutz, R.: Analyzing software requirements errors in safety-critical, embedded systems. In: Proceedings of IEEE International Symposium on Requirements Engineering, pp. 126–133, January 1993
4. Davis, A.M.: Operational prototyping: a new development approach. IEEE Softw. **9**, 70–78 (1992)
5. Goguen, J., Meseguer, J.: Rapid prototyping: in the obj executable specification language. SIGSOFT Softw. Eng. Notes **7**, 75–84 (1982)
6. Fickas, S., Feather, M.S.: Requirements monitoring in dynamic environments. In: Proceedings of the Second IEEE International Symposium on Requirements Engineering, RE 1995, pp. 140–147. IEEE Computer Society, Washington, DC (1995)

7. Noda, N., Kishi, T.: Aspect-oriented modeling for embedded software design. In: 14th Asia-Pacific Software Engineering Conference, APSEC 2007, pp. 342–349, December 2007

8. Karsai, G., Neema, S., Sharp, D.: Model-driven architecture for embedded software: a synopsis and an example. Sci. Comput. Program. **73**(1), 26–38 (2008)

9. Choi, K., Jung, S., Kim, H., hwan Bae, D.: Uml-based modeling and simulation method for mission-critical real-time embedded. In: System Development, IASTED Conference on Software Engineering 2006, pp. 160–165. Mittal, Zeigler and De la Cruz. (2006)

10. Kreiner, C., Steger, C., Weiss, R.: Improvement of control software for automatic logistic systems using executable environment models. In: Proceedings of 24th Euromicro Conference, vol. 2, pp. 919–923, August 1998

11. Auguston, M., Michael, J.B., Shing, M.T.: Environment behavior models for automation of testing and assessment of system safety. Inf. Softw. Technol. **48**(10), 971–980 (2006). Advances in Model-based Testing

12. Heisel, M., Hatebur, D., Seifert, T.S.D.: Testing against requirements using uml environment models. In: Fachgruppentreffen Requirements Engineering und Test, Analyse and Verifikation, pp. 28–31 (2008)

13. du Bousquet, L., Ouabdesselam, F., Richier, J.L., Zuanon, N.: Lutess: a specification-driven testing environment for synchronous software. In: Proceedings of the 21st International Conference on Software Engineering, ICSE 1999, pp. 267–276. ACM, New York (1999)

14. IEEE Standard: IEEE Standard Glossary of Software Engineering Terminology. IEEE Std 610. 12-1990, pp. 1–84, December 1990

15. Sommerville, I., Sawyer, P.: Requirements Engineering: A Good Practice Guide, 1st edn. Wiley, New York (1997)

16. Méry, D., Singh, N.K.: Formalization of heart models based on the conduction of electrical impulses and cellular automata. In: Liu, Z., Wassyng, A. (eds.) FHIES 2011. LNCS, vol. 7151, pp. 140–159. Springer, Heidelberg (2012)

17. Singh, N.K.: Using Event-B for Critical Device Software Systems. Springer, London (2013)

18. Méry, D., Singh, N.K.: Closed-loop modeling of cardiac pacemaker and heart. In: Weber, J., Perseil, I. (eds.) FHIES 2012. LNCS, vol. 7789, pp. 151–166. Springer, Heidelberg (2013)

Modeling of a Virtual Open Platform for Human Cranium Simulation

Pedro Perestrelo[✉], Maurício Torres, Pedro Noritomi, and Jorge Silva

Division of Three-Dimensional Technologies, Centre for Information Technology – Renato Archer, Rodovia Dom Pedro I (SP-65) Km 143, 6 Amarais, Campinas, SP 13069-901, Brazil
pedro.perestrelo@cti.gov.br

Abstract. To prevent, detect and treat trauma brain injuries (TBI) one must understand them and know how they occur. With the integration of biomechanical and clinical theories, as well as research cases, a new era of cooperation must be initiated. For that reason, our proposal of developing a virtual platform based on the BioCAD protocol through computed tomography (CT) software, computer aided design (CAD) software and finite element method (FEM) analysis software, represents a joined effort in that direction. Results obtained with the resultant model were in line with maxillary expansion results from the literature, thus validating it. This model must be adaptable to the user and/or patient, leading to an innovative tool for research, prevention and treatment of TBI.

Keywords: BioCAD · Brain · Finite element method · Simulation · Trauma

1 Introduction

The human head is one of the most critical area of the human body, so with severe trauma to the head comes a possible death situation or long-term disability [1]. From an anatomical point of view, the scalp, skull, sub-arachnoidal space and dura matter are natural protections for the brain but they cannot withstand the dynamical loading conditions of today's accidents [2]. The current methods to analyze the kind of injury sustained by the head in a trauma situation are mostly based on translational acceleration [3]. Since there are other parameters that cause injuries, such as rotational acceleration, the need to improve current test procedures is required [4]. As a result, our proposal to improve the approach to the classification of TBI is based on an interdisciplinary work group comprising engineers and a neurosurgeon with the objective of developing a virtual open platform to study these events. With this work group concept, problems that once were studied separately can be analyzed together allowing for faster and solid advances on TBI problems, such as, subdural haematoma (SDH), diffuse axonal injury (DAI) and strain rate on the cerebral tissue [5, 6]. Consequently, an extensive study to the anatomy of the human head was conducted, so that it could be correctly represented even if some simplifications had to be made. The development of this virtual platform, or computational model, leans on the premise that it must simulate TBI situations and for that, it is constructed using the BioCAD protocol with a specific patient modeling (SPM) method [7]. This protocol comprises a

© Springer International Publishing Switzerland 2015
V.G. Duffy (Ed.): DHM 2015, Part II, LNCS 9185, pp. 358–366, 2015.
DOI: 10.1007/978-3-319-21070-4_36

series of sequentially coordinated tasks in different softwares. It starts with the loading of a computerized tomography (CT) scan in a medical image processing software, then the resulting file is imported to a computer aided design (CAD) software and in the end a finite element method (FEM) analysis software is used. This proposed computational model is in the development stage an assessment was made to the stress distribution through the geometry, so that it could be verified if the behavior was consistent with other validated studies in the literature.

In the end, this virtual platform has to be adaptive to the user and/or patient, in order to simulate TBI close to reality. This will lead to an important tool for the study, treatment and prevention of TBI, which will be publicly available.

2 Materials and Methods

Since the main objective of this study is to develop a TBI platform, the head anatomy was studied. It was important that the geometry to obtain would not be too simplified nor too detailed, in order to reproduce coherent results in the simulations. Therefore, it was made a choice to use a compromised solution. An analysis to the basic structures of the human head was conducted with an outward to inward direction. First, appears the scalp with a thickness varying from 5 to 7 mm, followed by the skull and the meninges. The membranes that compose the meninges are the dura mater, arachnoid and the pia mater, having cerebrospinal fluid (CSF) in the subdural and subarachnoid space. This fluid creates a disconnection between them and has an important role in absorbing shock to the head, according to the scientific community [8].

Next, in our analysis, came the brain structure divided, by the invaginations, in three parts, which are the cerebrum, cerebellum and the brain stem (Fig. 1) [8].

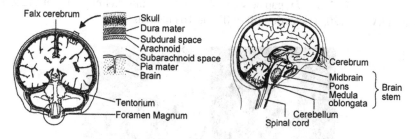

Fig. 1. Image portraying cutting planes of the human head [8]

Once understood the basic head anatomy, the next step was to study the types of injuries that could occur. In light of this, the head injuries are classified as open and closed. Open injuries relate to skull fracture but can also be linked to damage to the soft intracranial tissue, while in the presence of a skull fracture. Closed injuries do not have a skull fracture but have trauma inflicted to the intracranial contents. The most challenging injury to understand and replicate is the closed injury [8].

Nonetheless there were more structures and specific injuries to describe, an extensive anatomical analysis, as well as physiopathological, will be postponed since our model only contemplates, in this phase, bony structures.

Generally, the study of TBI has taken two separate approaches to the problem, the bioengineers view and the medical view. The bioengineers view leans specially on the input variables that cause the injuries, usually being those the linear acceleration, strain and strain rate in the brain tissue [6]. In the other hand, the medical view consists in the study of the consequences of the trauma, such as, diffuse axonal injury (DAI) and/or brain edema (BE) [9]. Despite of this, advances in the TBI research area have been achieved regarding, for example, head impact situations with or without helmets, skull fracture and the behavior of the human brain under impact conditions, as well as other studies [3, 4, 10, 11].

What is proposed with our study is a third approach by joining the previous two approaches, consequently, reinforcing the potential for research. This integration led to an interdisciplinary team formed by engineers and a neurosurgeon. In addition to this integration, there has been an objective of creating a computational model based on a SPM method with the ability to be adjusted to different purposes or situations. This means that this model will result into a virtual platform with the most important anatomical characteristics of the human head. For this to be possible, the model development followed a protocol called BioCAD. The BioCAD protocol was developed in the Division of Three-Dimensional Technologies (DT3D) in the Center for Information Technology – Renato Archer (CTI), Campinas, São Paulo, Brazil [12]. It comprehends a sequence of tasks executed in various softwares, starting with the loading of CT scans into the InVesalius® software, also developed in CTI [13]. This operation had the purpose of processing these CT images, suppressing imperfections and soft tissues, generating a stereo lithography (STL) mesh of the bony structures (Fig. 2a). The CT scan equipment used to acquire the images was a GE LightSpeed16 with a threshold parameter of −1024 to 3071, gap between slices of 1.25 mm, an image size of 512 × 512 pixels, a kVp of 120, a detection tilt of 0° and 16 channels.

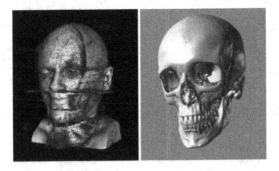

Fig. 2. In the lef, a CT scan loaded into the InVesalius® software and, in the right, a STL mesh generated in the same software and loaded into Rhinoceros® CAD software.

Next, the STL mesh file was imported into the CAD software Rhinoceros® because of the ability of this tool to combine surface modeling with complex geometries, as are the ones present in the human head (Fig. 2b).

With this STL mesh as a modeling guide, a geometry can be created having an anatomical accuracy in line with what is necessary for this specific case. In other words, this particular condition allows for the preservation of the skull anatomy and, at the same time, adjusts the detail depending of the area that needs to be represented and the importance to achieve a correct simulation. As mentioned above, all of these conditions depend on an accurate anatomical study of the human head.

Once the geometric model was created, it was imported to the FEM simulation software Hypermesh®. A mesh was created and optimized, in order to simulate the intended situation (Fig. 3) [14].

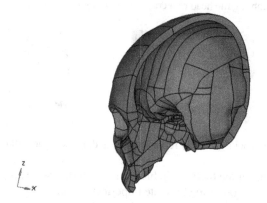

Fig. 3. Image of the geometry loaded into Hypermesh®

3   Discussion

One of BioCAD advantages is the fact that it is able to maintain the anatomical coherence of the models. This capability differs from other models found in the literature.

Models with a lack of detail, as seen in Fig. 4(a), for example, lead to incomplete results or difficulty to simulate due to a very rough mesh detail. On the other hand, the models with excess of detail can impose difficulties with a high need of processing power and a difficulty in presenting a correct solution. This excess of detailing, in the whole model, also makes impossible to have local detail adjustment. Example of such a model can be seen in Fig. 4(b). Differing from this first two examples, are models which resemble themselves to crash-test dummies heads. These models, due to their shape, have a different energy distribution on its geometry than a human head, leading to incorrect results. It can be observed in Fig. 4(c), an example of that kind of model.

During the development of the model, problems with the anatomy of the human head have been raised. For example, the bone inside the eye socket, that comprehends parts of the ethmoid, sphenoid, lacrimal and maxillary bones, was not totally represented by the CT scan due to its low thickness (Fig. 5a). Another problem, also because of low thickness and the anatomical geometries, was the generation of the 3D mesh that had, as an example, collapsed elements (Fig. 5b).

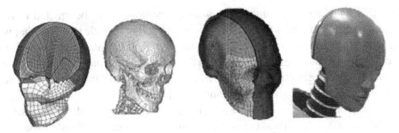

Fig. 4. Model (a) has little geometrical detail, model (b) has an excess of detail and a model (c) has an anatomy resembling the head of a crash-test dummy (d) [17–20].

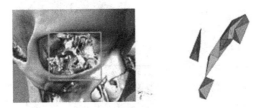

Fig. 5. In the left, a poor geometry representation and, in the right, collapsed 3D elements

A refinement, using the tools available in Hypermesh® software, was performed to the 2D surface mesh in order to eliminate imperfections in the elements and generate a 3D mesh close to simulation stage. Nonetheless, it was still necessary to perform a refinement to the 3D mesh.

Aside from these development obstacles, there is a constant evaluation of the work strategy due to the challenge of modeling complex anatomical geometries.

4   Simulation and Results

The current state of development of the computational model represents the skull structure with the cortical interior and exterior bone (Fig. 3).

The geometry exported for the simulation had half of the skull because it saves computer processing power and time, maintaining the ability of achieving similar results which do not threaten the validity of the model. This geometry was exported in the IGES (.igs) format from Rhinoceros® to Hypermesh®. Inside Hypermesh®, it was generated a 2D triangular surface mesh with an element size of 3.5 mm. From this 2D mesh was generated a 3D tetrahedral mesh with linear elements that was used in the simulation (Fig. 6).

A material for the cortical bone was created as linear isotropic with a Young's Modulus of 13700 MPa, a Poisson Coefficient of 0.35 and a Density of 2e-6 kg/mm^3. All of these are average values found in publications, regarding the cortical bone [15, 16]. For these initial simulations the bone was considered solid, meaning that the space between the exterior and interior cortical bone is filled with pyramidal elements.

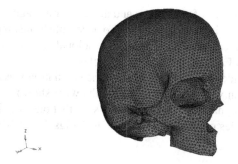

Fig. 6. Final 3D mesh

Since it was intended to verify if the model behavior was correct, the situation to simulate was a maxillary expansion. To emulate the stress distribution characteristic to this process, a pressure of 1 MPa was applied to a small area in the maxilla near the midsagital suture, as can be seen in Fig. 7. This pressure was applied normal to the surface. In Fig. 8, with blue color triangles, it can be seen the fixed support located in the foramen magnum.

This pressure value did not represent any real value obtained in this kind of procedures because, as mentioned earlier, the only aim is to observe the stress distribution in the geometry. Given that in such procedures there is a maxillary separation in the midsagital suture and that it was being used half of the skull, the sagital surfaces near the

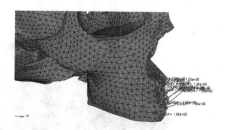

Fig. 7. Representation of the pressure application

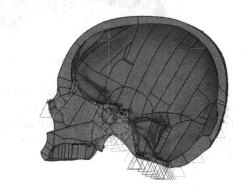

Fig. 8. Image showing the constraint present in the foramen magnum (Color figure online)

midsagital suture were free of constraints and the remaining sagital surfaces were given restrictions, in order to simulate symmetry. To accomplish this, these surfaces did not have translational movement in the x axis and rotational movement in the y and z axis, as can be observed in Fig. 8 in green color triangles.

Once all the considerations where in place the simulation was configured as linear static and the situation was replicated. The results were shown in a color map format regarding the absolute maximum principal stress, so that one could be able to compare its behavior with studies presented in the literature (Figs. 9 and 10).

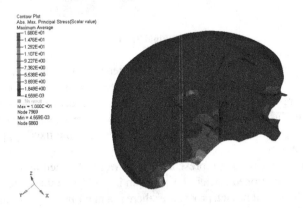

Fig. 9. Outer stress distribution map

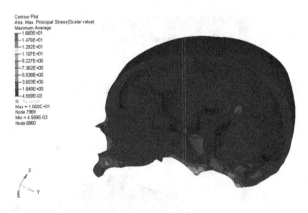

Fig. 10. Inner stress distribution map

The stress distribution is in line with what is referred in the literature, that is to say that there is an occurrence of stress in the skull base, in the sphenoid bone and in the zygomatic arch [21]. Furthermore, a propagation of stress takes place near the eye socket and in the palatal bone [22]. These patterns of stress dispersion are all in accordance with what is already confirmed.

5   Conclusion

Our model behaved as expected in the simulation of a maxillary expansion. The fact that it was possible to validate our model in this simulation strengthens the premise that models with poor anatomical representation, with excess of detail, rough or too refined meshing produce less accurate results. Nonetheless, that more simulations are to be made and that the model needs further development, the possibility of achieving breakthrough results has been reinforced. The application of the BioCAD protocol plays a very important role in the modeling as well as in the simulation, for example, due to its ability to create the conditions to reproduce anatomical geometries and to refine the mesh in specific areas of interest to the project. Although, it is important to refer that these tests do not have a clinical purpose but the objective of confirming that the model has achieved a state that is closer to the intended virtual platform.

As future works, steps must be taken to model the brain, simulate the model with a brain geometry inside and validate the results. When finished, this virtual platform will be an important advance in the study, prevention and treatment of TBI because of its qualities but also because it is intended to be made available publically.

References

1. Long, J., Yang, J., Lei, Z., Liang, D.: Simulation-based assessment for construction helmets. Comput. Methods Biomech. Biomed. Eng. (2013). doi:10.1080/10255842.2013.774382
2. Deck, C., Willinger, R.: Head injury prediction tool for protective systems optimisation. Paper Presented at the 7th European LS-DYNA Conference, Salzburg, Austria, 14–15 May 2009
3. Lashkari, M., Frahmand, F., Kangarlou, K.: Finite element modeling of the human brain under impact conditions. Int. Res. J. Appl. Basic Sci. **6**(6), 875–881 (2013). Science Explorer Publications
4. Fernandes, F., Sousa, R., Willinger, R., Deck, C.: Finite element analysis of helmeted impacts and head injury evaluation with a commercial road helmet. Paper Presented at the IRCOBI Conference 2013, Gothenburg, Sweden, 11–13 September 2013
5. Whyte, T., Gibson, T., Milthorpe, B., Stanford, G.: Head injury and effective motorcycle helmets. Paper Presented at the 23rd Enhanced Safety of Vehicles Conference, Seoul, Korea, 27–30 May 2013
6. King, A., Yang, K., Zhang, L. Hardy, W.: Is head injury caused by linear or angular acceleration? Paper Presented at the IRCOBI Conference, Lisbon, Portugal, 25 September 2003
7. Castellano-Smith, A.D., Hartkens, T., Schnabel, J.A., Hose, D.R., Liu, H., Hall, W.A., Truwit, C.L., Hawkes, D.J., Hill, D.L.: Constructing patient specific models for correcting intraoperative brain deformation. In: Niessen, W.J., Viergever, M.A. (eds.) MICCAI 2001. LNCS, vol. 2208, pp. 1091–1098. Springer, Heidelberg (2001)
8. Brands, D.: Predicting brain mechanics during closed head impact: numerical and constitutive aspects. Dissertation, Technische Universiteit Eindhoven (2002)
9. Marmarou, A.: Pathophysiology of traumatic brain edema: current concepts. Acta Neurochir. Suppl. **86**, 7–10 (2003)
10. Yan, W., Pangestu, O.: A modified human head model for the study of impact head injury. Comput. Methods Biomech. Biomed. Eng. **14**(12), 1049–1057 (2011). doi:10.1080/10255842.2010.506435

11. Asgharpour, Z., Baumgartner, D., Willinger, R., Graw, M., Peldschus, S.: The validation and application of a finite element human head model for frontal skull fracture analysis. J. Mech. Behav. Biomed. Mater. **33**, 16–23 (2013). doi:10.1016/j.jmbbm.2013.02.010. Elsevier
12. Kemmoku, D., Noritomi, P., Roland, F., Silva, J.: Use of BioCAD in the development of a growth compliant prosthetic device for cranioplasty of growing patients. In: Bártolo, P. et al. (ed.) Innovative Developments in Design and Manufacturing. 4th Advanced Research in Virtual and Rapid Prototyping, Leiria, Portugal, 6–10 October, pp. 123–144. CRC Press/Balkema, London (2010)
13. Camilo, A., Amorim, P., Moraes, T., Azevedo, F., Silva, J.: InVesalius: medical image edition. Paper Presented at the PROMED 2012, Brescia, Italy, 2–4 May 2012
14. Noritomi, P., Xavier, T., Silva, J.: A comparison between BioCAD and some know methods for finite element model generation. In: Bártolo, P. et al. (ed.) Innovative Developments in Virtual and Physical Prototyping. 5th Advanced Research in Virtual and Rapid Prototyping, Leiria, Portugal, 28 September–01 October, pp. 685–690. CRC Press/Balkema, Leiden (2012)
15. Acka, K., Cehreli, M.: Biomechanical consequences of progressive marginal bone loss around oral implants: a finite element stress analysis. Med. Biol. Eng. Comput. **44**(7), 527–535 (2006). doi:10.1007/s11517-006-0072-y. Springer, Heidelberg
16. Kleiven, S., Hardy, W.: Correlation on a FE model of the human head with local brain motion – consequences for injury prediction. Stapp Car Crash J. **46**, 123–144 (2002)
17. Yan, W., Pangestu, O.: A modified human head model for the study of impact head injury. Comput. Methods Biomech. Eng. **14**(12), 1049–1057 (2001). doi:10.1080/10255842.2010.506435
18. Watanabe, D., Yuge, K., Nishimoto, T., Murakami, S., Takao, H.: Head impact analysis related to the mechanism of diffuse axonal injury. High-Tech Research Center Project for Private Universities – Mext Japan (2008)
19. Ghajari, M., Deck, C., Galvanetto, U., Iannucci, L, Willinger, R.: Development of numerical models for the investigation of motorcycle accidents. Paper Presented at the 7th European LS-DYNA Conference, Salzburg, Austria, 14–15 May 2009
20. Connolly, C.: Instrumentation used in vehicle safety testing at Milbrook Proving Ground Ltd. Sens. Rev. **27**(2), 91–98 (2007). doi:10.1108/02602280710731641. Emerald Group Publishing Limited
21. Holberg, C.: Effects of rapid maxillary expansion on the cranial base – an FEM analysis. J. Orofac. Orthop. **66**(1), 54–66 (2005). doi:10.1007/s00056-005-0439-y
22. Boryor, A., Geiger, M., Hohmann, A., Wunderlich, A., Sander, C., Martin Sander, F., Sander, G.: Stress distribution and displacement analysis during an intermaxillary disjunction – a three-dimensional FEM study of a human skull. J. Biomech. **41**(2), 376–382 (2008). doi:10.1016/j.jbiomech.2007.08.016

Influence of Proficiency on Eye Movement of the Surgeon for Laparoscopic Cholecystectomy

Hisanori Shiomi[1], Masamori Notsu[2], Tomoko Ota[2], Yuka Takai[3], Akihiko Goto[3(✉)], and Hiroyuki Hamada[4]

[1] Shiga University of Medical Science, Otsu, Japan
Shiomi@belle.shiga-med.ac.jp
[2] Chuo Business Group, Chuo-Ku, Japan
Tomoko.ota@k.vodafone.ne.jp
[3] Department of Information Systems Engineering, Osaka Sangyo University, Daito, Japan
gotoh@ise.osaka-sandai.ac.jp
[4] Advanced Fibro-Science, Kyoto Institute of Technology, Kyoto, Japan
hhamada@kit.ac.jp

Abstract. In this study, a training system of laparoscopic cholecystectomy combined surgical instrument simulation and eye movement analysis was established. The surgical tool usage also was recorded by video cameras during the whole training process. The eye track information and utilization information of surgical tool were provided to interns as a study reference. The expert's information also was showed to interns in order to make a comparison after practice. The system had been shown to be effective in a variety of practices.

Keywords: Eye movement · Laparoscopic cholecystectomy · Surgeon · Expert · Non-expert

1 Introduction

In the field of a surgical operation technology has been developing in recent years. Moreover, since the acquisition method of the technology in a surgical operation has the main system with "studies technique by seeing" it requires long time for an expert's training. Furthermore, when there is little an advising doctor's number, or when an advising doctor's instruction capability is low, it further delays during an expert's rearing period. Operation under laparoscopy has many advantages such as the point and duration of hospitalization because operative wound is smaller than a laparotomy and end are comparatively short. These reasons are mostly desired by the patient. Since it is necessary to do the operation by only the information acquired from the image of a laparoscope while making full use of a special machine and instrument to relian, the operation technique should have high difficulty, and then the operated should have advanced technique [1, 2]. Although it can also train by using a simulator for the technical acquisition method besides the method of "studies technique by seeing" in

© Springer International Publishing Switzerland 2015
V.G. Duffy (Ed.): DHM 2015, Part II, LNCS 9185, pp. 367–373, 2015.
DOI: 10.1007/978-3-319-21070-4_37

order to raise a level of skill, it is indispensable to train repeatedly and to gain much experiences [3].

In this research, eye movement measurement was performed for the process of the operation under laparoscopy to two or more persons. The knack of advanced technique was understood through numerical method and the difference in technology were evaluated, and it aimed at showing the influence of years of experience on eye movement by comparing the operation for the operators with different level of skill. The target operation was laparoscopic cholecystectomy. We decided to carry out under the same conditions using a simulator, and the subject was taken as two experts and one unskilled operator from which years of experience differ so that comparison between two or more subjects might be attained. According to the procedure in which it is most worked by the whole operation by actual laparoscopic cholecystectomy, it classified into five items and measured the factor about working hours and a view at each process. As a result, when its attention was paid to the gaze rate to the internal organs and the surgical instrument at the time of inserting a surgical instrument and a surgical instrument was inserted, the look of unskilled operator from operating part was separated in many cases. And the look was repeated frequently between internal organs and a surgical instrument from the start of an operation before the end. Therefore, it is in the tendency to require many working hours. On the other hand, the expert is gazing at operating part in most operation processes, even if he is a time of operating the instrument, a look does not separate him from the operating part. This is the reason of shorten working hours in well trained operated case.

It became clear from this result that the working hours of an operation differ greatly by the difference in operator level of skill.

2   Experiment

2.1   Participants

Three doctors who work at department of gastroenterological surgery from Shiga University of Medical Science were selected as experts and non-expert in this study. Among of them, three doctors were divided into two groups, two experts, and one non-expert. The non-expert (female, right-handed) had six years of clinical experience with 29 years old. One of experts (male, right-handed) had fourteen years of clinical experience with 36 years old. Another expert was 47 years old (male, right-handed), who had 22 years of clinical experience.

2.2   Experimental Process

The simulative surgery of laparoscopic cholecystectomy based on a virtual reality endoscopic surgical training simulator (LapVR, manufactured Gadelius Medical Corporation) was focused on this research. The training system of virtual reality endoscopic surgical training simulator was aim to provide a training platform for laparoscopic cholecystectomy surgery and cultivate user's basic skills, such as three-dimensional space cognitive ability, eye-hand coordination ability and monitoring both hands and feet during endoscopic surgery. This system was consisted of 20 inches flat LCD monitor, haptic (tactile) devices, surgery forceps handle, and a camera. The camera illuminates the surgical location and sends a real-time picture from inside the body to the monitor, giving the surgeon a close-up view of the organs and tissues. The surgeon watches the monitor and performs the operation by manipulating the surgical instruments through the operating ports.

The characteristics of eye movement track during the whole training process were measured by eye movement measuring device with 60 Hz sampling frequency (Talk Eye, manufactured by Takei equipment Industrial Co., Ltd.). The experimental landscape of eye movement measurement was illustrated on Fig. 1.

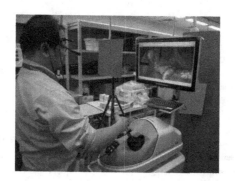

Fig. 1. Experimental landscape of eye movement measurement

2.3 Surgical Process

Laparoscopic cholecystectomy requires at least two small incisions in the abdomen to allow the insertion of operating ports, through which surgical instruments and the laparoscope camera are put into the abdominal cavity with around 30 degrees outward from patient's body (simulator).

The whole process of laparoscopic cholecystectomy surgery was divided into five steps as following:

(Step.1), Strip the cystic duct and cystic artery from the gallbladder neck.
(Step.2), Cut and clean cystic duct.
(Step.3), Cut and clean cystic artery.
(Step.4), Strip the gallbladder from the side cholecystopathy part.
(Step.5), Cleaning the operative field, (Based on procedural requirements).

Above surgical steps was the most popular procedure in the world based on clinical experience. The characteristics of working time and visual field for each step were measured in this research.

3   Results and Discussions

3.1   Results of Eye Movement

Both expert and non-expert's proportion time of gaze location during the whole process was illustrated in Fig. 2. According to Fig. 2, the gaze location focused the effective part of organs and surgical instruments were represented at black areas against time series. In case of non-expert, the gaze location was switched between organs and surgical instruments frequently during the whole surgery process. However, in case of expert, (An example of expert 2 was shown in Fig. 2), subject's gaze location didn't transform between target elements frequently.

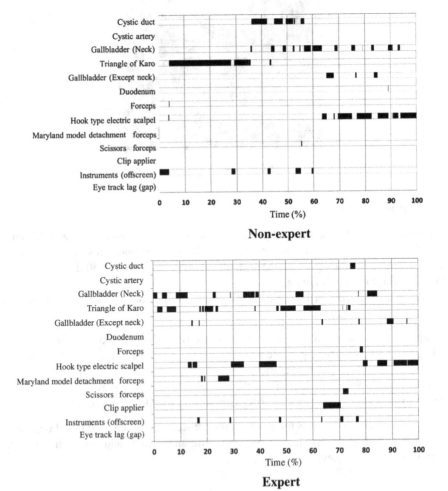

Fig. 2. Gaze location comparison between expert and non-expert

3.2   Results of Forceps Movement

The forceps movements also was summarized and presented at black areas against time series in Fig. 3. The forceps movement was defined as the moment of forceps touching organ while organ was occurring deformation according to image from eye movement's monitor.

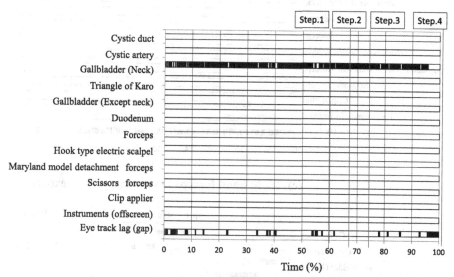

(a). Left hand forceps movement for non-expert

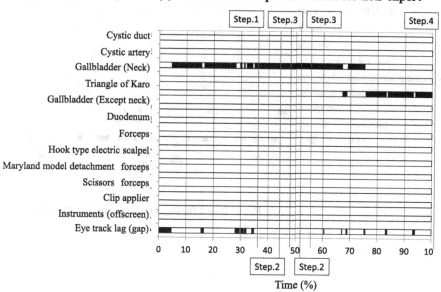

(b). Left hand forceps movement for expert

Fig. 3. (Continued)

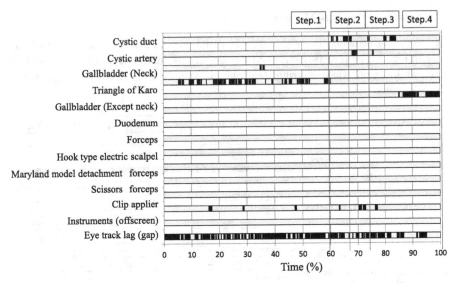

(c). Right hand forceps movement for non-expert

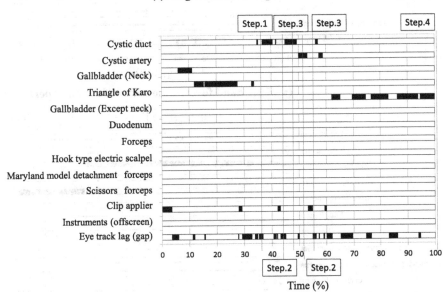

(d). Right hand forceps movement for expert

Fig. 3. Forceps movement

The Fig. 3 was shown the characteristics of the forceps movements held on left hand and right hand between non-expert and expert 2. (Fig. 3(a), Non-expert, left hand; Fig. 3(b), Expert, left hand; Fig. 3(c), Non-expert, right hand; Fig. 3(d), Expert, right hand). According to Fig. 3, normally, the gallbladder was clamped by left hand. The non-expert always clamped the gallbladder neck from step1 to step4. However, the non-expert clamped the gallbladder neck before the first half of stage4, afterwards clamped other parts of gallbladder. On the other hand, focused on right hand, the non-expert had unstable movements compared with expert. It was revealed that forceps held on right hand was always repeated or non-touch the organs during the whole process.

3.3   Collaboration Application of Eye Movement and Surgical Instrument

Additionally, the non-expert's sight always followed the surgical instruments. The eye move track focused the surgical instruments more than organs. However, eye move track of expert 2 main focused on the organs. Even eye movement track stop on organs when change surgical instruments. The expert will jump back to organs immediately.

4   Conclusions

In a word, the correct way of eye movement focused on five steps was clarified in this paper, which had a great influence on the whole process of laparoscopic cholecystectomy. The eye move way of expert can provide a reference, which had been suggested to be effective in the early learning process of laparoscopic surgery. Further work on collaboration application will comprise based on greater amounts of data of eye move track and surgical instrument movement, the achievement of training improvements in order to establish a effective teaching and learning system.

References

1. Goto, A., Takai, Y., Ota, T., Hamada, H., Tsuji, K.: Analysis of operation and eye movement concerning master of wire net. In: Proceedings of 4th International Conference on Applied Human Factors and Ergonomics, AHFE (2012)
2. Yoshida, H., Takai, Y., Goto, A., Sato, H.: Eye movement analysis of expert and non-expert on plastering Kyoto style earthen wall. In: Proceedings of 13th Japan International Sampe Symposium and Exhibition (2013)
3. Oka, Y., Oka, I., Narita, C., Takai, Y., Goto, A., Hamada, H.: Eye movement analysis and adhesive properties on the backing process of scrolls with different career craftsman. In: Proceedings of 13th Japan International Sampe Symposium and Exhibition (2013)

Formalizing the Cardiac Pacemaker Resynchronization Therapy

Neeraj Kumar Singh$^{(\boxtimes)}$, Mark Lawford, Thomas S.E. Maibaum, and Alan Wassyng

McMaster Centre for Software Certification, McMaster University, Hamilton, ON, Canada
{singhn10,lawford,wassyng}@mcmaster.ca, tom@maibaum.org

Abstract. For many years, formal methods have been used to design and develop critical systems in order to guarantee safety and security and the correctness of desired behaviours, through formal verification and validation techniques and tools. The development of high confidence medical devices such as the cardiac pacemaker, is one of the grand challenges in the area of verified software that need formal reasoning and proof-based development. This paper presents an example of how we used previous experience in developing a cardiac pacemaker using Event-B, to build an incremental proof-based development of a new pacemaker that uses Cardiac Resynchronization Therapy (CRT), also known as biventricular pacing or multisite pacing. In this work, we formalized the required behaviours of CRT including timing constraints and safety properties. We formalized the system using Event-B, and made use of the included Rodin tools to check the internal consistency with respect to safety properties, invariants and events. The system behaviours of the proven model were validated through the use of the ProB model checker.

Keywords: Pacemaker resynchronization therapy · Event-B · Refinement · Formal methods · Verification · Validation

1 Introduction

Patient safety is a global challenge that requires practical knowledge and technical skills in clinical assessments, embedded systems, and software engineering including human factors and systems engineering (HFE). Many incidents related to patient safety are due to lack of attention to HFE in the design and implementation of technologies, processes, and usability. The main objective of HFE is to improve system performance including patient safety and technology acceptance [1]. The USA Food and Drug Administration (FDA) has reported several recalls in which pacemaker and implantable cardioverter-defibrillator (ICD) failures are responsible for a large number of serious illnesses and deaths. According

Partially supported by: The Ontario Research Fund, and the National Science and Engineering Research Council of Canada.

© Springer International Publishing Switzerland 2015
V.G. Duffy (Ed.): DHM 2015, Part II, LNCS 9185, pp. 374–386, 2015.
DOI: 10.1007/978-3-319-21070-4_38

to the FDA, 17,323 devices (8834 pacemakers and 8489 ICDs) were explanted during 1990-2002, and 61 deaths (30 pacemaker patients, 31 ICD patients) were found to be due to device malfunction. The FDA found that these deaths and other adverse-events were caused by product design and engineering flaws including firmware problems [2]. Critical systems such as the pacemaker need to be better designed to provide the required level of safety and dependability.

Software plays a vital role in developing and controlling medical devices. In order to make sure that medical devices are safe, secure and reliable, regulatory agencies like the FDA, require evidence based criteria to approve these devices. Over the past twenty years, formal techniques have shown some promising results in the health care domain through identifying abnormal behaviours or possible errors by applying mathematical reasoning.

In 2003 Tony Hoare suggested a verification grand challenge for computing research. In similar vein, a real ten year-old, sanitized pacemaker specification [3] was used by the Software Quality Research Laboratory at McMaster University, to issue the *PACEMAKER Challenge* to the software engineering community. The challenge is characterized by system aspects emphasizing the development and certification of dependable and safe pacemakers, and is now managed by the McMaster Centre for Software Certification. Many researchers have worked and are working on the PACEMAKER Challenge [4], but most of them are focusing on 1-and 2-electrode pacemakers. In this paper, we demonstrate the results of our new work on the formalization of the system requirements for the *Cardiac Resynchronization Therapy (CRT)* pacemaker, or multi-site pacing pacemaker that can be used to help certify the CRT pacemaker. Our main objectives and contributions are as follows:

- To build on experience in the PACEMAKER Challenge in using Event-B to develop a CRT pacemaker;
- To further develop principles of how to use refinement in Event-B effectively, to model the required behaviour of a medical device;
- To formalize and analyze the behavioural requirements for the CRT pacemaker;
- To define a list of safety properties;
- To verify and validate the system requirements of the CRT pacemaker;
- To demonstrate how we can help to meet FDA requirements for certifying the CRT pacemaker using formal methods;

To formalize the CRT device we selected the Event-B modelling language [5], so that we could use previous experience to guide the refinement steps, and also because of the formal tools that were then available to us. Event-B supports traditional refinement in which each refinement step adds detail to existing functionality. It also supports (horizontal) refinement in which the steps add new functionality in the solution of the problem. This (horizontal) refinement allows us to develop an incremental approach to building these safety-critical medical devices. The incremental steps to use are not always obvious, and this is where previous experience plays an important role.

This incremental development preserves the required behaviour of the system in the abstract model as well as in the correctly refined models. The Event-B language is supported by the Rodin platform, which provides a rich set of provers and other supporting tools for developing the specifications. The Rodin platform helps us guarantee the preservation of safety properties. We use the ProB model checker tool [6] to analyze and validate the developed models of the CRT pacemaker.

The remainder of this paper is organized as follows. Section 2 presents preliminary information about the CRT pacemaker. The CRT pacemaker control requirements are presented in Sect. 3. Section 4 explores an incremental proof-based formal development of the CRT pacemaker. Brief discussion is provided in Sect. 5. Section 6 presents related work. Section 7 concludes the paper and presents future work.

2   Preliminaries

The cardiac pacemaker is an electronic device equipped with a microprocessor, and is designed to maintain regular heart beats. The pacemaker generally serves two main functions: *sensing* and *pacing*. Sensors are used to sense the intrinsic activities of the heart chambers, and when appropriate, actuators are used to deliver a short intensive electrical pulse into the heart chambers.

A CRT or multi-site pacing device is an advanced pacemaker that is designed to treat a specific form of heart failure – poor synchronization of the two lower heart chambers. This device sends a very low power electrical impulse to both lower chambers of the heart to help them beat together synchronously. As we said, it is an advanced pacemaker, so it carries all the functional behaviours of a simple pacemaker including these more advanced features to synchronize the lower chambers of the heart. The basic elements of a pacemaker system [7] are:

- **Leads:** A set of insulated flexible wires, used to transmit electrical impulses between the microprocessor and the heart for sensing and pacing purposes.
- **The CRT Generator:** The main unit consisting of battery and microprocessor to control the entire functionality of the system.
- **Device Controller-Monitor (DCM):** An external device that interacts with the implanted CRT using wireless for configuration and for setting new parameters.
- **Accelerometer:** A motion sensor to measure body motion to allow modulated pacing and sensing.

2.1   Event-B

Event-B [5,8] is a modelling language that enables us to formalize a system through stepwise refinement. We can thus build a complex system incrementally by introducing more detail in each refinement step, where each step is verified by generated proof obligations with respect to an abstract model. This refinement process finally culminates in a concrete implementation. The basic system modelling components are *context* and *machine*. The *context* describes static behaviour, while the *machine* describes the dynamic behaviour of the system using events. At each refinement step, the events can be refined by: (1) keeping the event as it is; (2) splitting an event into several events; or (3) refining by introducing another event to maintain state variables. Importantly, new refinement levels allow the introduction of new events. Refinement in Event-B is an essential component of the methodology. It is important to realize that many of the refinement steps in Event-B represent a decomposition of the strategy, while other refinement steps (more traditional refinement) are a decomposition of the system itself. A set of tools, the *Rodin* [8] *tools*, support model development, proof obligation generation for refinement steps and state predicates, and the discharging of generated proof obligations using automated theorem provers. Due to page limitations, we have not presented a detailed introduction to Event-B. There are numerous publications and books available for an introduction to Event-B and related refinement strategies [5,8].

3   CRT Pacemaker Control Requirements

The focus of this work is the formalization of biventricular sensing with biventricular pacing (BiSP) of CRT devices. There are various situations, where a CRT device can be used to control the heart rhythm. However, we are interested in formalizing the most complex mode (BiSP) since it also covers the other less complex modes. BiSP allows pacing and sensing in the right atrium, right ventricle, and left ventricle chambers (see Fig. 1) and this section only describes the control requirements of BiSP.

Biventricular pacing coordinates the left ventricle (LV) and right ventricle (RV), and intra-ventricular regional wall contractions. It also synchronizes pacing with the sinus rhythm sensed in the right atrium. There are various intrinsic events for LV and RV, like sensing and pacing occurrences, which can reset pacing intervals that produce several variations of the atrioventricular interval (AVI).

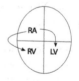

Fig. 1. Biventricular pacing.

Biventricular pacing controls the heart rate using various combinations of the timing from events in either LV or RV. For instance, the first ventricular sense either from the left or right ventricular chamber can reset the ventriculoatrial interval (VAI) and the heart rate depends on intervals between the first ventricular events in each cycle. However, heart rate intervals can vary due to stimulation in the opposite chambers.

Delays between RV and LV pacing introduce complications in biventricular timings. These timings allow multiple definitions of atrioventricular (AV) and ventriculoatrial (VA) escape intervals. The pacing rate is the sum of the VA and AV escape intervals for dual chamber timing. This definition can be preserved for biventricular timing if the VAI and AVI refer to pacing either the RV for RV-based timing or the LV for LV-based timing. Then the pacing delay can be represented by the RV-LV interval. This interval can be negative, positive or zero as per the occurrence order of the stimulations in both ventricles.

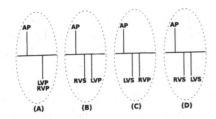
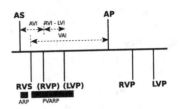

Fig. 2. Possible scenarios of the biventricular sensing and pacing. AS = atrial sensed; AP = atrial paced; LVS = left ventricular sensed; LVP = left ventricular paced; RVS = right ventricular sensed; RVP = right ventricular paced.

Fig. 3. Biventricular sensing and pacing (BiSP) with a RVS event

Figure 2 depicts the possible scenarios in a sequential order for biventricular sensing and pacing [9]. The possible scenarios are described as follows, assuming normal pacing and sensing activities in the right atrium chamber:

- **Scenario A** shows a situation in which the pacemaker paces in both ventricles after an AV interval in which no intrinsic heart activity is detected.
- **Scenario B** shows a situation in which the pacemaker paces in LV only after an AV interval, while RV pacing is inhibited due to sensing of an intrinsic activity in RV.
- **Scenario C** shows a situation in which the pacemaker paces in RV only after an AV interval, while LV pacing is inhibited due to sensing of an intrinsic activity in LV.
- **Scenario D** shows the case where pacing activities are inhibited in the ventricles due to sensing of intrinsic activities in both LV and RV.

There are various possible scenarios to show biventricular sensing and pacing in order to capture possible behavioural requirements. For example, Fig. 3 presents a scenario for biventricular sensing and pacing, in which an event sense related to the right ventricle resets all the pacing intervals for both the right and left ventricles, so pacing is not allowed in the right ventricle or in the left ventricle following a RVS, and a RVS event resets the timing cycle and starts a new VAI. Other requirements are omitted here.

4   Formal Development of CRT

Abstract Model: An abstract model of the CRT pacemaker specifies only pacing and sensing behaviour of three electrodes for each chamber (RA, RV, LV). In order to start the formalization process, we need to define some static properties of the system using Event-B context. The first context declares an enumerated set *Status* as *partition(Status, {ON}, {OFF})*. This enumerated set is used to specify the *ON* and *OFF* states of the actuators and sensors of the CRT pacemaker.

The CRT pacemaker delivers a pacing stimulus in the RA, RV, and LV as per the patient needs through sensing the intrinsic activities of the heart. The CRT is much more complex than the 1- or 2-electrode pacemaker, because the CRT pacing behaviour intelligently maintains the synchronicity between RV and LV. The Event-B model declares a list of variables for defining actuators and sensors. $PM\_Actuator\_A$, $PM\_Actuator\_LV$, and $PM\_Actuator\_RV$ are actuators for each chamber, and PM_Sensor_A, PM_Sensor_LV, and PM_Sensor_RV are sensors for each chamber, which are defined as the type of $Status$ using invariants.

At this stage the system describes only discrete functional behaviour for changing between two states (ON and OFF) without considering any timing requirements. We introduce twelve new events for specifying the pacing and sensing activities in terms of changing states. These events include a guard related to the current state of actuators and sensors, and the action changes the states of the actuators and sensors. An Event $PM\_Pacing\_On\_A$ is used to set ON for the right atrium actuator, when the right atrium actuator is OFF. Similarly, another event $PM\_Sensing\_On\_A$ is used to set ON of the right atrium sensor, when the atrium sensor is OFF. The other events are formalized in a similar way.

EVENT PM_Pacing_On_A
WHEN
    grd1 : $PM\_Actuator\_A = OFF$
THEN
    act1 : $PM\_Actuator\_A := ON$
END
	EVENT PM_Sensing_On_A
	WHEN
	    grd1 : $PM\_Sensor\_A = OFF$
	THEN
	    act1 : $PM\_Sensor\_A := ON$
	END

4.1   First Refinement: Timing Requirements

This refinement introduces the timing requirements by defining a logical clock. A list of constants are defined in a new *context* for specifying the desired timing requirements for controlling the pacing and sensing behaviours. We define four constants AVI, VAI, LVI, and RVI. The AVI allows a value within a range (50 .. 350). The VAI allows a value within a range (350 .. 1200). The RVI and LVI have similar timing intervals (0 .. 50). An extra axiom specifies that the RVI should be greater than or equal to LVI. In this study we consider all times to be in milliseconds.

A variable now is defined to represent the current clock counter in $inv1$, which progresses by 1 millisecond every clock tick. The next variable $PSRecord$ is used to store a time when a pacing or sensing activity occurs using $inv2$. The stored time can be used for deciding future pacing or sensing activity in any chamber. A few variables are defined to synchronize the pacing and sensing activities by capturing the different states of sensors and actuators for the atrium and ventricular chambers in order to define the desired behaviour.

$inv1 : now \in \mathbb{N}$
$inv2 : PSRecord \in \mathbb{N}$
$inv3 : now = 0 \Rightarrow PM\_Sensor\_RV = OFF \land PM\_Actuator\_RV = OFF$
$inv4 : now = 0 \Rightarrow PM\_Sensor\_LV = OFF \land PM\_Actuator\_LV = OFF$
$inv5 : now = 0 \Rightarrow PM\_Sensor\_A = OFF \land PM\_Actuator\_A = OFF$
$inv6 : PM\_Actuator\_RV = ON \Rightarrow now \geq AVI \lor Immd\_Pace\_RV = 1$
$inv7 : PM\_Actuator\_LV = ON \Rightarrow$
$\quad now \geq AVI + (RVI - LVI) \lor Immd\_Pace\_LV = 1 \lor Delay\_Pace\_LV = 1$
$inv8 : PM\_Actuator\_A = ON \Rightarrow$
$\quad now \geq PSRecord + VAI \lor now \geq AVI + VAI$

A list of safety properties can then be introduced using invariants. Invariants ($inv3$, $inv4$, and $inv5$) state that when the current clock counter is zero then all the actuators and sensors are OFF. It means, the sensor and actuator of each chamber should be OFF at the beginning of the pacing cycle. The next safety property $inv6$ states that the actuator of the right ventricle must pace when the AVI is elapsed or an immediate pacing is required. The next safety property $inv7$ shows that the actuator of the left ventricle must pace when the total duration of the atrioventricular interval and pacing delay is elapsed, an immediate pacing is required, or a delay pacing is detected in the left ventricle. The last safety property $inv8$ states that the actuator of the right atrium must pace when the VAI is elapsed after detecting the last pacing or sensing activity, or the total duration of AVI and VAI is elapsed.

```
EVENT PM_Pacing_On_A Refines PM_Pacing_On_A
  WHEN
    grd1 : PM_Actuator_A = OFF
    grd2 : (now = AVI + VAI ∧ No_Pace_LV_RV = 0 ∧ Delay_Pace_LV = 0)
           ∨
           (now = PSRecord + VAI ∧ (Delay_Pace_LV = 2 ∨ Delay_Pace_LV = 1∨
           No_Pace_LV_RV = 1 ∨ RV_Delay_AVI = 1 ∨ Immd_Pace_RV = 1
           ∨Immd_Pace_LV = 1))
    grd3 : PM_Sensor_A = OFF
    grd4 : Pace_A = 0
  THEN
    act1 : PM_Actuator_A := ON
    act2 : Pace_A := 1
  END
```

In this refinement, we introduced several new events to specify the desired behaviour of actuators and sensors according to the given timing requirements. The complete formal specification can produce an algorithm for implementation purpose. There are eighteen events in total, in which seventeen events refine the events of the abstract model. For example, the event $PM\_Pacing\_On\_A$ refines the abstract event $PM\_Pacing\_-On\_A$ by adding new guards and adding a new action.

The pacing and sensing events update a state every millisecond. We model this increment by a new event tic, that increments time by 1 ms. The event tic progressively increases the current clock counter now. The event tic has no guard in this

```
EVENT tic
  WHEN
  THEN
    act1 : now := now + 1
  END
```

refinement, but in further refinements, we introduce a guard to control the pacing and sensing activities within restricted time intervals.

4.2   Second Refinement: Threshold

An intrinsic activity of a chamber can be sensed by using the inbuilt sensor of an electrode. The pacemaker can deliver stimulation to the heart chamber based on monitored values and according to the selected safety margin. Each chamber of the heart contains a range of standard threshold values that can be pre-specified by a physiologist[1] for comparing with monitored values to detect the intrinsic

---

[1] Standard threshold constant values of atria and ventricular chambers are different.

activities. A set of constants (STA_THR_A, STA_THR_LV, STA_THR_RV) is defined to hold a range of standard threshold values for each chamber.

The pacemaker sensor starts sensing intrinsic activities during certain intervals to avoid sensing errors. A pacemaker actuator delivers a small intense electric pulse whenever the natural pace is absent and intrinsic activity is not detected by the sensor. A sensor can detect an intrinsic activity when the threshold value of the detected signal is greater than or equal to the standard threshold constant. In this refinement, we introduce the threshold for right atrium, left ventricle and right ventricle. An invariant ($inv1$) is defined for the right atrium, right ventricle and left ventricle to indicate the boolean states for synchronization purpose to maintain the order of sensing activities in the right atrium and both right and left ventricles. Three safety properties are introduced using invariants ($inv2$, $inv3$ and $inv4$) that state the sensor of each chamber is OFF when the detected sensor value is greater than or equal to the standard threshold value and boolean state of the chamber is TRUE.

---

inv1 : $Thr\_State\_A \in BOOL \wedge Thr\_State\_LV \in BOOL \wedge Thr\_State\_RV \in BOOL$
inv2 : $\forall i \cdot i \in \mathbb{N}_1 \wedge i \geq STA\_THR\_A \wedge Thr\_State\_A = TRUE \Rightarrow PM\_Sensor\_A = OFF$
inv3 : $\forall i \cdot i \in \mathbb{N}_1 \wedge i \geq STA\_THR\_LV \wedge Thr\_State\_LV = TRUE \Rightarrow PM\_Sensor\_LV = OFF$
inv4 : $\forall i \cdot i \in \mathbb{N}_1 \wedge i \geq STA\_THR\_RV \wedge Thr\_State\_RV = TRUE \Rightarrow PM\_Sensor\_RV = OFF$

This refinement step enriches the previously defined events through strengthening guards without introducing any new events. The new added guards are used to acquire the intrinsic activity by comparing the sensed threshold value with a standard threshold value for all chambers (right atrium, right ventricle, and left ventricle).

```
EVENT PM_Sensing_Off_A Refines
        PM_Sensing_Off_A
ANY Thr_A
  WHERE
    grd1 : PM_Sensor_A = ON
    grd2 : PM_Sensor_RV = OFF
    grd3 : PM_Actuator_A = OFF
    grd4 : PM_Actuator_RV = OFF
    grd5 : PM_Sensor_LV = OFF
    grd6 : PM_Actuator_LV = OFF
    grd7 : Thr_A ∈ N
    grd8 : Thr_A ≥ STA_THR_A
  THEN
    act1 : PM_Sensor_A := OFF
    act2 : PS Record := 0
    act3 : now := 0
  END
```

For example, the event $PM\_Sensing\_Off\_A$, refinement of an abstract event, is strengthened by introducing a new variable Thr_A and guards ($grd7$, $grd8$). The guard ($grd7$) defines the type of variable (Thr_A), while the next guard ($grd8$) compares the threshold value with the standard threshold value of the right atrium. The new introduced guards allow to monitor an activity of the right atrium by comparing a sensed value with the selected standard threshold value of the atrial chamber. We have modified several other events in similar fashion to model the desired behaviour of sensors.

4.3   Third Refinement: Refractory and Blanking Periods

This refinement introduces refractory and blanking periods[2] for atrial and ventricular chambers. These blanking and refractory periods are used to suppress device-generated artifacts and unwanted signal artifacts. These periods are designed to

---

[2] https://www.bostonscientific.com/content/dam/bostonscientific/quality/education-resources/english/ACL_Cross-Chamber_Blanking_20081219.pdf.

promote appropriate sensing of intrinsic activities, and to prevent over sensing activities in another chamber. In this refinement, we define eight constants Atrial Refractory Period (ARP), Right Ventricular Refractory Period (RVRP), Left Ventricular Refractory Period (LVRP), Post Ventricular Atrial Refractory Period (PVARP), Right Ventricular Blanking Period (RVBP), Left Ventricular Blanking Period (LVBP), A-Blank after Right Ventricular Activity (ABaRV), and A-Blank after Left Ventricular Activity (ABaLV).

We introduce six new safety properties using invariants ($inv1$ - $inv6$). The first two safety properties state that during the refractory periods and blanking periods, the sensor and actuator must be OFF, and these sensor and actuator can be ON only after the refractory and blanking periods are elapsed. To check the refractory period after pacing or sensing activity, we need to store the time of pacing or sensing activity of ventricular chambers. We use a variable $PSRecord$ for this. The next four safety properties state that sensing and pacing of both ventricular chambers can occur only after blanking periods and refractory periods. Here we do not need an additional variable because after pacing or sensing in the atrial chamber, the clock resets.

$$
\begin{aligned}
inv1 : \ & PM\_Actuator\_A = ON \Rightarrow now \geq PSRecord + PVARP \wedge \\
& now \geq PSRecord + RVRP \wedge now \geq PSRecord + LVRP \wedge \\
& now \geq PSRecord + ABaLV \wedge now \geq PSRecord + ABaRV \\
inv2 : \ & PM\_Sensor\_A = ON \Rightarrow now \geq PSRecord + PVARP \wedge \\
& now \geq PSRecord + RVRP \wedge now \geq PSRecord + LVRP \\
& \wedge now \geq PSRecord + ABaLV \wedge now \geq PSRecord + ABaRV \\
inv3 : \ & PM\_Actuator\_RV = ON \Rightarrow now \geq ARP \wedge now \geq RVBP \\
inv4 : \ & PM\_Actuator\_LV = ON \Rightarrow now \geq ARP \wedge now \geq LVBP \\
inv5 : \ & PM\_Sensor\_RV = ON \Rightarrow now \geq ARP \wedge now \geq RVBP \\
inv6 : \ & PM\_Sensor\_LV = ON \Rightarrow now \geq ARP \wedge now \geq LVBP
\end{aligned}
$$

In this refinement we introduce a new guard in the event tic to formalize the guard conditions that progress the current time (now), and to model the desired system behaviours of sensing and pacing activities correctly. The provided guard synchronizes all pacing and sensing activities by considering intrinsic activities of pacing and sensing according to the BiSP. We do not have space to show the complete timing requirements as the guard conditions of tic event, but as an example we present that portion that shows the progress of tic corresponding to Fig. 3.

```
EVENT tic
  WHEN
    grd1: (now < AVI ∧ PM_Sensor_LV = OFF ∧ PM_Sensor_RV = OFF∧
          No_Pace_LV_RV = 1)
          ∨
          (now ≥ AVI ∧ now < PSRecord + PVARP ∧ PM_Sensor_LV = OFF∧
          PM_Sensor_RV = OFF ∧ No_Pace_LV_RV = 1∧
          (Pace_RV = 2 ∨ Thr_State_RV = TRUE))
          ∨
          (now ≥ PSRecord + PVARP ∧ now < PSRecord + VAI ∧ PM_Sensor_LV = OFF∧
          PM_Sensor_RV = OFF ∧ No_Pace_LV_RV = 1 ∧ PM_Sensor_A = ON)
          ∨
          . . .

          . . .
  THEN
    act1 : now := now + 1
  END
```

4.4   Model Validation and Analysis

In this section, we present the proof statistics by presenting detailed information about generated proof obligations, and validity of the models using ProB [6]. Validation refers to gaining confidence that the developed models are consistent with requirements.

Table 1. Proof Statistics

Model	Total number of POs	Automatic Proof	Interactive Proof
Abstract Model	0	0(0%)	0(0%)
First Refinement	102	101(99%)	1(1%)
Second Refinement	23	23(100%)	0(0%)
Third Refinement	59	57(98%)	2(2%)
Total	184	181(98.37%)	3(1.63%)

Event-B supports two types of validation activities namely *consistency checking* and *model analysis*. Consistency checking shows that a list of events preserves the given invariants, and refinement checking makes sure that one machine is a valid refinement of previous machines. Model analysis is done with the help of ProB, which explores traces of Event-B models. The ProB tool supports *automated consistency checking* and *constraint-based checking*. ProB may help to find possible deadlocks or hidden properties that may not be expressed by generated proof obligations. In our work, ProB animation helps to identify the desired behaviour of the CRT pacemaker in different scenarios and validates the developed formal models. This tool assists us in finding potential problems, and to improve the guard predicates of events. The ProB model checker was able to animate all the possible machines from abstract to concrete level, and to prove the absence of errors (no counter example exist). It should be noted that ProB uses all the described safety properties during model checking process to report any violation of safety properties against the formalized system behaviour. Table 1 shows the proof statistics of the development in the RODIN tool. This development results in 184(100 %) proof obligations, in which 181(98.37 %) are proved automatically, and the remaining 3(1.63 %) are proved interactively using the Rodin prover. These proofs are quite simple, and can be achieved with the help of simplifying predicates.

5   Discussion

Stepwise refinement played an important role in our effort to develop a CRT pacemaker. Stepwise refinement in various forms has long been a suggested approach in the development of dependable systems, and was championed by Harlan Mills in his work on Box-Structures [10]. As mentioned earlier, refinement is a core concept in Event-B development. Of interest to practitioners is how we decide on what to introduce in each new refinement. There may be no universally 'correct' pattern to follow. However, building on experience with earlier development of pacemaker models we chose the order of: (1) Introduce all possible hardware elements at the abstract level like actuators and sensors; (2) Introduce a clock; (3) Include thresholds; and (4) Include refractory and blanking periods by introducing a guard on the clock.

We have designed our CRT pacemaker using a *correct by construction* approach. We described the system requirements using set theoretical notations abstractly, that can be further refined incrementally to reach a concrete level similar to code. Event-B has very good tool support that allows us to prove given properties (mostly) automatically. Other formal modelling tools like VDM, Z, Alloy can be used in place of the Event-B modelling language without considering refinement notions. However, Simulink and SLDV modelling techniques cannot be used in place of these formal modelling languages, because Simulink and SLDV do not allow us to build a system abstractly. The developed formal model contains all the possible ranges for each constant and variable used in describing the system behaviour, so the Event-B concrete model can be used for different implementation purposes. Therefore we can use the concrete Event-B models of the CRT pacemaker for implementing an actual system considering hardware requirements using Simulink and SLDV. The tool support of Simulink and SLDV can help guarantee a correct implementation.

As far as we know, there are no published formal system requirements for the CRT pacemaker, but several research publications and clinical books provide informal requirements and discussion on clinical practices. We used such informal descriptions as a basis for this work. We also identified a list of safety properties in the refinement process to verify the correctness of overall formalized system behaviour, including newly introduced features. These safety properties guarantee that all possible executions of the system are safe, if the generated proof obligations are successfully discharged – and if we our list of safety properties is correct and complete. We have considered only the main safety properties (see all invariants) related to actuators and sensors under timing requirements. We can introduce additional safety properties in further refinements which may or may not include new features.

6   Related Work

The pacemaker has been formalized by several researchers around the world. There is a distributed real-time model of the pacemaker formalized in VDM by Macedo et al. [11], in which they addressed selected behaviour of the pacemaker. Gomes et al. [12] formalized the sequential model of the pacemaker using Z, and then they used Perfect Developer tool to produce source code. In [13], authors used the dual chamber implantable pacemaker as a case study for modelling and verification of control algorithms for medical devices in UPPAAL. Tuan et al. [14] designed a real-time model of the pacemaker using CSP, and the developed model was verified by a model checker Process Analysis Toolkit (PAT) in order to verify system properties. A detailed formalization of the one- and two-electrode pacemaker was presented in [15,16], where the models were developed in an incremental way using refinements in the Event-B modelling language. In this work, the authors developed operating modes considering advanced features like *threshold*, *hysteresis* and *rate adaptive*. A closed-loop model of the pacemaker and heart was presented in [15,17]. Méry et al. used EB2ALL [15,18] to generate executable source code from the pacemaker specification in multiple programming languages.

7 Conclusion and Future Challenges

The CRT pacemaker is a complex medical device for sensing and pacing in the heart chambers. An actuator delivers a brief electrical stimulus when there is an absence of intrinsic heart activity within a bounded time interval, and the sensing and pacing activities of each chamber are synchronized so that the heart functions as normally as possible. Timing requirements are crucial to building a correct and effective model for the CRT pacemaker. However, the timing requirements for this sensing and pacing are extremely complex to analyze manually. Our proposed refinement based formal development of the CRT pacemaker captures what we think are the essential requirements, and enables us to verify that the model complies with the primary safety properties we derived. In the future we intend to augment these safety properties.

This paper presents a formal development of a CRT pacemaker using incremental refinement. As far as we know, this is the first formal model of the CRT pacemaker to analyze that the functional behaviour complies with its safety requirements. We used the Event-B modelling language, together with its associated tools, to develop the proof-based formal model using a refinement technique. Our incremental development reflects not only the many facets of the problem, but also that there is a learning process involved in understanding the problem and its ultimate possible solutions.

This formal model (or rather, future refinements of it) can be used to help certify CRT or multisite pacing devices. Our goal is to integrate formal models of CRT pacemakers and the heart, to model the closed-loop system for verifying the desired behaviour under relevant safety properties, and be able to guarantee the correctness of the functional behaviour of the CRT. We also intend to implement a CRT algorithm for a hardware platform by generating source code using EB2ALL from the formal model.

This work not only delivers a formal model of the CRT pacemaker, it builds on previous Event-B development of the 2-electrode pacemaker as described in the PACEMAKER Challenge. This is important because as we use the same technology/methodology to develop related medical devices we can begin to see principles for how to use that methodology so that development is more efficient. In our case, one of the principles we are starting to understand better is how to use stepwise refinement (in the Event-B sense) to build the requirements model.

Finally, whatever system we use to model the behaviour, the safety and dependability of the device depends on the *correctness* of our requirements model. We believe that we can use Event-B tools to validate these requirements with the help of clinical specialists, and correct any mistakes we may have in the current model.

References

1. Carayon, P., Wood, K.E.: Patient safety. Inf. Knowl. Syst. Manage. **8**(1–4), 23–46 (2009)
2. Maisel, W.H., Moynahan, M., Zuckerman, B.D., Gross, T.P., Tovar, O.H., Tillman, D.B., Schultz, D.B.: Pacemaker and ICD generator malfunctions: Analysis of food and drug administration annual reports. JAMA **295**(16), 1901–1906 (2006)
3. Boston scientific: pacemaker system specification. Technical report (2007). http://www.cas.mcmaster.ca/sqrl/SQRLDocuments/PACEMAKER.pdf
4. Dagstuhl seminar 14062: The pacemaker challenge: developing certifiable medical devices (2014)
5. Abrial, J.R.: Modeling in Event-B: System and Software Engineering, 1st edn. Cambridge University Press, New York (2010)
6. Leuschel, M., Butler, M.: ProB: A model checker for B. In: Araki, K., Gnesi, S., Mandrioli, D. (eds.) FME 2003. LNCS, vol. 2805, pp. 855–874. Springer, Heidelberg (2003)
7. Barold, S.S., Stroobandt, R.X., Sinnaeve, A.F.: Cardiac Pacemakers Step by Step. Futura Publishing (2004). ISBN 1-4051-1647-1
8. Project RODIN: Rigorous open development environment for complex systems (2004). http://rodin-b-sharp.sourceforge.net/
9. Wang, P., Kramer, A., Mark Estes, N.A., Hayes, D.L.: Timing cycles for biventricular pacing. Pacing Clin. Electrophysiol. **25**, 62–75 (2002)
10. Mills, H.D.: Stepwise refinement and verification in box-structured systems. IEEE Comput. **21**(6), 23–36 (1988)
11. Macedo, H.D., Larsen, P.G., Fitzgerald, J.S.: Incremental development of a distributed real-time model of a cardiac pacing system using VDM. In: Cuellar, J., Sere, K. (eds.) FM 2008. LNCS, vol. 5014, pp. 181–197. Springer, Heidelberg (2008)
12. Gomes, A.O., Oliveira, M.V.M.: Formal Specification of a cardiac pacing system. In: Cavalcanti, A., Dams, D.R. (eds.) FM 2009. LNCS, vol. 5850, pp. 692–707. Springer, Heidelberg (2009)
13. Jiang, Z., Pajic, M., Moarref, S., Alur, R., Mangharam, R.: Modeling and verification of a dual chamber implantable pacemaker. In: Flanagan, C., König, B. (eds.) TACAS 2012. LNCS, vol. 7214, pp. 188–203. Springer, Heidelberg (2012)
14. Tuan, L.A., Zheng, M.C., Tho, Q.T.: Modeling and verification of safety critical systems: A case study on pacemaker. In: Secure System Integration and Reliability Improvement, june 2010, pp. 23–32 (2010)
15. Singh, N.K.: Using Event-B for Critical Device Software Systems. Springer GmbH, London (2013)
16. Méry, D., Singh, N.K.: Functional behavior of a cardiac pacing system. Int. J. Discrete Event Control Syst. **1**(2), 129–149 (2011)
17. Méry, D., Singh, N.K.: Formalization of Heart Models Based on the Conduction of Electrical Impulses and Cellular Automata. In: Liu, Z., Wassyng, A. (eds.) FHIES 2011. LNCS, vol. 7151, pp. 140–159. Springer, Heidelberg (2012)
18. Méry, D., Singh, N.K.: Automatic code generation from Event-B models. In: Proceedings of the Second Symposium on Information and Communication Technology, SoICT 2011, pp. 179–188. ACM, New York (2011)

Stepwise Formal Modelling and Reasoning of Insulin Infusion Pump Requirements

Neeraj Kumar Singh[1]([⊠]), Hao Wang[2], Mark Lawford[1], Thomas S.E. Maibaum[1], and Alan Wassyng[1]

[1] McMaster Centre for Software Certification, McMaster University, Hamilton, Canada
{singhn10,lawford,wassyng}@mcmaster.ca, tom@maibaum.org
[2] Faculty of Engineering and Natural Sciences, Aalesund University College, Alesund, Norway
hawa@hials.no

Abstract. An insulin infusion pump (IIP) is a critical software-intensive medical device that infuses insulin satisfying patient needs under safety and timing constraints that are appropriate for the treatment of diabetes. This device is used by millions of people around the world. The USA Food and Drug Administration (FDA) has reported several recalls in which IIP failures were responsible for a large number of serious illnesses and deaths. The failures responsible for this harm to people who are dependent on external insulin were caused by the introduction of hardware or software design errors during the system development process. This paper presents an incremental proof-based development of an IIP. We use the Event-B modelling language to formalize the given system requirements. Further, the Rodin proof tools are used to verify the correctness of functional behaviour, internal consistency checking with respect to safety properties, invariants and events.

Keywords: Insulin Infusion Pump (IIP) · Event-B · Refinement · Formal methods · Verification · Validation

1 Introduction

Patient safety is a major concern and an always challenging goal in the design and manufacture of medical devices. It requires knowledge and skill in both the medical and engineering domains, especially in human factors and systems engineering (HFE). The main reasons for recalls related to medical systems are the lack of attention to HFE in the design and implementation of technologies, processes, and usability. The primary use of HFE is to enhance system performance, including patient safety and technology acceptance [1].

An insulin pump is a small, complex, safety-critical software-intensive medical device that allows controllable continuous subcutaneous infusion of insulin to patients for diabetes treatment. This device is used by millions of people around the world. The

Partially supported by: The Ontario Research Fund, and the National Science and Engineering Research Council of Canada.

V.G. Duffy (Ed.): DHM 2015, Part II, LNCS 9185, pp. 387–398, 2015.
DOI: 10.1007/978-3-319-21070-4_39

safety of IIPs has been a major concern in health care for a number of years. The USA Food and Drug Administration (FDA) has reported several recalls in which IIP failures are responsible for a large number of serious illnesses and deaths. According to the FDA, 17000 adverse-events were reported during 2006–2009, where 41 deaths were found to be due to malfunctioning IIPs. The FDA found that these deaths and adverse-events were caused by product design and engineering flaws including firmware problems [2,3].

Formal methods can, and should play a significant role in verifying the system requirements, and in guaranteeing the correctness, reliability and safety of developed system software. Since software plays an important role in the medical domain, regulatory agencies, like the FDA, need effective means to evaluate the software embedded in the devices in order to certify the developed systems, and to assure the safe behaviour of each system [2,4–6]. Regulatory agencies are striving for rigorous techniques and methods to provide safety assurance. Many people believe that formal methods have the potential to develop dependable, safe and secure systems that are also more amenable to certification with required features that can be used to certify dependable medical systems [6–9]. We also note that many formal techniques need to be much better targeted at practical software development and certification than they seem to be at present [10].

This paper contributes to the formalization and verification of an IIP using incremental refinement in Event-B [11]. We previously formalized pacemakers using Event-B [8], and this work now helps us to formulate more general strategies for developing medical devices using formal techniques. It should be noted that in the pacemaker case study, we investigated only a refinement strategy that was used to formalize required behaviours and operating modes incrementally by adding various safety properties. In the IIP case study, we are verifying functional behaviours including various system operations, which are required to maintain insulin delivery, user profile management, and the calculation of required insulin. The complete formal development builds incrementally-refined models of IIP formalizing the required functional behaviour by preserving its required safety properties. The primary use of the models is to assist in the construction, clarification, and validation of the IIP requirements. We use the Rodin [12] tool to develop the formal models. This tool provides an Event-B integrated development environment, automated proof strategies, model checking and code generation.

The remainder of this paper is organized as follows. Section 2 presents related work. Section 3 gives preliminary information about an IIP including informal system requirements. The modelling framework is presented in Sect. 4. Section 5 explores an incremental proof-based formal development of an IIP. Section 6 concludes the paper along with an indication of our intended future work.

2   Related Work

Masci et al. [13] presented the model-based development of user interface behaviour of an infusion pump in the Prototype Verification System (PVS). The developed model was verified against relevant safety requirements provided by the FDA. Finally, the PVS code generator was used to produce executable code from the verified specifications.

In [14], a prototype of the Generic Patient-Controlled Analgesic (GPCA) infusion pump controller was formalized using the UPPAAL model checker, and then this model was used to generate platform-independent C code. In [15], Structured Object-Oriented Formal Language (SOFL), a formal software engineering method was applied to develop a prototype of an insulin pump, in which the prime motivation was to use SOFL's data-driven, comprehensible, graphical notations for describing the specifications. A generic model for an IIP was developed in the Event-B modelling language to verify the safety requirements related to timing issues [16]. An insulin pump has been used as a case study in [17] for formalizing system behaviours using the Z modelling language.

3   The Insulin Infusion Pump

An insulin pump is a small, complex, software-intensive medical device that allows controllable, continuous subcutaneous infusion of insulin to patients. It delivers physiological amounts of insulin between meals and at meal times. An insulin pump consists of the physical pump mechanism, a disposable reservoir, and a disposable infusion set. The pump system includes a controller, and a battery. The disposable infusion set includes a cannula for subcutaneous insertion, and a tubing system to interface the insulin reservoir to the cannula. At present, open-loop and closed-loop insulin pumps exist. A closed-loop insulin pump is also known as an *artificial pancreas*, which automatically monitors and controls the blood glucose level of a patient. For an open-loop insulin pump, patients need to monitor the blood glucose level manually. An insulin pump can be programmed to release small doses of insulin continuously (basal), or one shot dose (bolus) before a meal, to control the rise in blood glucose.

3.1   Informal IIP Requirements

In this section, we describe briefly the high-level informal functional system requirements of an IIP, that forms the basis of our formal model described in Sect. 5. As far as we know, there are no published system requirements for an IIP, but several research publications provide informal requirements [13, 14, 16]. We used such informal descriptions as a basis for this work to identifying the system requirements by applying *use case* and *hazard analysis*. These system requirements focus on the functional behaviour of an IIP without addressing design requirements, and human computer interaction (HCI) requirements. Our prime objective is to use formal methods to check consistency and required safety properties of the IIP requirements. The informal IIP requirements are described as follows:

REQ1: *The device must suspend all active basal delivery or bolus deliver during pump refilling and in the case of system failure.*

REQ2: *The device must undergo a power-on-self-test (POST) whenever device power is turned on.*

REQ3: *The device shall allow the user to manage system functionalities related to: stopping insulin delivery; validating basal profiles parameters; reminder management; and validating bolus preset parameters.*

REQ4: *The device shall allow the user to define a basal profile that consists of an ordered set of basal rates, ordered over a 24 hour day, as well as a temporary basal,* *that consists of a basal rate for a specified duration of time within a 24 hour day.*

REQ5: *The device can contain several basal profiles, but only one basal profile can be active at any single point in time.*

REQ6: *The device must allow the user to override an active basal profile with a temporary basal, without changing the existing basal profile.*

REQ7: *The device shall resume the active basal profile after the temporary basal terminates.*

REQ8: *The device shall enforce a maximum dosage for the normal bolus or extended bolus.*

REQ9: *The user shall be able to stop the active normal or extended bolus.*

REQ10: *The device must maintain an electronic log of every operation associated with an user alert, such as an audio alarm.*

REQ11: *The device shall maintain a history of basal and bolus dosages over the past n days. The n always differs among brands, though most store up to 90 days of data.*

REQ12: *The device shall enable the user to create a food database that can be used to store food or meal descriptions and the carbs associated with them.*

REQ13: *The device shall allow to the user to change parameter setting basal profile, bolus preset, and temporary basal.*

REQ14: *The device shall provide feedback to the user regarding system and delivery status.*

4   The Modelling Framework

In this section, we summarize the Event-B modelling language [11]. The Event-B language has two main components: *context* and *machine*. A *context* describes the static structure of a system, namely *carrier sets* and *constants* together with *axioms* and *theorems* stating their properties. A *machine* defines the dynamic structure of a system, namely *variables, invariants, theorems, variants* and *events*. Terms like *refines, extends*, and *sees* are used to describe the relation between components of Event-B models. Events are used in a *machine* to modify state variables by providing appropriate *guards*.

4.1   Modelling Actions over States

The event-driven approach of Event-B is borrowed from the B language. An Event-B model is characterized by a list of *state variables* possibly modified by a list of *events*. An invariant $I(x)$ expresses required safety properties that must be satisfied by the variable x during the activation of events. An event is a state transition in a dynamic system that contains *guard(s)* and *action(s)*. A *guard*, predicate built on the state variables, is a necessary condition for enabling an event. An *action* is a generalized substitution that describes the ways one or several state variables are modified by the occurrence of an event. There are three ways to define an event e. The first is BEGIN $x : |(P(x, x')$ END, where the *action* is not guarded and the action is always enabled. The second is WHEN $G(x)$ THEN $x : |(Q(x, x'))$ END, where the *action* is guarded by G, and the *guard* must be satisfied to enable the *action*. The last is ANY t WHERE $G(t,x)$ THEN $x : |(R(x,x',t))$ END, where the *action* is guarded by G that now depends on the local state variable t for describing non-deterministic events.

The proof obligations (POs) are generated by the Rodin platform [12]. Event-B supports several kinds of POs like invariant preservation, non-deterministic action feasibility, guard strengthening in refinements, simulation, variant, well-definedness etc. Invariant preservation (INV1 and INV2) ensures that each invariant is preserved by each event; non-deterministic action feasibility (FIS) shows the feasibility of the event e with respect to the invariant I; guard strengthening in a refinement ensures that the concrete guards in the refining event are stronger than the abstract ones; simulation ensures that each action in a concrete event simulates the corresponding abstract action; variant ensures that each convergent event decreases the proposed numeric variant; and well-definedness ensures that each axiom, theorem, invariant, guard, action, or variant is well-defined.

$$
\begin{aligned}
&INV1 : Init(x) \Rightarrow I(x) \\
&INV2 : I(x) \;\wedge\; BA(e)(x,x') \Rightarrow I(x') \\
&FIS \;\; : I(x) \;\wedge\; Grd(e)(x) \Rightarrow \exists y.BA(e)(x,y)
\end{aligned}
$$

4.2 Model Refinement

A model can be refined to introduce new features or more concrete behaviour of a system. The Event-B modelling language supports a stepwise refinement technique to model a complex system. The refinement enables us to model a system gradually and provides a way to strengthen invariants thereby introducing more detailed behaviour of the system. This refinement approach transforms an abstract model to a more concrete version by modifying the state description. The refinement process extends a list of state variables (possibly suppressing some of them) by refining each abstract event to a corresponding concrete version, or by adding new events. These refinements preserve the relation between an abstract model and its corresponding concrete model, while introducing new events and variables to specify more concrete behaviour of the system. The abstract and concrete state variables are linked by *gluing invariants*. The generated POs ensure that each abstract event is correctly refined by its concrete version. For instance, an abstract model AM with state variable x and invariant $I(x)$ is refined by a concrete model CM with variable y and gluing invariant $J(x,y)$. e and f are events of the abstract model AM and concrete model CM respectively. Event f refines event e. $BA(e)(x,x')$ and $BA(f)(y,y')$ are predicates of events e and f respectively. This refinement relation generates the following PO:

$$
I(x) \;\wedge\; J(x,y) \;\wedge\; BA(f)(y,y') \Rightarrow \exists x' \cdot (BA(e)(x,x') \;\wedge\; J(x',y'))
$$

The new events introduced in a refinement step are viewed as hidden events, that are not visible to the environment of the system being modelled. These introduced events are outside the control of the environment. Newly introduced events refine *skip* and are not observable in the abstract model. Any number of executions of an internal action may occur in between each execution of a visible action. This refinement relation generates the following PO:

$$I(x) \; \wedge \; J(x,y) \; \wedge \; BA(f)(y,y') \; \Rightarrow \; J(x,y')$$

The refined model reduces the degree of non-determinism by strengthening the guards and/or predicates. The refinement of an event e by an event f means that the event f simulates the event e, which guarantees that the set of traces of the refined model contains (up to stuttering) the traces of the resulting model. The Rodin platform provides rich tool support for model development using the Event-B language. The tool support includes project management, model development, proof assistance, model checking, animation and automatic code generation.

5 Formalizing the Insulin Infusion Pump

To cope with the inherent complexity of an IIP, we will use the stepwise refinement approach mentioned in Sect. 4. In our work, we will use this stepwise incremental approach to specify the IIP requirements by introducing new safety properties at each refinement level. The complete development of the IIP using this approach, required eight phases (the initial abstract model followed by seven refinement steps): power status (initial abstract model); basal profile management; temporary basal profile management; bolus preset management; bolus delivery; reminder management; and insulin output calculator. It should be noted that there is no specific order required in which to apply the refinements. Any order can be chosen after developing the initial abstract model. The abstract model can be further refined by introducing new components, enriching the existing behaviours or strengthening the guards.

Since the length of this paper is limited to 12 pages, we only include a brief description of the model development and refinements. We invite readers to use a detailed version of this work [18] to understand the formal development and related refinements of the case study including formally proved Event-B models.

5.1 Abstract Model: Power Status

An abstract model of an IIP specifies only power status and related functionality that controls the power status, i.e. turning *on/off* the system (REQ2). In order to start the formalization process, we need to define static properties of the system. An Event-B context declares three enumerated sets *e_pwrStatus*, *e_basicResp*, and *e_postResult* defined using axioms ($axm1$ - $axm3$) for power status.

$axm1 : partition(e\_pwrStatus, \{Standby\_pwrStatus\}, \{POST\_pwrStatus\},$
$\qquad \{Ready\_pwrStatus\}, \{OffReq\_pwrStatus\})$
$axm2 : partition(e\_basicResp, \{Accept\_basicResp\}, \{Cancel\_basicResp\})$
$axm3 : partition(e\_postResult, \{Pass\_postResult\}, \{Fail\_postResult\})$

An abstract model declares a list of variables defined by invariants ($inv1$ - $inv5$). A variable *POST_Res* is used to state the result of *power-on-self-test (POST)*, where the result 'pass' ($Pass\_postResult$) means system is safe to turn *on*, and the result 'fail' ($Fail\_postResult$) means system is unsafe to start. The next variable *post_completed* is used to show successful completion of POST of an IIP.

The variable *c_pwrStatus* shows the current power status of the system. The variable *M_pwrReq* is used to model a request for power *on/off* from the user, and the last variable *M_pwrResp* is used for modelling user responses to system prompts.

$inv1 : POST\_Res \in e\_postResult$
$inv2 : post\_completed \in BOOL$
$inv3 : c\_pwrStatus \in e\_pwrStatus$
$inv4 : M\_pwrReq\_A \in BOOL$
$inv5 : M\_pwrResp \in e\_basicResp$

We introduce 10 events for specifying the desired functional behaviour for controlling the power status of an IIP. These events include guard(s) for enabling the given action(s), and the actions that define the changes to the states of the power status (*c_pwrStatus*) and power-on-self-test (*POST_Res*). Here, we provide only two events related to the power status and power-on-self-test in order to demonstrate the basic formalization process. An event *POST_Completed* is used to assign pass result (*Pass_postResult*) to *POST_Res*, when *post_completed* is *TRUE*. Similarly, another event *PowerStatus1* is used to set $POST\_pwr - Staus$ to *c_pwrStatus*, when power status is *standby*, and there exists a power request from the user. The remaining events are formalized in a similar way.

```
EVENT POST_Completed
  WHEN
    grd1 : post_completed = TRUE
  THEN
    act1 : POST_Res := Pass_postResult
  END
```

```
EVENT PowerStatus1
  WHEN
    grd1 : c_pwrStatus = Standby_pwrStatus
    grd2 : ∃x·x ∈ BOOL ∧ x = M_pwrReq
  THEN
    act1 : c_pwrStatus := POST_pwrStatus
  END
```

We now present summary information about each refinement step in the IIP development, since we do not have space for the detailed formalization and proofs.

5.2   A Chain of Refinements

First Refinement: User Operations. This refinement introduces a set of operations that is performed by the user to operate/program the system for delivering insulin. These user operations create, remove, activate and manage the basal profile, bolus profile, and reminders (REQ3, REQ12, REQ13). These system operations are allowed when an IIP is *on* and we want to deliver an insulin amount in a controlled manner according to the physiological needs of a patient. This refinement formalizes the possible interactions for each system operation to make sure that the given requirements are consistent. For example, if no basal profile exists in the system, then the user will not be allowed to perform any operation other than to create a basal profile, and a notification will appear on the screen to direct the user. This step implements all user interactions with the system, including user initiated commands and system responses. This also includes all safeguards generated by safety constraints resulting from the hazard analysis.

In this refinement, we define an enumerated set and a list of variables to formalize user operations. This refinement step introduces 35 events to specify all the possible user operations related to the given requirements. All these new events refine *skip*. For example, an event *CurrActiUserOper_Idle1* refines *skip* that allows a user to create a new basal profile. The guards of this event state that power status is ready, system is in idle state (means no user operation is currently being performed) and there exists an operation requested by a user to create a new basel profile. We omit the formalization of the rest of the events, which are formalized in a similar way.

```
EVENT CurrActiUserOper_Idle1
WHEN
    grd1 : c_pwrStatus = Ready_pwrStatus
    grd2 : c_operation = Idle_operations
    grd3 : ∃x·x ∈ BOOL ∧ x = M_basCreateReq
THEN
    act1 : c_operation := CreateBasProf_operations
END
```

Second Refinement: Basal Profile Management. This refinement introduces basal profile management (REQ4, REQ5) to maintain a record and to store basal profiles defined by the user. The operations of interest are: create a basal profile; remove a basal profile; check the validity of a selected basal profile; activate a basal profile; and deactivate a basal profile. The basal activation process must allow activation only of a valid non-empty basal profile that is stored in the IIP's memory. When a new basal profile is activated then the old basal profile is automatically deactivated, since only one basal profile is allowed to be active at any time. The new profile activation is always confirmed by the user before it can take effect. These operations are introduced in this refinement along the lines seen in the First Refinement, above.

Third Refinement: Temporary Basal Profile Management. This refinement introduces temporary basal profile management (REQ6, REQ7) that allows for activating, deactivating and checking the validity of a selected temporary basal profile. The temporary basal profile management is similar to the basal profile management. As soon as the elapsed period is finished, the paused basal profile resumes after notifying the user. In this refinement, we formalize the possible operations related to the temporary basal management by introducing several new events just as in the previous refinement steps.

Fourth Refinement: Bolus Preset Management. This refinement introduces bolus preset management (REQ3, REQ9) that allows for creating a new bolus preset, removing an existing bolus preset, checking the validity of a created bolus preset, and activating the selected bolus preset. Using new events in a similar way to previous refinement steps, we can formalize the required behaviour. For example, scheduling a bolus has different states like 'no' bolus, 'normal' bolus, and 'extended' bolus. We define transitions between these states to inform the user by notification to confirm a proper bolus status.

Fifth Refinement: Bolus Delivery. This refinement introduces bolus delivery that includes events to start bolus delivery, to calculate the required dose for insulin delivery, and to check the validity of the calculated bolus and manually entered bolus. The bolus delivery formalization step describes how the system will calculate and behave when the user requests a bolus (REQ9, REQ11). When an IIP is *on*, the requested bolus is compared against an average bolus size. The bolus standard deviation must always satisfy the given range. The bolus notification process informs the user whether the bolus is within the regular bolus size, or whether it is larger/smaller than normal. At the time of bolus delivery, an IIP needs confirmation from the user. If the user does not confirm the bolus delivery confirmation, the bolus delivery is unchanged. This refinement formalizes the calculation of bolus delivery and other controlling operations to make sure that an IIP always delivers a correct amount of bolus at the scheduled time.

Sixth Refinement: Reminder Management. This refinement introduces reminder management (REQ10, REQ14) that allows for creating a new reminder, checking the validity of a newly entered reminder, and for removing an existing reminder. The reminder management is a complex task to control several user operations. It includes events to store and maintain reminders defined by the user. Invalid reminders will not be accepted. This refinement step introduces all the events necessary to model all the elements and operations for describing the reminder management, and to verify the requirements of reminder management.

Seventh Refinement: Insulin Output Calculator. This is the last refinement that models the insulin output calculator (REQ8, REQ11). It calculates the insulin required over the course of the day, the appropriate time segment, and the time steps for delivering the insulin. It also keeps track of the insulin delivered within the time segment. The infusion flow rate can be 0, if the system is *off*, and there is no active profile or the maximum amount of insulin has already been delivered.

In this refinement, we introduce 26 events to model the insulin calculator and 14 events to refine other previously abstractly defined events. Again, as an example to demonstrate the refinement process, a new event *InsulinOutputCalculator1* is defined to calculate the amount of insulin to output. It depends on both basal and bolus that are formalized in actions ($act1$-$act2$). The guards of this event are: power status is ready ($grd1$); temporary basal is active ($grd2$); there exists an active temporary basal in which the rate of temporary basal is less than or equal to the maximum allowable rate ($grd3$); bolus delivery is in progress ($grd4$); and there exists an active bolus in which the bolus amount to be delivered is greater than the remaining allowable maximum amount for the next time step ($grd5$). The generated proof obligations also guarantee that an IIP does not deliver excess insulin to a patient.

```
EVENT InsulinOutputCalculator1
  WHEN
    grd1 : c_pwrStatus = Ready_pwrStatus
    grd2 : TemporaryBasalIsActive = TRUE
    grd3 : ∃x, y, z·x ↦ y ↦ z = f_activeTmpBasal∧
           y ≤ k_maxOutputRate ∧ val = y ∧ val ∈ ℕ
    grd4 : BolusDeliveryinProgress = TRUE
    grd5 : ∃s, t·s ↦ t = f_activeBolus∧
           t > (k_maxOutputRate − val)/k_msPerHr * Delta_T
  THEN
    act1 : f_basalOut := (val/k_msPerHr) * Delta_T
    act2 : f_bolusOut := ((k_maxOutputRate − val)/k_msPerHr) * Delta_T
  END
```

5.3 Safety Properties

Informally, a safety property stipulates that *"bad things"* do not happen during system execution. A formalized specification that satisfies a safety property involves an invariance argument. This section presents a list of safety properties using invariants ($spr1$ - $spr9$). These safety properties are introduced to make sure that the formalized IIP system is consistent and safe. The first safety property ($spr1$) ensures that when *EnteredBasProfValid* is TRUE, the entered basal delivery rate is within the safe range. Similarly, when *EnteredBasProfValid* is TRUE, $spr2$ ensures that the total amount of insulin delivered over a day is within the state limit. $spr3$ and $spr4$ perform the same checks for the selected basal rate and amount when *SelectedBasalProfileIsValid* is *TRUE*. $spr5$ and $spr6$ perform the same checks for the temporary basal profile when *EnteredTemporaryBasalIsValid* is *TRUE*. $spr7$ states that when *SelectedPresetIsValid* is *TRUE*, the bolus rate of a selected bolus profile must be within the range of minimum bolus bound and maximum bolus bound. $spr8$ ensures that when *EnteredBolusIsValid* is *TRUE*, the bolus rate of the entered bolus profile must be within the range of minimum bolus bound and maximum bolus bound. The last safety property ($spr9$) states that the total amount of insulin to output over the next time unit is less than or equal to the maximum daily limit of insulin that can be delivered.

$$
\begin{aligned}
spr1 : \ & EnteredBasProfValid = TRUE \Rightarrow (\exists x, y \cdot x \mapsto y = M\_basProf \wedge \\
& (\forall i \cdot i \in index\_range \wedge i \in dom(y) \Rightarrow y(i) \geq k\_minBasalBound \\
& \wedge y(i) \leq k\_maxBasalBound)) \\
spr2 : \ & EnteredBasProfValid = TRUE \Rightarrow (\exists x, y, insulin\_amount \cdot x \mapsto y = M\_basProf \wedge \\
& insulin\_amount \in y\_insulinValue \wedge (\forall i \cdot i \in index\_range \wedge i \in dom(y) \Rightarrow \\
& insulin\_amount = insulin\_amount + y(i) * k\_segDayDur) \wedge \\
& insulin\_amount \leq k\_maxDailyInsulin) \\
spr3 : \ & SelectedBasalProfileIsValid = TRUE \Rightarrow (\exists x, y \cdot x \mapsto y = M\_basActSelected \wedge \\
& (\forall i \cdot i \in index\_range \wedge i \in dom(y) \Rightarrow y(i) \geq k\_minBasalBound \\
& \wedge y(i) \leq k\_maxBasalBound)) \\
spr4 : \ & SelectedBasalProfileIsValid = TRUE \Rightarrow \\
& (\exists x, y, insulin\_amount \cdot x \mapsto y = M\_basProf \wedge \\
& insulin\_amount \in y\_insulinValue \wedge \\
& (\forall i \cdot i \in index\_range \wedge i \in dom(y) \Rightarrow \\
& insulin\_amount = insulin\_amount + y(i) * k\_segDayDur) \wedge \\
& insulin\_amount \leq k\_maxDailyInsulin) \\
spr5 : \ & EnteredTemporaryBasalIsValid = TRUE \Rightarrow \\
& (\exists x, y, z \cdot x \mapsto y \mapsto z = M\_tmpBas \wedge \\
& y \geq k\_minBasalBound \wedge y \leq k\_maxBasalBound) \\
spr6 : \ & EnteredTemporaryBasalIsValid = TRUE \Rightarrow \\
& (\exists x, y, z \cdot x \mapsto y \mapsto z = M\_tmpBas \wedge y * z \leq k\_maxDailyInsulin) \\
spr7 : \ & SelectedPresetIsValid = TRUE \Rightarrow (\exists x, y \cdot x \mapsto y = M\_bolSelected \wedge \\
& y \geq k\_minBolusBound \wedge y \leq k\_maxBolusBound) \\
spr8 : \ & EnteredBolusIsValid = TRUE \Rightarrow (\exists x, y \cdot x \mapsto y = M\_bolus \wedge \\
& y \geq k\_minBolusBound \wedge y \leq k\_maxBolusBound) \\
spr9 : \ & c\_insulinOut \leq k\_maxDailyInsulin
\end{aligned}
$$

5.4   Model Analysis

In this section, we present the proof statistics by presenting detailed information about generated proof obligations. Event-B supports *consistency checking* which shows that a list of events preserves the given invariants, and *refinement checking* which makes sure that a concrete machine is a valid refinement of an abstract machine.

Table 1. Proof Statistics

Model	Total number of POs	Automatic Proof	Interactive Proof
Abstract Model	3	3(100%)	0(0%)
First Refinement	22	22(100%)	0(0%)
Second Refinement	98	82(83%)	16(17%)
Third Refinement	26	25(100%)	1(0%)
Fourth Refinement	52	45(87%)	7(13%)
Fifth Refinement	54	54(100%)	0(0%)
Sixth Refinement	66	60(91%)	6(9%)
Seventh Refinement	123	51(42%)	72(58%)
Total	444	342(77%)	102(23%)

This complete formal specification of an IIP contains 263 events, 16 complex data types, 15 enumerated types, and 25 constants for specifying the system requirements. The formal development of an IIP is presented through one abstract model and a series of seven refinement models. In fact, the refinement models are decomposed into several sub refinements. Therefore, we have a total of 43 refinement levels for describing the system behaviour. In this paper, we have omitted the detailed description of the 43 refinements by grouping them into the main components we used to present the formal specification of an IIP.

Table 1 shows the proof statistics of the development in the Rodin tool. To guarantee the correctness of the system behaviour, we established various invariants in the incremental refinements. This development resulted in 444 (100 %) proof obligations, of which 342 (77 %) were proved automatically, and the remaining 102 (23 %) were proved interactively using the Rodin prover (see Table 1). These interactive proof obligations are mainly related to the complex mathematical expressions, which are simplified through interaction, providing additional information for assisting the Rodin prover. Other proofs are quite simple and were achieved by simplifying the predicates.

6 Conclusion and Future Challenges

An insulin pump is a critical software-intensive medical device for delivering controllable continuous subcutaneous infusion of insulin to patients. An insulin delivery process can be programmed by monitoring the patient's condition. Every year recalls are reported by FDA related to insulin pump malfunctions, and many of these recalls are a result of software issues. These software issues include unexpected controller behaviour for delivering insulin, incorrect measurement of insulin dose, overdose of insulin delivery, incorrect inputs for configuration management, etc. To address these software issues, we have proposed a refinement based formal development of an insulin pump to capture the essential requirements and to verify the required safety properties.

To formalize the requirements of an IIP, we used the Event-B modelling language [11] that supports an incremental refinement approach to design a complete system using several layers from an abstract to a concrete specification. Each refined model was proven to guarantee the preservation of required (safety) properties in that model. The initial model captured the basic behaviour of IIP in an abstract way. Subsequent refinements were used to formalize the concrete behaviour for the resulting IIP that covers user operations, basal profile management, temporary basal management, bolus preset management, reminder management, and insulin calculation. In order to guarantee the 'correctness' of the system behaviour, we established various invariants in the incremental refinements. Our complete formal development of this IIP is available in the appendix of report [18], which is more than 1500 pages long. In summary, our main contributions are:

1. Formalizing the requirements of an IIP.
2. Verifying and validating the required behaviour of an IIP.
3. Defining a list of safety properties.
4. Demonstrating how we can help to meet FDA requirements for certifying IIPs using formal methods.
5. Showing how to use Event-B's refinement process to retain intellectual control of the modelling process, formalization, and analysis.

The prime objective of this IIP model is to verify the requirements of an IIP, to check that all the system operational and functional behaviours are consistent that may help to certify the IIPs. In the future, we will use this model to produce source code using

EB2ALL [8]. Moreover, we have plans to develop a closed-loop system using our glucose homeostasis model [3] to verify the correctness of system behaviour, to analyze system operations, and to provide the required safety assurances to meet certification standards.

References

1. Carayon, P., Wood, K.E.: Patient safety. Inf. Knowl. Syst. Manag. **8**(1–4), 23–46 (2009)
2. Chen, Y., Lawford, M., Wang, H., Wassyng, A.: Insulin pump software certification. In: Gibbons, J., MacCaull, W. (eds.) FHIES 2013. LNCS, vol. 8315, pp. 87–106. Springer, Heidelberg (2014)
3. Singh, N.K., Wang, H., Lawford, M., Maibaum, T., Wassyng, A.: Formalizing the glucose homeostasis mechanism. In: Duffy, V.G. (ed.) DHM 2014. LNCS, vol. 8529, pp. 460–471. Springer, Heidelberg (2014)
4. Keatley, K.L.: A review of the FDA draft guidance document for software validation: guidance for industry. Qual. Assur. **7**(1), 49–55 (1999)
5. A reseach and development needs report by NITRD: high-confidence medical devices: cyber-physical systems for 21st century health care. http://www.nitrd.gov/About/MedDevice-FINAL1-web.pdf
6. Lee, I., Pappas, G.J., Cleaveland, R., Hatcliff, J., Krogh, B.H., Lee, P., Rubin, H., Sha, L.: High-confidence medical device software and systems. Computer **39**(4), 33–38 (2006)
7. Bowen, J., Stavridou, V.: Safety-critical systems, formal methods and standards. Softw. Eng. J. **8**(4), 189–209 (1993)
8. Singh, N.K.: Using Event-B for Critical Device Software Systems. Springer GmbH, London (2013)
9. Méry, D., Singh, N.K.: Real-time animation for formal specification. In: Aiguier, M., Bretaudeau, F., Krob, D. (eds.) Complex Systems Design and Management, pp. 49–60. Springer, Berlin Heidelberg (2010)
10. Wassyng, A.: Though this be madness, yet there is method in it? In: Proceedings of FormaliSE, pp. 1–7. IEEE (2013)
11. Abrial, J.: Modeling in Event-B - System and Software Engineering. Cambridge University Press, Cambridge (2010)
12. Project RODIN: rigorous open development environment for complex systems (2004). http://rodin-b-sharp.sourceforge.net/
13. Masci, P., Ayoub, A., Curzon, P., Lee, I., Sokolsky, O., Thimbleby, H.: Model-based development of the generic PCA infusion pump user interface prototype in PVS. In: Bitsch, F., Guiochet, J., Kaâniche, M. (eds.) SAFECOMP. LNCS, vol. 8153, pp. 228–240. Springer, Heidelberg (2013)
14. Kim, B.G., Ayoub, A., Sokolsky, O., Lee, I., Jones, P., Zhang, Y., Jetley, R.: Safety-assured development of the GPCA infusion pump software. In: 2011 Proceedings of the International Conference on Embedded Software (EMSOFT), pp. 155–164, October 2011
15. Wang, J., Liu, S., Qi, Y., Hou, D.: Developing an insulin pump system using the SOFL method. In: 4th Asia-Pacific Software Engineering Conference (APSEC), pp. 334–341 (2007)
16. Xu, H., Maibaum, T.: An Event-B approach to timing issues applied to the generic insulin infusion pump. In: Liu, Z., Wassyng, A. (eds.) FHIES 2011. LNCS, vol. 7151, pp. 160–176. Springer, Heidelberg (2012)
17. Sommerville, I.: Software Engineering, 7th edn. Pearson Addison Wesley, New Jersey (2004)
18. Singh, N.K., Wang, H., Lawford, M., Maibaum, T.S.E., Wassyng, A.: Report 18: formalizing insulin pump using Event-B. Technical report 18, McSCert, McMaster University, October 2014. https://www.mcscert.ca/index.php/documents/mcscert-reports

Quality in Healthcare

Later Life: Living Alone, Social Connectedness and ICT

Alma L. Culén(✉)

Department of Informatics, University of Oslo, Oslo, Norway
almira@ifi.uio.no

Abstract. The paper presents a qualitative, interview-based study that seeks to describe participants' perceptions and experiences with information and communication technology. The participants in the study were active people, aged 67 and over, who live alone in an urban setting. Interactionist theory of loneliness was used to guide the inquiry, in particular regarding the perception of the relation between the quality and quantity of connections, loneliness, and technology. A set of visual tools such as communication maps and cards were made to aid reflections and associations during interviews.

Keywords: Loneliness · Social connectedness · Communication technology · Elderly

1 Introduction

In 1960, life expectancy at birth in Norway was 71 years for men and 76 for women. The projection for 2030 was 79 for men and 85 for women, as reported in the Active Aging report for 2003 [1]. In 2013, these numbers were already somewhat higher than predicted for 2030: 79,6 for men and 86,5 for women [2]. In 2014, 11 % of the population was over the age of 67, but that number is growing fast and is predicted to double by 2025 [2]. Many of those over 67 are, and will be, living alone [3], increasingly so in urban areas [4].

The living arrangements of elderly have clear implications for policy makers. They affect the need for care and resources. Those elderly who live alone tend to require more of both. In the National Council for Senior Citizens' action plan [5], it is stated that three out of ten people who live alone suffer from depression. Loneliness and depression are among the main reasons for elderly living alone to move into care homes [6]. Furthermore, a positive correlation between loneliness and functional decline and death is reported [7].

An extensive cross-cultural study of loneliness in Europe was conducted recently [8]. The study included 14 countries and tested several types of explanations for observed differences in loneliness: differences in demographic characteristics, wealth and health, and social networks. It showed that frequent contacts with adult children, social participation, and providing support to family members were important in

© Springer International Publishing Switzerland 2015
V.G. Duffy (Ed.): DHM 2015, Part II, LNCS 9185, pp. 401–412, 2015.
DOI: 10.1007/978-3-319-21070-4_40

preventing and alleviating loneliness in almost all countries. The study suggested further that increasing social connectedness is an important factor for reducing loneliness. A systematic overview of the literature on an effectiveness of interventions aiming to increase social connectedness was presented in [9]. It showed that there was no evidence for many of interventions that they worked, or, were transferable to different settings. The findings further suggested that the most effective interventions were based on educational or support oriented group activities. The most ineffective types of interventions were based on one-to-one social support, advice giving, health assessment or information sharing.

Recognizing effects of loneliness on the aging population and the need for solutions to the social isolation problem also engages the human-computer interaction (HCI) community. Design, often co-design with elderly, of new interfaces, interaction modes and new technologies, is seen within the HCI community as a powerful possibility for the field to contribute to solving growing challenges related to aging populations [10]. However, studies show that the use of information and communication technology (ICT) among elderly is still controversial, see, for example, [11–14]. Despite inconclusive results, many studies end on a technology deterministic note that future, easier to use technologies are going to solve problems they considered.

A look at statistics on the ICT use among elderly in Norway, provides the following data: in 2014, according to the Norwegian Statistical Bureau [15], the use of PCs for the age group 65–74 was 76 %. In contrast, 95 % of those under the age of 65 used computers. The Internet use was reported to be similar. However, the use of mobile and smartphones to connect to the Internet outside of a home was only 20 % among those over 65. The corresponding percentage for those under 65 was 92 %. These numbers imply that age-related digital divide still exists. How does this divide affect elderly living alone? Can technology help to solve or diminish challenges related to social connectedness for those living alone?

This paper presents a qualitative study based on in-depth interviews with six elderly over 65 who are living alone. The interviews were conducted using tools developed to facilitate and visualize reflections around the use of ICT and connectedness to others.

The primary aim of the study was to explore how well-educated, active elderly living alone view the potential of present and future technologies to support social connectedness and possibly reduce the sense of loneliness. The secondary aim was to explore whether tools that were made to assist reflections during interviews were effective in soliciting rich responses from interviewees.

The results of the study show that while the participants were not technology shy, they did not have technology deterministic views either. Personal contacts still mattered the most. In some cases, the choice to not use the technology was motivated by an ideological stance that it still should be possible to do things through human interaction, i.e. walk to the bank or the library and talk to a human rather than the Internet. Further, it was found that tools supported introspective and reflective processes to a varying degree, but that the social mapping has worked well.

The paper is structured as follows: the next section provides a brief description of the interactionist theory that guided the inquiry. In Sect. 3, the method, the choice of participants, the interview guide and the tools designed to aid interviews are presented. The analysis and the discussion are presented in Sect. 4, followed by a conclusion.

2 Interactionist Theory of Loneliness

The term loneliness indicates a subjective perception of an individual that the number of relationships is smaller than the individual considers desirable, or that the level of intimacy that the individual wishes for, has not been realized. Living alone does not automatically imply the loneliness. It is possible to live alone and not feel lonely, due to the presence of meaningful relations with, for example, adult children [16]. The reverse, being surrounded by others and still feeling lonely [17], is also possible. Thus, the link between living alone and loneliness is not a strong one. Many studies explore how the elderly experience their social situation, e.g., [18]. Various psychological theories have been formulated, among them existential, cognitive, psychodynamic and interactionist. The latter guided the research presented in this paper. Interactionist theory, see Weiss [19], suggests that there are two main components to loneliness: emotional loneliness and social loneliness. The first one arises in the absence of attachments, such as the absence of a meaningful relation with an adult child. The social loneliness is viewed as a lack of an appropriate network. Thus, individuals may evaluate their emotional and social loneliness subjectively, not only in terms of the quality, but also the quantity of social connections. If so, what and how could ICT support? A hypothesis could be made that the technology-supported communication is inferior to in-person connection and an impeding factor for the quality of connections. At the same time, it could be hypothesized that it could be a positive influence on increasing a number of connections. How elderly, living alone actually think about the role of technology in relation to social connectedness is of interest.

3 Method

The study takes a qualitative approach, seeking to describe the participants' perceptions and experiences of living alone, and their communication patterns with others that may or may not include the technology. Qualitative research is well suited to inquiry about human behavior, motives, views and challenges [20]. It can complement well quantitative studies on aging, loneliness and quality of life that abound in the literature in nursing, gerontology, psychology and even human-computer interaction (HCI) design.

When it comes to studies on the use of technology, HCI researchers frequently use ethnographic approaches. However, as described in [21], ethnography in HCI is often misused and in order to be perceived as having relevance for the field, such research is often forced to conclude with some 'implications for design'. Furthermore, in this study, the observations would need to take place in participants' homes. This could give rise to a number of other problems, among them ethical. Thus, in-depth interviews were chosen as the main approach. In addition, a set of tools consisting of communication maps, cards, and vignettes, inspired by participatory and co-design techniques [22, 23], was developed as an aid for reflection during the interview.

The following sections describe the tools, the choice of participants and finally, provide an interview plan.

3.1   Tools Made to Support the Interviews

Communication Maps. Inspired by the social mapping and, in particular, a technique described in [24], communication maps were developed, see Fig. 1 and [25]. The communication maps consist of three maps (friends and family, contacts and services and future technology), colored pens and images representing different communication platforms (e.g., phones, tablets, laptops, desktops), communication channels (e.g., Skype, email, call, SMS, chat, social media) and images of some future technologies (e.g., holographic phones, sensors, implant chips). The participants could, in addition, draw anything else they thought was relevant directly to the map. The maps, see Fig. 1, had an individual (represented by the word '*me*') positioned at the bottom of the map. Two circles were drawn to separate connections that are very close, close and not close. The participants were instructed to show their connections accordingly. Whether closeness was understood as intimacy or a physical proximity was left to each of the participants to decide. Alternatively, they could also arrange contacts by the frequency of communication. The other maps were used in a similar way.

The process of making and reflecting over these maps, in particular the first one, served as an opening for the conversation.

Communication Cards. Instead of using the maps, one interview utilized a set of cards, with the same idea of being able to represent close and distant relations (both geographically and in terms of intimacy) and the technology supporting those connections. The reason for making and testing cards in addition to the maps was that they worked well in other situations, e.g., [26] for broad explorations. Furthermore, images on cards were large and could make viewing easier for participants, see Fig. 2.

The cards were tested using a quick and dirty technique with three university students in order to ensure that images conveyed the meaning clearly and quickly.

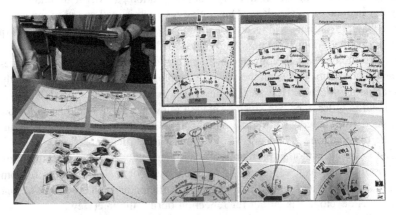

Fig. 1. A participant used the iPad to repeatedly take pictures of her maps. She did not consider looking at her relations in this way before. The image on the right shows examples of maps made by other participants.

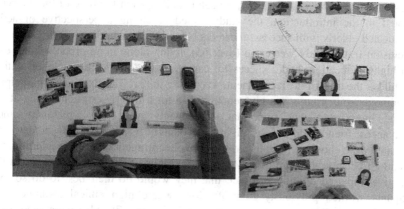

Fig. 2. An interviewee working with cards while talking about the role of ICT and her social connections.

The concepts used in this process are those of immediacy and impedance, see [27]. This was done by allowing viewing of the image for a second or two, asking a tester for their immediate understanding of the image, recording the answer and then presenting the same image, with a word or two of the explanatory text. If the image was not understood correctly, inquiry into what impeded the correct understanding was made. Then a decision was made whether to include the image into the card set.

Vignettes. Vignettes were used to provide a context, a very short scenario for participants to reflect over when contemplating the future technologies. Depending on the interviewee's responses, one or more vignettes were introduced. If the interviewee did not wish to reflect over the future technologies, vignettes were skipped. Two sample scenarios are provided bellow. An image representing the first scenario was included with both maps and cards.

Vignette 1. *Kaya is 83 and lives alone. In order to stay in touch, the family convinced her to get a tiny implant for the arm. When touched, the implant projects small hologram bubbles, with an image of a family member in each. Touching the bubble establishes a call to the person whose image it had.*
Vignette 2. *Ole is 93. He lives alone and spends much time watching TV. Alongside his TV, there is a large basket and on the sofa table there are two soft balls. One has the image of his son, and the other his brother. Choosing the one with the image of his son, Ole throws the ball into the basket. This establishes Skype connection and the TV now shows the Skype interface with an active call to his son. The son does not answer, the Skype shuts down and the TV re-starts.*

3.2   Choosing Participants

In contrast to many studies focusing on vulnerable groups of elderly [25], such as demented [23, 28], bereaved [29], or those with physical disabilities [30], this study focuses on active elderly without major health challenges at the time of the interview. As stated in the introduction, the study aimed at taking a perspective of active, well-educated elderly with successful careers behind them, who live alone. The criteria for inclusion in the study were: age (over 65), living alone in an urban setting, completed higher education, had a successful career, and had a positive relation with an adult child at the time of the recruitment. According to [31, 32], six to eight participants from homogeneous groups can give enough data for a rich description. Being at ease with the interviewer was important. Participants were, thus, recruited among acquaintances, friends and family, giving surprisingly many possible candidates. Six participants were chosen who satisfied the above recruitment criteria. In addition, they were chosen because they are usually candid, and thus, it could be expected that they would give unbiased opinions, in fact, that they would do their best to do so. Four participants worked previously in professions where high ethical awareness was expected. The age distribution for women was 71, 73 and 76. Men were aged 67, 74 and 83. Career wise, two participants have practiced medicine (W73 and M74), one psychology (W71), one was an academic (M67), and two worked in business (W76 and M83). Five participants were retired, while one, (M67), was still partly employed. One man (M74) and one woman (W71) were ethnically Norwegian. Including participants who are not ethnically Norwegian, was seen as interesting in terms of social loneliness and connectedness. Four of the interviews were conducted in English and two in Norwegian; the author translated the latter.

3.3   Interview Plan

The interviews were conducted on one-to-one bases, with two exceptions. In one case, the interviewee brought along a friend, who remained unengaged during the interview. In the second case, another researcher was present. On that occasion, the use of communication cards was tested. All interviews were conducted in quiet locations within the university (four interviews), or home (2 interviews), always with ample space for maps and cards. The shortest interview took about an hour, while the average length was about an hour and a half. The following interview plan was implemented:

1. Can you tell a bit about technology that you use to communicate with others?
2. Please take a look at maps in front of you. Let us start with communication with friends and family map (or cards). Can you draw your communication network on that map? And then, add icons representing the kind of devices that you use for each?
3. How do you experience this map?
4. Repeat questions 2. and 3. for the contacts and services map and the future technology map (or cards).
5. Use a vignette. What are your reflections around this vignette?
6. Any other reflections on social connectedness?

4   Analysis and Discussion

The interviews were coded and analyzed based on categories related to interactionist theory, i.e. perception of quality and quantity of social connectedness. It was evident from interviews that access to services was important for connectedness and the personal safety. Only basic services such as banking, health services,, and social services were explicitly mentioned, leaving it up to participants to add any additional services that could be important for them. Some have added travel related services, while others were concerned with alarms that could notify someone in the case of a medical emergency. Finally, the future needs were explored, in the same categories.

4.1   General Use of ICT

Although many studies exist on the general use of ICT among elderly, e.g., [11, 33], the use among interviewees is described briefly.

All participants had a phone and used it regularly. Four of the participants had smartphones. One of them got a brand new iPhone 6 plus as soon as it became available (M74). Two participants had ordinary phones (W71, M83). All were able to make a call, receive an SMS, and all but one could also send an SMS. *"See, this is my mobile* [note: shown in Fig. 2]. *It is not some kind of a smart mobile; it is a completely idiotic one. I can call, and I can get SMSs, but I cannot answer. I never bothered to learn"* (W71).

Further, all interviewees were able to take pictures and send or receive them. Three persons with smartphones used a much broader set of features and apps, such as dictation, voice over Internet, advanced photo editing, Dropbox and so on. One of the participants, upon seeing HD Recording app used during the interview, said: *"It is an app, right? How do I get it?"*(M67).

All participants either owned a PC (M74, M67), a laptop (M83, W71, M67) or a tablet (W73, W76, M67). They used these to varying degrees. One woman barely used her laptop, another used her tablet daily while the third used it only occasionally. The men used their devices for work or hobby daily, two of them extensively so. The participants showed no signs of dislike or fear of new technology, although some (W71 and W76) expressed a wish to preserve a lifestyle with as little technology in it as possible.

4.2   The Quality of Connectedness

Personal. Phone calls seemed to be an acceptable way to connect to friends and family.

"I call my family and friends in the States all the time. It is the best I can do from here [note: Norway], *and it is OK"* (M67).

"I have four people that I speak to more or less daily. Every day. It is comforting, and when somebody skips a call, I miss it" (W76).

However, the interviewee also remarks that while phones enable staying in touch, aging does reduce desire for face-to-face connections, as they require effort.

"I have 2 sisters living far away. I talk to them almost every Sunday. I wished to see them in person much more when I was younger, but now, I think that the phone is what I have the energy for, even if we lived in the same city. It is all right to just check in with them" (W76).

While recognizing that technology helps stay in touch, another participant raises a concern that it makes it easier to miss the opportunity for face-to-face contact.

"The communication, what is it? I think that talking to my child is a real connection. So when I want that connection, I pick up the phone. I find the reason to call. So we communicate, using technology. It does not replace the real ting. It helps to keep it going. One can get addicted to technology and try to replace the real care with it. It does not work" (W73).

Sometimes, the quality of face-to-face contact is interrupted by technology.

"When I am with my son, he often plays with his phone. Sometimes there is too little human contact" (W71).

One participant expressed that technology may serve the purpose of making the connection, extending it, even when the physical body is no longer there.

"I have a laptop. I am not really good at using it. But I started this project of organizing my pictures. It is fun. I have this young man who comes twice a week for 4 h, so we organize pictures and write a bit of text together. Perhaps, it all turns into a book, or something for my family when I am no longer here. This is also communication. Using technology to stay in touch, in a way, even when I am gone" (M83).

"It is the quality of friendships, it is the sense of community that counts" (M74).

This last sentence summarizes prevailing sentiments about the technology. While it may be fun, especially when used in active and constructive, even creative manner, it was not experienced as a tool that helps the quality of a contact. Rather, it was helping to 'stay in touch' and to prevent loss of existing connections.

Services. Looking into services, for two of the female participants (W73 and W76), safety was important. One had an alarm installed in her flat, while the other remarked:

"I also want to have a fast and reliable communication with someone [note: in case of an emergency]. *If one gets a stroke, the response needs to be really fast"* (W73).

The remaining participants did not talk about alarms or medical emergencies. A participant, who travels a lot, expressed a need for personalized travel services, perhaps also better food services.

A female participant tells a story:

"I wanted to extend my passport and I was trying to find the phone number to the police. There are no phone books any longer. I had to call my son to ask for the number. So, I called to make an appointment. The person who answered the call said that I have to book online. ... I was so angry. I went totally into an impotent rage. They must know that there still are people on the higher end of age that travel and are not Internet oriented. I see that I am becoming a museum object. I am a Stone Age woman, a Venus of Willendorf" (W71).

With only one exception, participants expressed a desire for all fashioned services to remain, sometimes in addition to electronic ones. One of the participants said:

"I like to find out what kinds of services am I entitled to get. When I do, I always inform my friends and family what they too can get. I do not learn this from the

Internet, but from human contacts. It is funny, I teach my friends how to fill forms so that they too can deny electronic services and have everything sent via *surface mail. I do not know for how long I can stay out of it, but I am fighting this online thing"* (W76).

The old fashioned services were part of the perception of being well connected:

"I like to go to the bank, or walk to my doctors office. I like to know people working there and I do not like to talk over the phone to people, or worse, machines, that I do not know" (M83).

This kind of personal connection to services, and people providing them, mattered. This way of connectedness was experienced as being in danger of disappearing, and the technology was to blame for it.

Future Technologies. Discussions on the fuure technology were mostly not very spirited.

"It is too late for me to consider the future technology. No point in thinking about it" (M83).

"No! Absolutely not. We are not talking about future technology. I am a cave dweller" (W71).

"I do not really want to think about any future technology" (W76).

"Holographic computing probably would not be interesting to me partly because I have a choice of voice or voice and video already. I often use voice only. This allows me to concentrate and really reach out to the person I am taking to, with voice. Using video, it tends to be the case that communication is a bit more superficial" (M67).

One woman had a different view. If the technology could help her overcome one of her personal barriers, the language, she would take a chance with technology:

"Those who moved out of their own country to Norway many, many years ago, are now getting old. So, as old people, perhaps they live alone, but they also really need to communicate. That chip should be used so that they do not feel isolated. If one does not have the language, and can not express themselves clearly, then one is isolated. Isolation is an open prison for me. I would get that chip implanted in my brain, if I could speak different languages well at once" (W73).

4.3   The Quantity of Connections

The interactionist theory assumption that people would be interested in evaluating their connections also by quantity was evident, whether they had a large number of connections or a single one.

"I talk mostly to my son" (W71).

"I have acquaintances in Norway, probably 50, vs. about 20 in the US. But all of my close friends and family are in the US" (M67), [see Fig. 1, top row of maps, where the participant used the letter A for acquaintances, F for family and C for close friends, adding the number of such connections in parenthesis].

"I have a lot of connections, most numerous are acquaintances and my old clients, I really know a lot of people. They are a network, although perhaps not of a kind to

keep in close contact with. I cannot put them all here. But I would say that I have four primary close connections that I care most about" (M74).

The three male participants all expressed that the number of connections was important to consider, and were considering options to increase the number of meaningful connections by building a community, or moving into one. The three female participants were happy to have at least one strong close connection, and the number of connections was less important. This indicates that some gender differences may exist regarding the importance of emotional connectedness and the need for broader networks.

4.4   Tools Evaluation

Drawing their personal connections to the friends and family map was really interesting for all participants. Three participants kept taking pictures, as depicted in Fig. 1, while making their maps. One remarked: *"I have never thought about it this way"* (W73). In one case, seeing explicitly the map of the connections, brought about an insight that had a consequence for participant's life choice: *"I see that I am being at risk of isolation in Norway. That would be a major factor in wanting to, not just wanting, but actively building another life style and life in the US"* (M67).

Thus, the maps have worked well for inquiry into social connectedness, also to necessary services. The cards did not work as well as the maps. They seemed to obstruct drawing in connections and other things on the paper. Also, the act of drawing connections to the map seemed to lead to a deeper reflection over connections, than a more active approach involving browsing and placing the cards on a large sheet of paper did. Furthermore, the effect of a sense of a new perspective on their connections that the participants had with maps was not the same for the card user.

Vignettes had limited usefulness, as most of the participants were really not interested in discussing the future technology. Perhaps, the video approach as described in [34] could engage the participants better. Only two participants engaged:

"Actually, this implant on the hand is good, something like that would always be part of me. In all kinds of emergencies" (W73).

"I would like to have a ball to open the Skype on my TV. Only, I do not know who would pick up the ball all the time. My dog, perhaps. I like the playfulness of it, but would not really want anything like that" (M74).

Overall, the interview tool that best supported reflections, was the friends and family communication map.

5   Conclusion

The relative disinterest in technology that the participants showed through described interviews did not originate from any difficulty in understanding how today's, or future, technologies could support them. Rather, when it came to relations and services, most of them had preference for real, face-to-face contacts. Even if it required, as for one of the participants, the move to another continent, as the close relations were preferred to more numerous casual ones in Norway. The phones were an acceptable solution for keeping in touch, but the participants were aware that this was not the same as a real contact. Even casual contacts, such as those with service providers in banks, were more valued in person than online, and these service providers were experienced as parts of the individual's network, parts of their of social connectedness. In conclusion, the findings from interviews indicate that, even though they live alone, participants do not view the technology as a possible solution to social loneliness. This perception, of course, could change as their circumstances change. Several findings indicated some differences between male and female participants and those would warrant further exploration, e.g., relation between gender and the sense of social connectedness. This study is too small to have external validity, but clearly indicates that even when elderly could use the ICT for fulfillment of their social networking needs, they choose, or prefer, non-technological solutions, even when those may lead to increased loneliness.

References

1. Christensen, D.A.: Active ageing: country report Norway. (2003)
2. Syse, A., Pham, D.Q.: Befolkningsframskrivinger 2014-2100: Dødelighet og levealder - SSB, http://www.ssb.no/befolkning/artikler-og-publikasjoner/befolkningsframskrivinger-2014-2100-dodelighet-og-levealder
3. Keilman, N., Christiansen, S.: Norwegian elderly less likely to live alone in the future. Eur. J. Popul. **26**, 47–72 (2009)
4. Sundsli, K., Söderhamn, U., Espnes, G.A., Söderhamn, O.: Ability for self-care in urban living older people in southern Norway. J. Multidiscip. Healthc. **5**, 85–95 (2012)
5. The National Council for Senior Citizens' action plan - Nyheter – Seniorporten. http://www.seniorporten.no/Nyheter/The+National+Council+for+Senior+Citizens%27+action+plan.312320.cms
6. Russell, D.W., Cutrona, C.E., de la Mora, A., Wallace, R.B.: Loneliness and nursing home admission among rural older adults. Psychol. Aging **12**, 574–589 (1997)
7. Perissinotto, C.M., Cenzer, I.S., Covinsky, K.E.: Loneliness in older persons: a predictor of functional decline and death. Arch. Intern. Med. **172**, 1078–1083 (2012)
8. Fokkema, T., De Jong Gierveld, J., Dykstra, P.A.: Cross-national differences in older adult loneliness. J. Psychol. **146**, 201–228 (2012)
9. Cattan, M., White, M., Bond, J., Learmouth, A.: Preventing social isolation and loneliness among older people: a systematic review of health promotion interventions. Ageing Soc. **25**, 41–67 (2005)
10. Blythe, M.A., Monk, A.F., Doughty, K.: Socially dependable design: the challenge of ageing populations for HCI. Interact. Comput. **17**, 672–689 (2005)
11. Heart, T., Kalderon, E.: Older adults: are they ready to adopt health-related ICT? Int. J. Med. Inform. **82**, e209–e231 (2013)
12. Wiklund Axelsson, S., Melander Wikman, A., Näslund, A., Nyberg, L.: Older people's health-related ICT-use in Sweden. Gerontechnology **12**, 36–43 (2013)
13. Culén, A.L., Bratteteig, T.: Touch-screens and elderly users: a perfect match? In: ACHI 2013, The Sixth International Conference on Advances in Computer-Human Interactions. pp. 460–465 (2013)
14. Culén, A.L., Finken, S., Bratteteig, T.: Design and interaction in a smart gym: cognitive and bodily mastering. In: Holzinger, A., Ziefle, M., Hitz, M., Debevc, M. (eds.) SouthCHI 2013. LNCS, vol. 7946, pp. 609–616. Springer, Heidelberg (2013)

15. Bruk av IKT i husholdningene – SSB. http://www.ssb.no/ikthus
16. Mancini, J.A., Blieszner, R.: Aging parents and adult children: research themes in intergenerational relations. J. Marriage Fam. **51**, 275–290 (1989)
17. Hawkley, L.C., Cacioppo, J.T.: Loneliness matters: a theoretical and empirical review of consequences and mechanisms. Ann. Behav. Med. **40**, 218–227 (2010)
18. Victor, C., Scambler, S., Bond, J., Bowling, A.: Being alone in later life: loneliness, social isolation and living alone. Rev. Clin. Gerontol. **10**, 407–417 (2000)
19. Weiss, R.S.: Loneliness: The Experience of Emotional and Social Isolation. MIT Press, Cambridge (1974)
20. Neergaard, M.A., Olesen, F., Andersen, R.S., Sondergaard, J.: Qualitative description - the poor cousin of health research? BMC Med. Res. Methodol. **9**, 52 (2009)
21. Dourish, P.: Responsibilities and implications: further thoughts on ethnography and design. In: Proceedings of the 2007 Conference on Designing for User eXperiences, pp. 25:2–25:16. ACM, New York, NY, USA (2007)
22. Lindsay, S., Brittain, K., Jackson, D., Ladha, C., Ladha, K., Olivier, P.: Empathy, participatory design and people with dementia. In: Proceedings of the 2012 ACM annual conference on Human Factors in Computing Systems, pp. 521–530. ACM, New York, NY, USA (2012)
23. Sixsmith, A.J., Gibson, G., Orpwood, R.D., Torrington, J.M.: Developing a technology "wish-list" to enhance the quality of life of people with dementia. Gerontechnology **6**, 2–19 (2007)
24. Living Profiles » Map your social tree. http://livingprofiles.net/?page_id=99
25. Culén, A.L., van der Velden, M.: The digital life of vulnerable users: designing with children, patients, and elderly. In: Aanestad, M., Bratteteig, T. (eds.) SCIS 2013. LNBIP, vol. 156, pp. 53–71. Springer, Heidelberg (2013)
26. Culén, A.L., van der Velden, M., Herstad, J.: Travel experience cards: capturing user experiences in public transportation. In: The Seventh International Conference on Advances in Computer-Human Interactions. ThinkMind (2014)
27. Karabeg, A., Akkøk, N.: Visual representations and the web. In: Griffin, R., Chandler, S., Cowden, B.D. (eds.) Visual Literacy and Development: An African Experience, pp. 115–123. The International Visual Literacy Association, Toledo (2005)
28. Malinowsky, C., Almkvist, O., Kottorp, A., Nygård, L.: Ability to manage everyday technology: a comparison of persons with dementia or mild cognitive impairment and older adults without cognitive impairment. Disabil. Rehabil. Assist. Technol. **5**, 462–469 (2010)
29. Massimi, M., Baecker, R.M.: A Death in the family: opportunities for designing technologies for the bereaved. In: Proceedings of the SIGCHI Conference on Human Factors in Computing Systems. pp. 1821–1830. ACM, New York, NY, USA (2010)
30. Stefanov, D.H., Bien, Z., Bang, W.-C.: The smart house for older persons and persons with physical disabilities: structure, technology arrangements, and perspectives. IEEE Trans. Neural Syst. Rehabil. Eng. **12**, 228–250 (2004)
31. Holloway, I., Wheeler, S.: Qualitative Research in Nursing and Healthcare. Wiley-Blackwell, Chichester, Ames (2009)
32. Van der Velden, M., El Emam, K.: "Not all my friends need to know": a qualitative study of teenage patients, privacy, and social media. J. Am. Med. Inform. Assoc. **20**, 16–24 (2013)
33. Selwyn, N., Gorard, S., Furlong, J., Madden, L.: Older adults' use of information and communications technology in everyday life. Ageing Soc. **23**, 561–582 (2003)
34. Lindsay, S., Jackson, D., Schofield, G., Olivier, P.: Engaging older people using participatory design. In: Proceedings of the 2012 ACM Annual Conference on Human Factors in Computing Systems. pp. 1199–1208. ACM, New York, NY, USA (2012)

Effective Design of Traditional Japanese Tea Ceremony in a Group Home for the Elderly with Dementia

Teruko Doi[1](✉), Noriaki Kuwahara[2], and Kazunari Morimoto[2]

[1] Doi Clinic, 1-3-17 Nagaoka, NagaokaKyo City, Kyoto 617-0823, Japan
mialuna.conme.pino@gmail.com

[2] Kyoto Institute of Technology, 1 Hashigami-cho, Matsugasaki, Sakyo-ku, Kyoto City, Kyoto 606-8585, Japan

Abstract. Our group home is based on the following concept: "With the collaboration of medical treatment and nursing care, we make it our goal to have everyone smile every day and live life in accordance with their true selves." There are many ways of inducing smiles, and one of them is providing recreation rooted in Japanese traditional culture. We arrange events according to the season. In this way we seek to arrange the environment and offer an individualized care plan for the care of elderly persons with dementia whom we make every effort to support every day. As dementia progresses, it becomes impossible to maintain relationships or to remember one's past. Vexation and antagonistic attitudes become prominent due to anxiety, and communicating becomes problematic. But we have discovered that elderly persons with dementia change through participation in a traditional Japanese tea ceremony, recovering their smiles and their dignity. The tea ceremony is a tool enabling them to concentrate and share information with staff. This record shows the gradual introduction of tea ceremony at our group home.

Keywords: Japanese traditional culture · Dementia care

1 Introduction

Last November in Tokyo an international conference was held as a follow-up to the G8 Dementia Summit. This year Prime Minister Shinzo Abe declared a "national strategy on dementia." Countermeasures against dementia require the attention of the entire nation. It is estimated that in Japan, by 2025 one out of every five elderly persons above age 65, or roughly seven million people, will have dementia.

The basic principle of the "Plan for Promotion of Measures against Dementia," also known as the New Orange Plan, is "to respect the wills of those who have dementia, and to realize a society where they can live in a familiar, good environment and continue living life in their own way." This principle overlaps with our principle, which is "With the collaboration of medical treatment and nursing care, to make it our goal to have everyone smile every day and live life in accordance with their true selves."

The group home "Nursing Care for Communal Living for Dementia Patients" is a nursing insurance service for those with dementia to receive care and live communally. It is specialized to offer care of those with dementia to support respect for the individual

© Springer International Publishing Switzerland 2015
V.G. Duffy (Ed.): DHM 2015, Part II, LNCS 9185, pp. 413–422, 2015.
DOI: 10.1007/978-3-319-21070-4_41

and decrease BPSD (Behavioral Psychological Symptoms of Dementia) including depression, paranoia, irritation, excitement, violence, wandering, etc.

At the group home, non-drug treatment is the main way of dealing with dementia. Specifically, the treatments include reminiscence therapy, music therapy, physical therapy, occupational therapy, recreational therapy, and horticultural therapy. In this paper we would like to introduce environmental maintenance and psychotherapy as methods. This is the concrete practice of Person Centered Care [1]. In one of the forms of reminiscence therapy which focuses on memory dysfunction, media therapy, the person reminisced with their family and staff about their life, and it was attempted to raise the quality of care and as a result there was a decrease in BPSD.

At the group home "Terado" records of conversations (process records) of patients with dementia were read before and after the practice of tea ceremony, which has been continued at the group home since its opening. The practice of tea ceremony at the group home has an effect towards unexpected emotional reactions, mood, and emotions, and not only does it allow patients to enjoy the activity at the moment, but was seen to be effective in the improvement of everyday living, feeling purpose in life, and creating a sense of belonging. For those with dementia whose ability to communicate verbally has deteriorated by their condition, the practice of tea ceremony provides the security of following a set pattern and also allows better relations with others through spending time together at the same place with the same purpose. Also it provides an occasion for family members and staff to understand the person with dementia, who they are and how their spirits are. This leads to greater respect for the individual with dementia and a consequent reduction of BPSD.

2   Practicing Tea Ceremony at "Terado": Tea Ceremony

The group home must provide time and space where people can smile from their heart and make full use of their survival ability. The care staff must respect those with dementia as "whole persons" and at all times acknowledge their personhood [1]. However, the amount of time is in fact limited in which each person with dementia is listened to and acknowledged as a whole person and their suffering is understood. Therefore, it is important to devise strategies for daily recreation.

Types of recreation rooted in traditional Japanese culture such as "*Ikebana*" (Japanese flower arrangement) and tea ceremony are more easily accepted by those with dementia and are popular among family members and care staff. As a practical matter, without the approval of family members continuation is difficult, and if the recreation is not interesting for the care staff then it does not last long.

Tea ceremony, along with "*Ikebana*", was first among arts young ladies were expected to master, and "*Kaiseki*" cuisine, served as part of the tea ceremony, has now been designated a world heritage. Honeymoon meals served at ryokan (Japanese style hotels) are probably a luxurious version of "*Chakaiseki*" (meals served during tea ceremony), and "*Wagashi*" (Japanese sweets) using bean-paste skillfully are beautiful to the eye and certainly delicious. Few people may have the morning habit of boiling water in a pot and enjoying a little powdered tea, but most Japanese people have had the experience of healing their fatigue with a little powdered tea and tea ceremony sweets at a temple in Kyoto or a tea store in Kamakura. Whether or not they were formally taught, most Japanese also know that it is proper to hold the tea ceremony bowl with both hands, not one; to raise it reverently over the head; and to slowly turn it before drinking.

"*Hare* and *ke*": From ancient times the Japanese called ordinary days "*ke*" and non-ordinary days, those celebrating festivities and annual events, "*hare*," thus differentiating the ordinary and the extraordinary. Japan, with its four seasons, has cherished annual events which give color to everyday living, and the Japanese people have enjoyed a lifestyle of variety with clear lines drawn. "*Hatsugama*" (the first tea ceremony of the year) at New Year's as shown in Fig. 1 and the practicing of tea ceremony with seasons in mind allows those with dementia to have rhythm in their lifestyle and encourages rehabilitation of the brain's ability to awaken and recover memory.

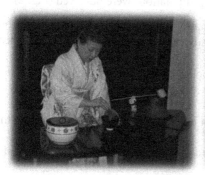 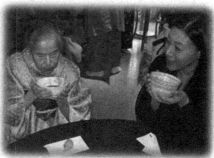

Fig. 1. "*Hatsugama*" in our group home

3 Method

3.1 Planning the Practicing of Tea Ceremony

Practicing tea ceremony with those with dementia requires different considerations from practicing it with healthy people. To determine what specific considerations were necessary, discussions were held among the staff in charge, the teacher, nurses, care workers, and care managers, and an appropriate environment was set in place.

1. "*Hatsugama*" was set as an occasion for the participation of all residents, nursing care workers, and members of the community.
2. To enable residents, nursing care staff, and members of the community to wear kimono (Japanese traditional clothing) when participating in "*Hatsugama*", a year-long kimono-wearing class will be held, thus building enthusiasm.
3. To gain their support, family members will be informed that tea ceremony is part of the care of dementia.
4. To heighten expectation, tea ceremony practice will be brought up in ordinary conversation.

5. Residents' general health will be improved. Leaving the main room and going to the tea room of the guest house creates a sense of being on an expedition, but if general health conditions are not good, this can become burdensome.

3.2 Method of Application of Practice of Tea Ceremony

Place, time, and frequency of tea ceremony practice are as follows.

- Place: tea room of group home "Terado"
- Time: from 2 pm until about 4:30 pm. People will be entering on their own so everyone can participate at their own pace
- Frequency: once a month

Regarding the actual practice, the following stipulations were observed (Fig. 2).

1. The purpose is not to have participants master the procedures for making tea but to allow them, as experts in life, to offer advice to younger nursing staff members practicing tea ceremony.
2. Equipment such as "*Fukusa*" (silk wrapping cloth), folding fans, and "*Kaishi*" (paper folded and tucked inside the front of the kimono) are to be made ready to be quickly used.
3. "*Mochi*" (glutinous rice cake) should not be the main snack as it can stick in the throat.
4. The temperature of the powdered tea must be monitored. Never say "Please be careful because it is hot."
5. The "*Fukusa*" is not to be handled by those with disability of the hand. Share information with the doctor beforehand.
6. Take existing friendships into consideration so that members of each table can enjoy their time together. Make sure that those who do not get along are not seated at the same Table
7. Pay careful attention to whether participants are tired or not, or if they are pushing too hard.
8. Make sure that residents are not getting bored with nothing to do. Try to talk to those who do not usually strike up conversations themselves when there are many people around.
9. On the day of tea ceremony practice, make announcements to the residents in the morning and repeat over and over that today is the day for tea ceremony practice. Prepare the tea room together for making sure no one is forced to participate.
10. When the delivery of "*Wagashi*" comes from the local store, receive it together with the residents, and ask about the origin of the name of the "*Wagashi*" and its ingredients.
11. The staff receives training in preparation of the tea. Participants will refine their manners as guests, and enjoy talking about the season and the sweets as well as the arrangement of the room, the hanging scroll, the teacher's comments, and the tea equipment.

12. The staff, as they practice preparing the tea, will maintain close coordination and adjust the entering of people from the main room.

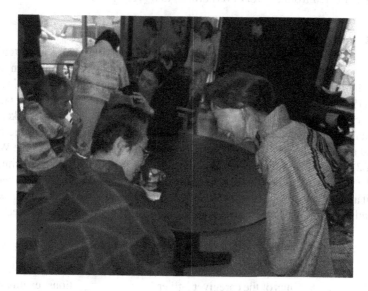

Fig. 2. A photograph taken during practice

3.3 Participants in the Tea Ceremony Practice

The average age of the group home residents is 85, and depending on the day they may or may not be able to participate. Also, it is difficult to maintain the same mood so the participants are not the same people each time. Besides residents, neighboring elderly people and local volunteers are also invited. At times a variety of guests may also participate, including local elementary school students, family members, kimono-wearing teachers, and staff of other offices.

– Group home residents 8–15 people
– Local elderly people 2–4 people
– Local volunteers 2–5 people
– Nursing care staff 3–5 people.

3.4 Evaluation Method

3.4.1 Method of Measuring the Effects of Tea Ceremony Practice
For the evaluation of tea ceremony practice, as regards to the psychological condition of the group home residents, to evaluate A before the practice, B during the practice, and C after the practice, the GBS scale [2], which is the scale used to evaluate the severity of different aspects of symptoms of dementia, was used and selections were made for the evaluation of emotion.

Specifically, the headings were "Emotional blunting", "Emotional liability", "Reduced motivation", "Anxiety", "Reduced mood" and "Restlessness," and the person recording evaluated from a level of 0 (normal) to 6 (very bad).

3.4.2   Record of Conversations (Process Record)

A process record, something put forward by Hildegard Peplau (1952), is a written record of interpersonal relationships, especially nurse and patient interactions, in clinical nursing. The format of this record, influenced by the nursing process discipline of Ida Orlando (1972), was refined to a method whereby after an event the nurse notes the patient's actions (interpersonal interaction), a percept analysis, and action taken based on that analysis, along with the nurse's introspective observations. When the process record and nurse's introspective observations were put into practice, Ernestine Wiedenbach (1962) standardized five self-evaluation categories, and clarified the technique of writing the process record so that a series of actions, or sequence, is taken as one undivided unit and each sequence is recorded as a chain of meaningful (i.e. analysis-worthy) actions and perceptions. Table 1 shows the example of the process record sheet.

Table 1. Example of the process record sheet

Patient behavior	Thoughts and feelings of the caregiver based on observation	Action of the caregiver	Analysis, observations, evaluations
Entry column 1	Entry column 2	Entry column 3	Entry column 4

3.5   Ethical Considerations

This investigation was carried out after we obtained consent, having explained using written documents that the gathered data will not be used for any purpose other than research, that when the research results are published no information that could identify individuals will be used, that participants' privacy will be carefully protected, and that if there is any change in the consent data will be deleted, etc. We also explained orally that participation in the study is optional, and based on the response gained we determined that consent was attained.

4   Results

4.1   GBS Scale

Figure 3 shows the average of the GBS scale of all subjects for before the practice, during the practice, and after the practice. For the sake of comparison, the scale for "Ikebana" practice which is done in Terado is shown in Fig. 4. Compared to Fig. 4 of "Ikebana", in Fig. 3 of tea ceremony the numbers for participants' condition before practice are low on the whole; in other words, the conditions were good, so no remarkable difference cannot be acknowledged for before, during, and after the practice, but as with the practicing of "*Ikebana*" there was a tendency of conditions to improve during and after the practice. But for people with relatively bad conditions, as Fig. 5 shows there was a tendency for notable amelioration during the practice. In Figs. 3 and 4 the limit of the vertical axis was at 3.5, but in Fig. 5 it is at 6.

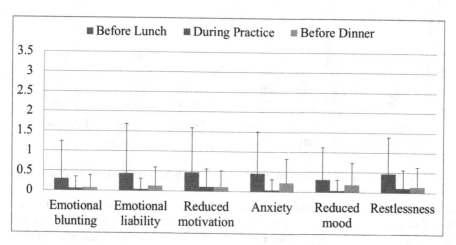

Fig. 3. Average of the GBS scale of all subjects in the tea practice (Color figure online)

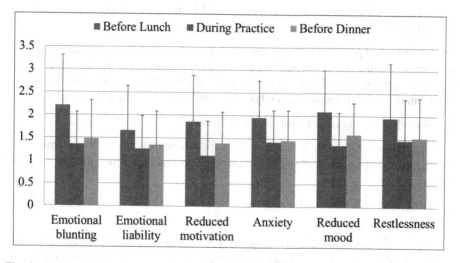

Fig. 4. Average of the GBS scale of all subjects in the "*Ikebana*" practice (Color figure online)

4.2 Records and Analysis of Utterance

As a characteristic of dementia, there is a frequent tendency to "cover up" from a desire that others not know one's illness-related suffering and anxiety, so it is usually quite difficult to hear the honest feelings of the person. This complicates communication

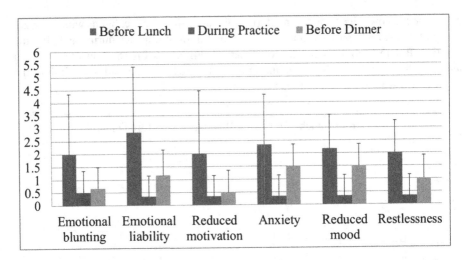

Fig. 5. Average of the GBS scale of the people with relatively bad conditions (Color figure online)

between the one with dementia and the care staff or family members. But this time, the record of utterances during the practice includes mention of the participant's anxiety and suffering. Below are typical utterances regarding anxiety and suffering about time, relationships, and independence, from the perspective of spiritual pain [3].

1. "Wow, January, when was New Year's? Did I eat mochi? I don't know anything anymore."

Uncertainty of previous memory leads to self-awareness of being forgetful and loss of the past; with the loss of the past, the present becomes uncertain and the future is also lost. There are no plans for the future or goals to shape the present. There is lack of understanding of why the person is where they are. (Spiritual pain with regard to time).

2. "Nobody from my family visits me. I feel lonely."

Impaired orientation leads to a loss of relationships with others. Even family and friends become enemies, resulting in loneliness. (Spiritual pain with regard to relationships).

3. "How long will this hand be functional? I don't want to live causing trouble to others."

Functional disorders mean the things the person was once able to do are no longer possible, leading to a loss of independence and productivity. (Spiritual pain with regard to independence).

5 Observations

At Terado, besides the practicing of tea ceremony, they do other recreational activities rooted in traditional Japanese culture like "Ikebana." But this time, with "Ikebana" and the practicing of tea ceremony, there was a measurable difference in effects. What could cause this difference, when both tea ceremony and "Ikebana" when are traditional forms of Japanese culture? Participants in the practice of tea ceremony included people who were relatively quieter and well-behaved, rather than those whose BPSD are more apparent, so the GBS scale was lower. In the practice of "Ikebana," attention is given to the flowers in front of one, and if there are scissors and a flower container ready then hands will move by themselves and start arranging flowers naturally. The activity utilizes experiences of the past. In nursing care, attention naturally goes to people who are loud, or to who simply have low ADL and need more intensive nursing care.

A dementia patient, who is paranoid, thinks their daughter-in-law is a thief, and insists someone call the police can focus on something interesting in front of them and enjoy themselves. Another person believes that their grandchild, who is now an adult, is still in elementary school and tries to go pick him/her up at the school. Others mumble meaningless words. Residents with severe symptoms who came in contact with an atmosphere different from the usual, for example the flowers with their various colors and fragrances, the flower teacher, and guests from the larger community, showed amelioration of their symptoms.

It would be incorrect to say that the tea ceremony had no discernible effects. This is because records of conversation during the practice include comments that get to the heart of caring for those with dementia. Usually, those who have a higher need for nursing care and those who speak with a loud voice do not have noticeable BPSD, but those with dementia experience spiritual pain. They feel that living is pointless and experience suffering, feelings of emptiness, purposelessness, vanity, and loneliness. In palliative medicine this is called "spiritual pain." The thoughts that filter out during the practice of tea ceremony suggest where the staff should direct their awareness and become involved, and are considered true words of the participants.

"Ichigo ichie," one of the teachings of the tea ceremony, means to value meetings that occur only once in a lifetime, and the non-ordinary place, atmosphere, and environment of the tea ceremony practice allows those words to come true. The shift from the main room to the tea room; the teacher and staff in kimono; the sound of the hot water boiling in the pot; the fragrance of incense; the attention poured on the tea server's every motion in a charged atmosphere; people giving strict admonishments to the care staff, who become students; people laughing: the space is definitely non-ordinary, and it is a world without barrier between givers and receivers of care. In this environment, whether one is aware of it or not, interpersonal communication is more easily established.

6   Conclusion

People can mind others and move towards independence once they are understood and attain a feeling of mutual understanding. What kind of care does not treat dementia patients as people who no longer know anything but acknowledges their individuality and treats them with according respect? Care eases suffering, makes it lighter, or makes it go away [4]. What is the anxiety and suffering of a person with dementia? Going beyond "cogito ergo sum (I think therefore I am)," there needs to be the mindset of "although I have dementia and I am different from who I once was, I desire, I feel, and I connect to other people; therefore I still exist." The suffering of those with dementia is the loss of meaning in life, loss of value, loss of purpose, loneliness, alienation, and emptiness which are all "suffering that comes from the loss of the meaning and existence of the self" [5].

Tea ceremony practice in the group home provided a chance to dig deeply into the idea of how and what to do for caregiving. Caregiving is based on relationship, and its purpose is to ease suffering and make it disappear through that relationship. The purpose of the tea ceremony is not to drink delicious tea. As demonstrated in the words *"Ichigo Ichie"* (once-in-a-lifetime encounter), the tea ceremony provides a setting for people to meet and understand one another. We showed that tea ceremony can be a "shape" that facilitates human relationships and that it can be effectively used in the frontlines of caring for those with dementia.

References

1. Kitwood, T.: Dementia Reconsidered: The Person Comes First, 1st edn. Open University Press, England (1997)
2. Gottfries, C.G., Brane, G., Gullberg, B., Steen, S.: A new rating scale for dementia syndrome. Arch. Gerontol. Geriatr. **1**(4), 311–330 (1982)
3. Murata, H.: Actual implementation of spiritual care in clinical settings (2) Detecting spiritual pain. Terminal Care **12**(5), 420–424 (2002). (In Japanese)
4. Murata, H.: Series Phenomenological Nursing 1: Delirium, 1st edn. Nihon Hyōronsha, Japan (2014). (In Japanese)
5. Murata, H.: Spiritual pain and its care in patients with terminal cancer, their care assessment, and construction of a conceptual framework for care. Jpn. J. Palliat. Med. **5**(2), 157–165 (2003). (In Japanese)

A Collaborative Change Experiment: Diagnostic Evaluation of Telecare for Elderly Home Dwellers

Suhas Govind Joshi and Anita Woll$^{(\boxtimes)}$

Department of Informatics, University of Oslo, Oslo, Norway
{joshi,anitwo}@ifi.uio.no

Abstract. This paper presents the diagnostic evaluation of a longitudinal collaborative change experiment that introduces telecare as a means for delivery of home care service to elderly home dwellers. The television is used as platform for delivery of care services from the home care nurses office to the private homes of the elderly home dwellers. We have included 34 participants in three sessions with evaluation and we use the results from the diagnostic evaluation to discuss how we can optimize the design of remote care in real environment. Our main findings concentrate on contextual factors that made impact on experienced usability issues, including timing and unstable network connection, complexity, and privacy and trust. In our study, we found that telecare is not for every elderly home dweller as it requires a high degree of functional capability in order to be experienced as appropriate and useful for the elderly users.

Keywords: Diagnostic evaluation · Usability issues · Elderly · Home telecare · Collaborative change experiment

1 Introduction

This paper reports from a diagnostic evaluation study of public home care service for the elderly by use of a video consultation system that builds on existing and familiar equipment in the home, i.e., the television. The study is a part of a larger collaborative change experiment, a longitudinal study set to last for 3 years. The motivation of the experiment is to study remote caring for active elderly people by transferring selected home care services to delivery through ICT. A challenge in the conventional home care service is that many active elderly are unable to start their day until the home care nurse has been on the daily visit, e.g., to give medications. The introduction of ICT-supported delivery of home care services allows active elderly people to receive home care services at more suitable and fixed times.

However, there is still a need to further explore how the care givers and care receivers experience ICT-supported care, especially bringing attention to usability according to the system's ability to perform selected care tasks by real users within their specific user context [1]. In our prior work [2], we presented findings from a usability testing study of the video consultation system. The study was conducted in controlled environments in our demonstration apartment in a building for care homes as the third phase of the long-term collaborative change experiment later illustrated in Fig. 1.

© Springer International Publishing Switzerland 2015
V.G. Duffy (Ed.): DHM 2015, Part II, LNCS 9185, pp. 423–434, 2015.
DOI: 10.1007/978-3-319-21070-4_42

Collaborative change experiment

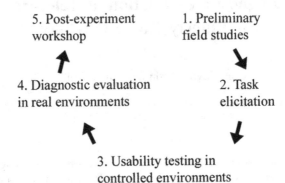

5. Post-experiment   1. Preliminary
workshop   field studies

4. Diagnostic evaluation   2. Task
in real environments   elicitation

3. Usability testing in
controlled environments

Fig. 1. Overview of the steps included in the collaborative change experiment

This paper presents findings from the fourth step of the collaborative change experiment, where the video consultation system has been refined and moved from controlled environments into the homes of the elderly home dwellers. Hence, this paper reports from a diagnostic evaluation of the video consultation system after being adopted into real environments.

The contribution of this paper adds to the existing HCI literature on caregiving through television by presenting findings from a longitudinal study of a video consultation system deployed and integrated into the work routines of the home care workers and as a part of the daily life activities of elderly home dwellers. Our research discusses both practical and methodical challenges when moving a system from controlled settings into real environments, and during the diagnostic evaluation, we emphasize on capturing the two-sided user experience of care including both the care givers (home care nurses) and care receivers (elderly home dwellers). Our results present users' assessment of system quality as well as discovered usability issues during delivery of home care via video consultation. Altogether, our diagnostic evaluation involved 34 participants, namely 16 home care workers and 18 elderly home dwellers.

The paper is organized as follows. Section 2 presents an overview of related work within the HCI-community. Section 3 briefly describes the longitudinal collaborative change experiment. Section 4 gives and overview of sessions and distribution of participants as well as our methodic approach, while Sect. 5 presents the results. In Sect. 6, we discuss usability issues based on our results and relate these to the previous work within HCI. Section 7 concludes the paper.

2   Related Work

Home telecare is a popular topic within the HCI community. However, few studies have addressed usability issues of incorporated telecare technologies between the home care nurses and their elderly care receivers directly. Milligan, Roberts and Mort [3] have studied how the move of telecare technologies affects the context of the private space, as well as the user experience of the care service. They state that *"Telecare affects the nature of care interactions within the home; hence the widespread adoption of these technologies is likely to have a significant impact on the broader landscape of care."* [3, p. 349]. The authors pinpoint that homes that are transformed into institutional context – with all kinds of medical devices and public regulations – conflicts with the gain of staying in the home for these home dwellers. They argue that designers have addressed these issues in recent time by developing and integrating telecare devices that match the layout of the home in order integrate assistive technologies in a subtle manner by providing *"invisible"* [p. 353] support in the home. Doyle, Bailey and Scanaill [4] confirm how few studies have looked into use of technology in practice, and further add that independent living technologies need to be moved into the homes of elderly people. This way, it can be tested in real environment in order to assess the real value of the design and to study the impact that the technology could have on their lives. Goodman-Deane and Lundell [5] continue the discussion on how the design of technology should meet the needs of the elderly by emphasizing the importance on capturing the user needs of *"real older people, including "baby boomers" still in employment, frail older people with disabilities and the full range in between* [6, p. 3]". Blythe, Monk and Doughty [6] explore the needs of the elderly people, and how these provide design implications for HCI. Their study is based on findings from structured interviews with health professionals and elderly people. The authors express concern about technologies used for monitoring bring very little attention to the social context of the home.

Other HCI studies report findings from collaborative or interactive services where elderly people use the television from their home as a platform to receive telecare or similar services [7]. Several studies have made contributions that concern age-related challenges when designing for the elderly generation [8–12]. Others have provided new knowledge on how to develop interfaces usable for older people, e.g., [13, 14]. For instance, Baunstrup and Larsen [13] point out that the television has evolved from a one-way monologue into a communications platform by offer increased dialogue-based services. They also argue that an iTV provides more *"complex interaction paradigm"* [13, p. 13] since it usually involves additional equipment such as set-top box, additional monitor and media streaming device. Other research contributions emphasize the importance of studying elderly people who already master the interface in the search for compensatory strategies that may be generally applicable to this user group in order to improve the user experience [15]. They point out that previous studies, e.g., [12], mainly deal with physical, sensory and cognitive limitations that come with aging, while they them-selves believe that one should also include aspects of *"privacy, acceptability, stigma, control, trust, choice and social alienation"* [15, p. 614] into the design process. Specifically, they believe that privacy and trust to be key elements when HCI research enters private homes and communities.

3 Collaborative Change Experiment

We have designed a collaborative change experiment consisting of five stepwise activities. Through these five activities, we aim to experiment with alternative solutions to the existing routines in the delivery of home care services. We emphasize that our goal is not to bring in a permanent change, but rather to explore underlying issues and gain a deeper insight that may contribute to a future permanent change. To address the inter-dependency, we have designed our collaborative change experiment in such a way that it captures usability issues on both sides of the service. Two traditional task-centered user evaluations make out the key activities in our change experiment: the usability testing reported in [2], and the diagnostic evaluation presented in this paper. Common for both of these activities is that they have been expanded from a traditional user-observer setup to a parallel experiment where we have users and observers on both sides of the service simultaneously. In addition to these two main activities, we have supplemented the collaborative change experiment with three supporting activities that we believe helps strengthen the design process, as well as make it more coherent. Through these auxiliary activities, we (1) address some of the challenges that are not directly covered by traditional usability testing, and we (2) gain important input that contribute directly towards the facilitation of the usability testing and diagnostic evaluation. Figure 1 illustrates the five activities and their order. A comprehensive description of the collaborative change experiment was previously presented in [2].

4 Diagnostic Evaluation

The diagnostic evaluation consisted of three different sessions and involved 34 participants altogether. The first session was held in the office of the home care workers over two days and included 12 home workers and administrators. The second session was conducted at the local care home with 14 elderly participants. The third session was a two-way test where we were present on both sides of the interaction and captured issues from both perspectives. This session involved 4 home care workers and 4 elderly participants. Table 1 gives an overview of the three sessions and the distribution of participants. The reason for the number of participant being considerably lower in the third test was that it required parallel presences and had to be coordinated beforehand so we could be ready in the homes of the elderly participants for the call. Nevertheless, all three sessions followed the same methodical procedure and used the same criteria and scale for the tests. Participants were asked to give an evaluation of how they perceived the quality of the system from a technical perspective by grading the image clarity, sound quality and light conditions. For each conversation, we kept track of usability issues by counting five particular values: number of attempts to establish the call, numbers of words repeated during the conversation, number of image freezes, number of drops in image quality, and number of instances with choppy sound.

Table 1. Overview of the three sessions in the diagnostic evaluation

Session	Participants	Site	Elderly participants	Home care workers
1	Home care workers	Home care office		12
2	Elderly participants	Local care home	14	
3	Both groups	Both sites	4	4

In order to capture a broader frame with environmental factors, e.g., lightning and tidiness, all participants, were equipped with 40-inch televisions with wide-angle HD-camera, as well as all necessary network facilities. The nurses called each home dweller, and they had to actively answer the call by using a remote controller in order to establish the connection.

The empirical setting for our study was a local care building with 87 care homes for elderly. The elderly participants were located in their private homes while the nurses were at their homecare service office. Figure 2 demonstrates how two of the home care nurses used the setup in their office, while Fig. 3 shows the setup at the homes of the 4 home dwellers that participated in session 3.

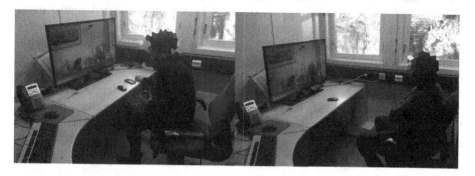

Fig. 2. Two home care workers talking to an elderly from their office

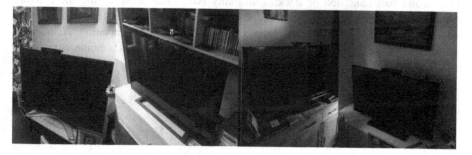

Fig. 3. The television setup in the apartments of the four elderly participants in session 3

5 Result

5.1 System Quality

One half of the evaluation consisted of participants assessing image clarity, sound quality and light conditions. Table 2 summarizes the average score reported by each group. As we can see from the table, the assessment of image clarity, sound quality and

Table 2. Average assessment of image, sound and light quality

Test #	Image clarity	Sound quality	Light conditions	Mean	SD
Group 1	8.86	7.57	8.57	8.33	0.55
Group 2	8.08	7.62	8.15	7.95	0.24
Group 3	8.07	7.93	8.36	8.12	0.18
Mean	8.34	7.71	8.36		
SD	0.37	0.16	0.17		

light conditions were very similar across the three groups. All three usability metrics had low internal standard deviation ($\sigma_{image} = 0.37$, $\sigma_{sound} = 0.16$, $\sigma_{light} = 0.17$), which indicates that the quality of image, sound and light were considered similar equal between the three groups. The average score given by each group for the three quality metrics ($\sigma_{session1} = 8.33$, $\sigma_{session2} = 7.95$, $\sigma_{session3} = 8.12$) suggests that the system is – from a technical perspective – capable of delivery all tasks listed in our previous paper [2], and that the overall assessment of the system itself was positive. Figure 4 illustrates the grades given on image clarity, sound quality and light conditions by each of the 34 participants that contributed to the three tests. The lowest grade given at any point was 5 out of 10. This suggest that there were no incidents at any time during the 34 tests – involving 95 min with real delivery of home care services – where the image, sound or light were considered to be worse than 5 out of 10.

5.2 Usability Issues

The second part consisted of tracking usability issues that arose during the conversation between the elderly person and the home care nurse. We kept track of five values in order to count the numbers of issues during each conversation. *Number of attempts to establish the call* helped us record how many times a home care nurse had to call before the elderly participant answered the call. *Number of words*

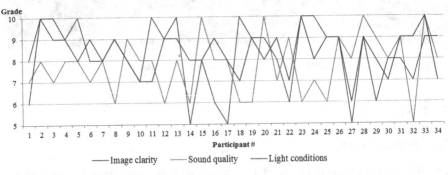

Fig. 4. Overview of grading on image, sound and light qualities from all participants

repeated during the conversation gave us an idea of how many times there was a miscommunication and one of the parties had to repeat a word or sentence. We only counted those issues that happened due to technical problems (e.g., choppy sound) as elderly people struggling to hear everything is still an issue with physical presence. *Number of image freezes* provided a count on how many times the screen froze or went black. While this often accompanied sound issues, there were instances of only image freezes without any sound issues. *Number of drops in image quality* was an indicator of how often the quality of the image would drop to a low-resolution, pixelated and blurry image. This usually happed when the Internet connection was slow or unstable. *Number of in-stances with choppy sound* captured all occurrences of unclear or dropping sound. Table 3 gives an overview of the average number of issues per conversation we registered in each session. The conversation time is included for all session in order to give an idea of error counts not only per conversation, but also per minute.

Table 3 presents the average number of issues registered per conversation. The number registered for each issue is fairly consistent between session 1 and 2 – with the biggest difference being 0.30 for sound chops. We registered a higher number of issues on per conversation during session 3, but that was only due to longer conversation time on average. In fact, the numbers of issues we registered during session 3 were lower than the number we registered during session 1 and 2. Since we were present at both sites simultaneously during session 3, the eight participants only yielded four conversations. Compared to session 1 and 2 with a total of 26 participants, we ended up with a much smaller selection this might have affected the number of errors we registered on average. However, being able to capture such issues on both sides of the interaction simultaneously allowed us to capture usability issues more accurately, thus we should expect the number to rise with additional two-sided evaluations. The average conversation time was 02:44 min, and the average numbers of errors per conversation was 8.10 (or 2.97errors/minute). As the deviation in errors/minute was low between these three sessions ($\sigma = 0.16$), we consider the diagnostic evaluation to have captured a representative understanding of usability issues experienced in real-life use rather than in laboratorial settings. As we can see from Fig. 5, the registered issues are for most part evenly distributed. The

Table 3. Average issue count for the three sessions

Issue (avg. count)	Session 1	Session 2	Session 3	Mean	SD
Attempts at calling	1.43	1.38	1.71	1.51	0.15
Repeated words	1.64	1.85	2.29	1.92	0.27
Image freeze	1.07	1.23	2.00	1.43	0.41
Quality drops	1.07	1.23	1.57	1.29	0.21
Sound chops	2.07	1.77	2.00	1.95	0.13
Total number	7.28	7.46	9.57	8.10	0.90
Conversation time	02:24	02:20	03:29	02:44	00:32
Issues per minute	3.03	3.19	2.75	2.97	0.16

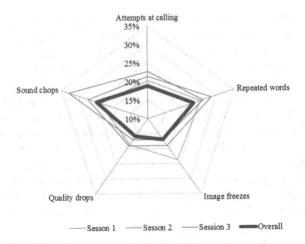

Fig. 5. Distribution of issues for each session and overall aggravated distribution

thick red polygon indicates the overall distribution, and on average, sound chops seem to be the biggest problem (25.0 %). This is one of the most common symptoms of Internet connectivity issues and was not unexpected.

5.3 Beyond the Usability Issues

As we can see in Table 2, the overall assessment of the system quality was positive. However, the use of the system is a part of a larger context, in which we have to consider the task, the flow, the complexity, as well as the very presence of the technology in their homes. First of all, usability issues were not symmetrical, i.e., they were not experienced the same on both sides. Session 3 revealed big differences in both what issued that occurred on each side, as well as how the elderly participant experienced them. Issues due to network instability may result in sound or image issues on both sides, however we registered that the symptoms were rarely similar or never happened simultaneously. The grading assessment was also different during the two-sided observation in session 3. The fact that the number of issues we registered per minute was very similar between the two groups (session 1 and 2) suggests that over time, the issues converge towards very similar levels despite there being individual anomalies. Nevertheless, the type of issue did not matter as much as how disturbing it was to the established flow. For instance, one person in the middle of an exercise may not be bothered if the image quality drops for a few seconds as long as they can still see the main movements and hear the instructions. However, if the sound drops just as the health care worker is about to give instruction on taking medicine, then it becomes a serious issue. Ultimately, it was not the actions of the users but rather the connectivity that decided the frequency and duration of these issues. While the users themselves reported high scores on the isolated technical capabilities of the system, once we counted the issues that arose during conversations, we saw how the experience and quality of the service was greatly reduced due to connectivity issues.

6 Discussion

The results display usability issues of home telecare in real environments. Doyle et al. [4] recommend studying technology use in practice by moving out of the comfortable computer laboratory. Our experiences as we moved from controlled to real test environments were that the underlying contextual factors became more evident compared to the technical capabilities of the system, and the contextual factors had a high impact on the results.

6.1 Timing and User Context

We experienced less control as facilitators when testing in real environment concerning both practical and methodical issues, e.g., we did not know if the participants were awake and ready; or even at home at the time the video consultation was supposed to find place. Neither did we have control over the infrastructure, e.g. the network capacity in the private spaces nor if the camera was still connected to the television. Thus, the results were more affected by the users' context than isolated technical capabilities, and the timing of the call had great impact on the user's ability to incorporate ICT-supported care into their daily life activities. Moreover we lost the ability to observe every usability issue at close up in the move from controlled to real environment. Therefore, we had to translate the users' problems as they reported them. In our previous usability study [2], we observed that the fixed position of the television screen and the camera within the living room were found helpful to compensate the participants' decline motoric skills [2]. However, in real environment, the fixed position were not experienced as flexible in use for elderly users who were unexpected bedridden or for those doing their morning bath or eating breakfast in the kitchen. All participants had various mobility issues, which resulted in extra time spent moving from one place to another in the home. Thus, we support Dolye et al. [4] who stress the importance of testing in real environment. It is only then, when real users adopt the technology into their everyday life activities, researchers can gain knowledge of the sustainability of their design, and whether it can work in everyday practice with regards to necessary infrastructure, design and simplicity of use.

Another experience we made according to the user context was our interruption of the television domain. As we found it constructive to build the home telecare services on existing and familiar technology in the home by using the participants own television as a platform for the HD camera. This among others to avoid according to Milligan et al. [3] to transform the home with alienating telecare technologies that can affect the participant's own perspective of the home, as well as the user's experiences of the care service. However, we found it in some occasions difficult when disturbing the participants while watching television as e.g. one participant expressed: *"Oh no, you just called me while the reporter interviewed Petter Northug (a famous ski athlete in Norway) – can you please switch the channel back."* The care giver may in traditional home care service use such an occasion to share the highlights in the news together with the care receiver in order to small talk. Thus, a care giver has to know the care receiver well in order to make a conversation beyond the set care tasks and context when moving the care interaction into a video conference. However, this could also imply that the participants may demand the home care nurses not to call them during their favorite television programs.

6.2 Complexity

A number of HCI researchers have pinpoint age-related challenges when designing for the elderly [8–14]. However, building services on familiar technology such as the television still require additional equipment for additional services - which are making the mastery of the television increasing in complexity. Our study participants have all a large and modern television in their living room, and a set up box for addition channels. Thus, the participants had to master an additional remote controller, and navigate to the correct hdmi source for video conference as we added the HD camera to their television. Moreover, the participants had to switch back to the correct hdmi source in order to return to their television services. This was experienced as troublesome for all of our elderly end-users. Moreover, a common user challenge for the majority of our participants was to locate the remote controller in order to operate the video conference. A universal or an integrated remote controller to the TV – chair may be a solution to this usability problem. Thus, the HD camera should be designed for manual operation as a backup option for lost remote controller. However, the participants need training and practice in order to fully see the potential and understand different use of a familiar technology – as well as they need to be allowed to get the necessary time in order to answer the video call.

6.3 Privacy and Trust

Niman et al. [16] emphasized the importance of including privacy and trust as central aspect of the design process [13], which are especially relevant for HCI researchers moving their test environment into private spaces. Two participants in our study asked if we as researchers could see them 24/7. Moreover, one of the participants pulled out the hdmi cable as she did not want us to see her half naked sitting at the kitchen table. Installing cameras in the homes of the elderly address both privacy and trust issues – and it is essential that we as researchers are aware of informing the participants thorough, and that we show humility and respect when entering private spaces. Moreover, we support that privacy and trust should be included in design, e.g. in our study we rather should have used a camera that had a "curtain" in front of the camera lens (when not in use) to avoid the end-users feeling that their privacy was intruded.

Additionally to contextual factors that were found present during diagnostic evaluation in real environment, we as well as experienced usability issues concerning deterioration of our participants health condition. We have over time experienced that the participants within our empirical setting have had increased need for health care services as a result of decreased functional capability. Blythe et al. [6] argue for the importance of capturing the broader range of user needs among elderly including users with high to low functional capabilities. However, home telecare is not for every elder, and merely for selected services that are experienced appropriate delivered as remote care. Thus, for elderly with complex health care needs, home telecare as delivery of health care services is not an option. However, if the home care nurses are able to reduce their overall work load by delegating some of their services via video conferences to those elderly who are more or less independent living, then the nurses can allocate their time more efficiently by providing traditional health care services to those care receivers who need them the most, and are depended on extended and local care in the home.

7 Conclusion

In this paper, we have studied the two-sided interaction of care between elderly home dwellers and home care nurses by use of video conference equipment in real environment. As we moved from controlled to real test environments, several contextual factors became evident and had a high impact on the usability issues. Despite positive experiences with the system's technical capabilities and potential, the circumstantial issues became predominant. These issues are as follows: First, the timing of the telecare call was essential in order for the participants to receive remote care as part of their everyday life activities. Second, adding services and additional equipment to the familiar television platform increased the complexity of its use for the participants. Third, privacy and trust were central concerns among the participants included in our study –these concerns should be supported in design of home telecare systems. Finally, home telecare is not for every elder home dweller, and merely for selected services that are experienced appropriate delivered as remote care. Thus, home telecare such as video conference requires a certain degree of functional capabilities in order to be experienced as appropriate and useful for the elderly participants.

References

1. Bevan, N.: Measuring usability as quality of use. Softw. Qual. J. **4**, 115–150 (1995)
2. Joshi, S.G., Woll, A.: A collaborative change experiment: telecare as a means for delivery of home care services. In: Marcus, A. (ed.) DUXU 2014, Part III. LNCS, vol. 8519, pp. 141–151. Springer, Heidelberg (2014)
3. Bevan, N.: Measuring usability as quality of use. Softw. Qual. J. **4**, 115–150 (1995)
4. Milligan, C., Roberts, C., Mort, M.: Telecare and older people: who cares where? Soc. Sci. Med. **72**(3), 347–354 (2011). doi:10.1016/j.socscimed.2010.08.014
5. Doyle, J., Bailey, C., Scanaill, C.: Lessons learned in deploying independent living technologies to older adults homes. Univ. Access Inf. Soc. **13**(2), 191–204 (2014)
6. Goodman-Deane, J., Lundell, J.: HCI and the older population. Interact. Comput. **17**(6), 613–620 (2005)
7. Blythe, M.A., Monk, A.F., Doughty, K.: Socially dependable design: the challenge of ageing populations for HCI. Interact. Comput. **17**(6), 672–689 (2005)
8. Miyazaki, M., Sano, M., Mitsuya, S., Sumiyoshi, H., Naemura, M., Fujii, A.: Development and field trial of a social TV system for elderly people. In: Stephanidis, C., Antona, M. (eds.) UAHCI 2013, Part II. LNCS, vol. 8010, pp. 171–180. Springer, Heidelberg (2013)

9. Carmichael, A., Newell, A.F., Morgan, M.: The efficacy of narrative video for raising awareness in ICT designers about older users' requirements. Interact. Comput. **19**(5–6), 587–596 (2007)
10. O'Neill, S.A., et al.: Development of a technology adoption and usage prediction tool for assistive technology for people with dementia. Interact. Comput. **26**(2), 169–176 (2014)
11. Sayago, S., Sloan, D., Blat, J.: Everyday use of computer-mediated communication tools and its evolution over time: an ethnographical study with older people. Interact. Comput. **23**(5), 543–554 (2011)
12. Weiner, M.F., Rossetti, H.C., Harrah, K.: Videoconference diagnosis and management of Choctaw Indian dementia patients. Alzheimer's Dement. **7**(6), 562–566 (2011)
13. Hawthorn, D.: Possible implications of aging for interface designers. Interact. Comput. **12** (5), 507–528 (2000)
14. Baunstrup, M., Larsen, L.B.: Elderly's barriers and requirements for interactive TV. In: Stephanidis, C., Antona, M. (eds.) UAHCI 2013, Part II. LNCS, vol. 8010, pp. 13–22. Springer, Heidelberg (2013)
15. van de Watering, M.: The impact of computer technology on the elderly. In: Human Computer Interaction (2005)
16. von Niman, B., et al.: User experience design guidelines for telecare services. In: Proceedings of the 8th Conference on Human-Computer Interaction with Mobile Devices and Services. ACM (2006)

A Mobile Visual Diary for Personal Pain Management

Tor-Morten Grønli[1(✉)], Gheorghita Ghinea[2,3], and Fotis Spyridonis[3]

[1] Faculty of Technology, Mobile Technology Lab (MOTEL), Westerdals Oslo School of Arts, Communication and Technology, Schweigaardsgt. 14, 0185 Oslo, Norway
tmg@westerdals.no

[2] Faculty of Technology, Westerdals Oslo School of Arts, Communication and Technology, Schweigaardsgt. 14, 0185 Oslo, Norway
george.ghinea@brunel.ac.uk

[3] School of Information Systems, Computing and Mathematics, Brunel University, Uxbridge, London, UB8 3PH, UK
fotis.spyridonis@brunel.ac.uk

Abstract. Back-pain is one of the most prolific health problems within the population and costs industry lost revenue due to the amount of days people have to take off in order to recover. In this paper, we have targeted this problem and suggested a mobile app for visually diarizing the pain experience of patients. The Android platform is utilized and its technology stack forms the basis for this 3D centric application. Positive evaluations obtained provide evidence of the promising nature of the approach and indicate several future directions of research within mobile pain management.

Keywords: Pain management · Pain diary · Interface · Mobile application · Android · 3D

1 Introduction

Chronic pain can be a debilitating condition; it affects men and women in equal measure, citizens of both developed and developing countries, impacting considerably on countries' GDP through reduced productivity and lost working days. Moreover, back-pain does not affect solely the adult population: studies across Europe show that back-pain is very common in children, with around 50 percent experiencing back-pain at some time [1]. Any improvement in the way that patients with back-pain can be analyzed (and subsequently treated) is therefore potentially capable of significantly saving both benefit expenditure and lost man-hours [2–6].

To this end, in this paper we propose the use of mobile application ('app') for visually diarizing a patient's experience of pain. Our solution is based on the use of a "pain drawing" – these are two dimensional representations of the contour of a human body, widely used in clinical settings, on which the patient indicates the location, spread and type of pain [3, 4, 6, 7]. Based on previous work of ours [8], we extend these traditional paper-based pain drawings not only into the digital realm, but, given the ubiquity of mobile phone technology, into an app through which patients can indicate on a 3D

© Springer International Publishing Switzerland 2015
V.G. Duffy (Ed.): DHM 2015, Part II, LNCS 9185, pp. 435–440, 2015.
DOI: 10.1007/978-3-319-21070-4_43

mannequin not only the type and position of the pain experienced, but also its intensity. This enables chronic pain sufferers to keep electronic diaries of their pain; given that the app is available on a mobile platform, the diarizing process can be performed anytime-anywhere. Moreover, in so doing, not only does the patient become an active stakeholder in the management of his/her pain, but, s/he builds a better understanding of the relationship between the pain experienced and the type of activities undertaken as well as the timing and quantity of the medication administered [9]. Indeed, by engaging in this process, chronic sufferers have reported a better pacing of medication intake, with a reduction of up to a third in the quantities of medication involved.

2   Application Architecture and Design

The application is developed for the Android platform [10]. By the nature of the Android platform, this enables the application to run on smartphone devices as well as tablets. The full benefit of the application is first reached when running on a 7″ or larger tablet device. In such a device we are able to facilitate full interaction and visualization for the user, emphasizing the interaction with the displayed 3D model as the main feature of the app. The application is built around a 3D toolkit implementation to allow cross device Android implementation, increase developer environment support and provide a robust, scalable architecture.

2.1   Platform Architecture

Google released Android in November 2007, under the framework of the Open Handset Alliance [11]. The goal was to provide a platform for open innovation for mobile solutions and that the source code should be provided free of charge and made available through open source arenas. Android is an open source mobile operating system based on the Linux kernel and facilitates developers to write managed code in Java using Google developed Java libraries [12]. The Android platform does not only provide the mobile operating system itself including the development environment, but also provides a custom built runtime environment, named the "Android Runtime Environment (ART)" starting from their 2014 release of the operating system codenamed "Lollipop" (This replaced the previous virtual machine runtime based on the Dalvik Virtual Machine). Applications can run independently as well as acting as the middleware between native code/API components and the operating system. For application development, Android facilitates the use of 2D and 3D graphic libraries, a customized, a media framework, onboard SQL engine for persistent storage, near field communication capabilities and advanced network capabilities such as 3G, 4G and WLAN (Fig. 1).

The API is constantly evolving and the current release (5 Lollipop) [12] is a huge increment compared with number of available features from release 1.0. The current version of the API facilitates not only programming for mobile devices, but also separate segments for TV, cars and wearables. Since Android is an open source mobile operating system, the community is welcomed to collaborate in the evolvement of the programming environment, the operating system and the API.

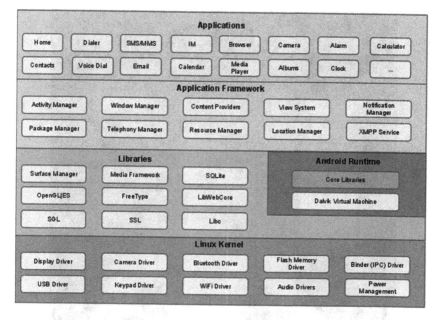

Fig. 1. Android system architecture [10]

2.2 Application Design

The Mobile Visual Diary for Personal Pain Management product reduces the cost of caring for patients suffering significant pain whilst improving their overall quality of life. It does this by replacing the current traditional 2 dimensional paper based pain indication methods during consultations with a system that records patient's pain profile over time, away from the clinic. The data collected by the patient can later very efficiently be presented for clinicians during their appointment. This reduces clinician/patient exposure time and increases the accuracy of determining prescription, saving significant costs and increasing the number of patients seen during clinics. By applying a mobile approach we take advantage of the everyday presence of mobile devices and empower the user to take control of his/her own situation. The native environment on the Android platform enables easily for integration of 3D based figures and everyday mobile gestures such as tap, pinch-to-zoom, drag and drop etc. are available in the platform software development kit.

On the screen (Fig. 2), the user is presented with five different pain types; numbness, stabbing, pins & needles, burning, and stiffness, which were arbitrary color-coded. These types were chosen carefully after consultation with clinical staff, and are well documented in the literature [2, 7].

User interaction is based both on touch and gesture input. For example, the user can tilt the device and engage the device accelerometer to rotate the 3D mannequin model. Additionally for pain selection, the user selects an appropriate pain type by tapping on the predefined list presented on the left of the screen, and then the location of the pain is selected, again by tapping on the desired body part of the model. Each color represents

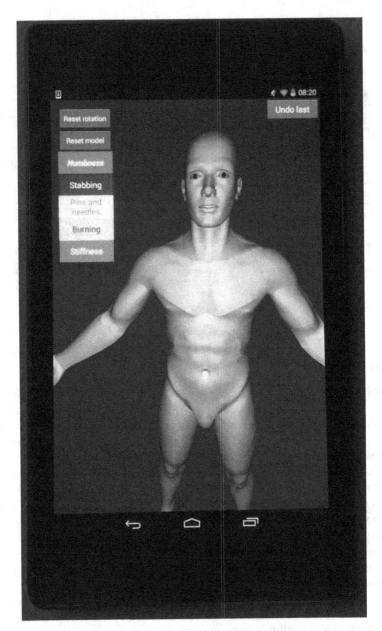

Fig. 2. App running on a Nexus 7″ tablet device

a pain type and the model is colored at the selected location (Fig. 3). With multi-tap (up till four times) the color is applied on the same body part, a darker color will be displayed for each tap, indicating a stronger pain.

When the user exits the model interaction screen, the application saves model history data about the selected body part (s) and pain type (s), timestamp and a comment. Later

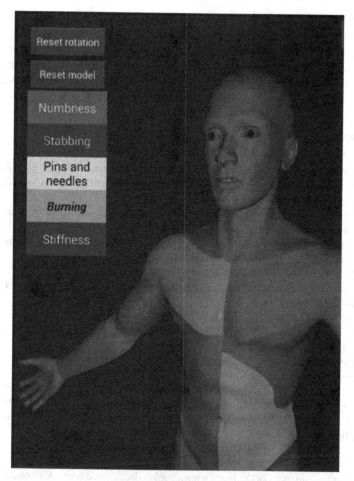

Fig. 3. User interface close up with the 3D model including pain indicator (Color figure online)

the user can revisit the saved models and play back the history of indicated pain levels for any period of his/her choosing.

3   Results and Conclusion

Preliminary evaluation of the application indicates a generally positive user experience when interacting with the app in respect of the apps usability and functionality (the features receives very positive feedback and commentary when presented and tested). The application shows how it can be a feasible alternative for users in conical pain in terms of self-management of the pain and possibly lead to positive benefits such as improved life quality, intake of medicines adjusted to pain development and daily control the personal pain levels.

Back-pain is one of the most prolific health problems within the population and costs industry lost revenue due to the amount of days people have to take off in order to recover. In this paper, we have targeted this problem and suggested a mobile app for visually diarizing the pain experience of patients. The positive evaluations obtained provide evidence of the promising nature of the approach described; this will however have to be confirmed by more extensive studies benefitting from clinical settings.

References

1. Baker, M., et al.: Improving the current and future management of chronic pain: A European Consensus Report (2014). http://www.mijnpijn.nl/pdf/PainProposalEuropeanReport.pdf. Last Accessed 10 June 2014
2. Lee, S.J.: Pain measurement: understanding existing tools and their application in the emergency department. Emerg Med. **13**, 279–287 (2001)
3. Mannion, A.F., Balague, F., Pellise, F., Cedraschi, C.: Pain measurement in patients with low back pain. Nat. Clin. Pract. Rheumatol. **3**, 610–618 (2007)
4. Haefeli, M., Elfering, A.: Pain assessment. Eur. Spine J. **15**, 17–24 (2006)
5. Ohnmeiss, D.D.: repeatability of pain drawings in a low back pain population. Eur. Spine. **25**, 980–988 (2000)
6. Jamison, R.N., Fanciullo, G.J., Baird, J.C.: Usefulness of pain drawings in identifying real or imagined pain: accuracy of pain professionals, non-professionals, and a decision model. Eur. J. Pain **5**, 476–482 (2004)
7. Masferrer, R., Prendergast, V., Hagell, P.: Colored pain drawings: preliminary observations in neurosurgical practice, in. Eur. J. Pain **7**, 213–217 (2003)
8. Spyridonis, F., Hansen, J., Gronli, T.-M., Ghinea, G.: PainDroid: an android-based virtual reality application for pain assessment. J. Multimedia Tools Appl. **72**(1), 191–206 (2014)
9. Serif, T., Ghinea, G.: Recording of time-varying back-pain data: a wireless solution. IEEE Trans. Inf Technol. Biomed. **9**(3), 447–458 (2005)
10. Google Developers (2015). Android development. http://developer.android.com/develop/index.html. Accessed 10 Feb 2015
11. Open Handset Alliance (2015). http://www.openhandsetalliance.com/. Accessed 20 Feb 2015
12. Google (2015). What is Android? http://developer.android.com/about/index.html. Accessed 20 Feb 2015

Usefulness of Ikebana a Nursing Care Environment

Yuki Ikenobo[1,2], Yusaku Mochizuki[1(✉)], and Akinori Kuwahara[1(✉)]

[1] Department of Advanced Fibro-Science, Kyoto Institute of Technology,
Matsugasaki, Sakyo-ku, Kyoto 606-8585, Japan
hanahana@ikenobo.jp, mczk0520@gmail.com,
nkuwahar@kit.ac.jp
[2] Ikenobo, 248 Donomae-cho, Nakagyo-ku, Kyoto 604-8134, Japan

Abstract. Japanese society is aging rapidly and currently one in four people of the population are the elderly. Due to the increasing number of the elderly who need nursing care, improvement of their QOL is required. As a recreation activity of the nursing care for the elderly, I implemented Ikebana, an aspect of Japanese traditional culture of life. There was no change in the test subject's NPI score, but in the GBS scale, which measures an immediate change, improvement in emotional state of the subject was found. Compared to popular recreation activities such as karaoke or viewing of DVD video, the subject's mental state was maintained in good condition for a long period of time even after making ikebana. The result suggested that ikebana has a healing effect, especially for reducing the anxiety or for recovering calmness. Enjoying a sense of season through flower materials, use of five senses by touching or seeing, thinking for oneself, hand working with tools such as scissors and having a dialogue with people are possible contributing factors. It is likely that ikebana gives the elderly mental stability and that it is useful for keeping them stay in good mental health, making a great contribution for the QOL in aging society in the future.

Keywords: Nursing care · Health · Recreation activity · Dementia

1 Introduction

Japan's population continues to increase in age, and as of October 2012, the percentage of elderly people was 24.1 %, the highest it has ever been. 1) It is believed that this trend will continue in the future. As a result of this, it is also predicted that the number of nurses, a necessity to the elderly, will also increase, and methods to maintain and improve elderly people's QOL (Quality of Life) are sought after. Up to now, various programs have been implemented as recreation in caring for the elderly. Examples of these programs include music concerts, karaoke and growing vegetable gardens, as well as calisthenics and exercise programs. Among these programs are also programs that increase effectiveness. For example, it has been reported that color-by-number pictures that use colored calligraphy pens have a fixed effect on reducing the amount of times nurses are called and the number of times residents have fallen over. 2) Up to

© Springer International Publishing Switzerland 2015
V.G. Duffy (Ed.): DHM 2015, Part II, LNCS 9185, pp. 441–447, 2015.
DOI: 10.1007/978-3-319-21070-4_44

now, a variety of programs have been introduced, yet due to management's desire for ease in caring for the elderly, using ikebana has been difficult. However, because the percentage of elderly ikebana teachers and students is large and examples of ikebana students staying healthy while maintaining their QOL during their elderly years have been observed, ikebana shows promise in maintaining and improving the QOL of elderly people. Ikebana uses different flower arranging materials in each of the four seasons. The students devise an arrangement and perform actions using their fingers, such as cutting and bending. It is also assumed that looking at the color and shapes of various plants, touching them with their hands, smelling them, and expressing using their five senses contribute to the benefits of ikebana.

In this paper we will report what effects ikebana activity had on residents of a nursing facility (Super Court Co., Ltd).

2   Methodology

2.1   Subjects

The two test subjects, neither of whom had previous experience with ikebana, included a woman aged 91 years (test subject 1) and a woman aged 86 years (test subject 2). Test subject one suffers from poriomania (the unconscious tendency to wander), and desired to go home. She would request that she be sent home up to 5 or 6 times a day. She has a short-term memory disorder and to stabilize her mood she is currently under psychiatric care. The second test subject has Alzheimer's disease and basically her mood is stable but she also has poriomania. Fantasizing and odd behavior occur sporadically (Table 1).

2.2   Experimental Protocol

We utilized ikebana as a part of recreation for two residents. Recreation at the facility includes many activities such as cards, karaoke, painting, ball-toss game, watching DVDs, calligraphy, Japanese karuta card game, tanka poetry, exercise, target-hitting game, collage of pieces of colored paper, bowling, and ikebana. 13 to 15 residents, including the 2 test subjects, participated in the recreation. The place for the experiment was a cafeteria, 5 m by 10 m in size. Two adjacent walls were completely white, and the other two were covered with large windows. A table and chairs were placed in the center of the room, and the experiment took place there from 2 pm to 3 pm. Ikebana

Table 1. Biological data of subjects

Subject	Age	Sex	Symptoms	Dominant-hand
Suject-1	91	Female	Poriomania, homesickness, short-term memory loss, currently receiving treatment at a department of psychosomatic medicine	Right
Suject-2	86	Female	Alzheimer's dementia	Right

was performed as part of recreational activity from January 2014 through December 2014, once a month. After the teacher explained the materials, the test subjects followed the teacher's example and arranged the flowers accordingly. The teacher and nursing care employee supported the effort. Each of the subjects engaged in ikebana gave positive feedback about the flowers e.g. "They're so pretty, it makes me happy," "I look forward to doing it once a month," and "It makes me happy having flowers I can decorate my room with. The exercise came to a close after the teacher made some adjustments to the subjects' arrangements. Nursing staff place the arrangements in the rooms of the subjects that were able to do the exercise and also tidies up afterwards. Furthermore, karaoke and watching DVDs, normal recreation that is conducted frequently, was used for comparison.

2.3   Materials

The material used for ikebana in January was *yukiyanagi* (Thunberg spirea), tulip, sweet pea, dracaena, and peacock aster. In February it was peach blossom, wild daffodil, sweet pea, ageratum, and Osmond. In this way we chose 4 to 5 different types materials per month from the most beautiful materials of the current season.

2.4   Neuropsychiatric Inventory

We evaluated the recreational activities including ikebana (ikebana, karaoke, watching a DVD) based on the condition of the test subjects before, during, and after the activity in a GBS scale with 6 mental states, and a NPI scale. In the GBS, scale we evaluated six conditions (emotional lethargy, emotional instability, loss of motivation, insecurity, depression, and anxiety) on a scale of six, ranging from zero (normal) to five (very bad). These 6 mental states refer to the condition of the residents and are necessary for nursing staff in caring for the residents. They also reduce the workload of nursing staff that can evaluate them effectively (Tables 2 and 3).

Table 2. GBS

Outcome measure	Symptoms
Emotional lethargy	Is unable to respond appropriately to the situation
Emotional instability	Is unable to control their emotions normally
Loss of motivation	Has no motivation for activities and work
Insecurity	Embraces feelings of anxiety
Depression	Has abnormal emotional levels that show signs of being disheartened or depressed
Anxiety	Is unable to sit still and do normal activities; wanders about

Table 3. NPI

Outcome measure	Symptoms
Delusions	Firmly believes things they know not to be fact
Hallucinations	Sees and hears things that are not there
Agitation	Gets too worked up and is unable to control their emotions.
Depression	Is unable to fend off feelings of concern and feels depressed
Insecurity	Is unable to relax and is excessively nervous.
Euphoria	Is in an excessively good mood
Apathy	Is disinterested in everyday activities and other people.
Disinhibition	Talks to other people they have never seen or met before as if they were an acquaintance and says things that hurt others
Irritability	Instantly gets into a bad mood over trivial things, becomes agitated and gets angry
Abnormal behavior	Continually repeats the same meaningless actions, such as walking around their house and playing with buttons and strings
Sleep	Does not have enough sleep and is seen being active at night time
Eating behavior	Regularly has changes in their appetite and eating style, experiences changes in body weight or becomes unwell

3   Results and Considerations

3.1   Process Analysis

Figure 1 shows the results of the evaluation of the condition of the two test subjects before, during, and after the ikebana activity. Emotional instability, loss of motivation, insecurity, and anxiety were ameliorated during the ikebana activity. After the ikebana

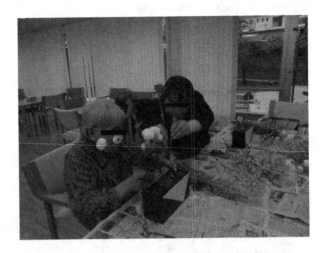

Fig. 1. Experimental circumstance

activity, there was similar amelioration to that during the ikebana activity, but compared to during the activity the condition had worsened.

Results of the evaluation of the conditions of the test subjects in a GBS scale before, during, and after the recreational activities of karaoke and watching a DVD are shown in Figs. 2 and 3. Figure 2 shows the amelioration of emotional lethargy during karaoke, but after the karaoke emotional lethargy and anxiety worsened compared to before the activity. In Fig. 3 we see that during the activity of watching a DVD, all conditions in the GBS scale ameliorated, but after the activity emotional lethargy, emotional instability, loss of motivation, insecurity, and anxiety had worsened. From the information above, we have confirmed that ikebana has a tendency to stabilize emotions. From the NPI scale, no change was observed from the normal condition of both of the subjects, and there was also no change in the workload in caring for them (Figs. 4 and 5).

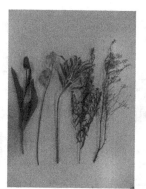
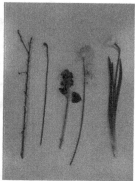

Fig. 2. Floral materials

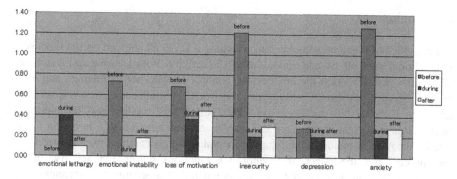

Fig. 3. GBS scale of Ikebana

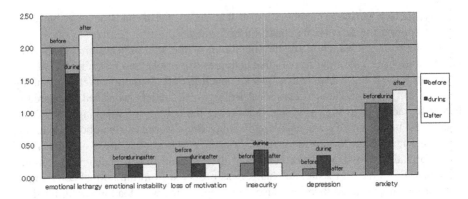

Fig. 4. GBS scale of Karaoke

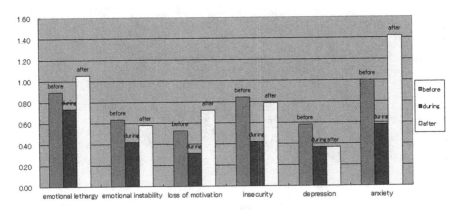

Fig. 5. GBS scale of watching DVDs

4   Conclusions

The activities of ikebana, karaoke, and watching a DVD all showed on the GBS scale an amelioration of all six conditions during the activity. With karaoke and watching a DVD, after the recreation the ameliorated conditions were not maintained and worsened to the state prior to the activity or even worse. A similar tendency was seen to a degree in ikebana, but the degree of exacerbation was smaller, and the emotional amelioration was clearer compared to karaoke and watching a DVD. In caring for the elderly, we need to maintain their current mental and physical condition. Recreation in nursing care has the effect of ameliorating emotions during the activity. In this experiment, we can observe that ikebana, compared to other forms of recreation (karaoke, watching DVDs), has a greater effect of ameliorating emotions during the activity and also can maintain the amelioration to a greater degree. We believe the reason to be that ikebana involves handling plants that differ according to season, using scissors and other tools, and communicating with others during the process. From this experiment we can expect that ikebana can be useful for the amelioration of the emotions of elderly people in need of nursing care, and can possibly ease the burden of the caregiver. From here on we would like to focus on and examine the utility of ikebana in a nursing care environment and the differences between ikebana and other forms of recreation. In the future, we would like to investigate what changes occur in the condition of the subjects through the continual engagement in ikebana, and how these changes correlate to the length the length it continues.

References

1. Ministry of Internal Affairs and Communications: The 2012 White Paper on Aging Society (2012)
2. Kawabata, S., Nasu, M., Yamamoto, T., Kita, N., Kuwahara, N., Hamada, H.: Researching and Developing Colored Calligraphy Pens for Color-By-Number Picture Recreation in High-Grade Nursing Care
3. Doi, T., Ikenobo, Y., Kuwahara, N.: Report on Usefulness of Traditional Japanese Culture in the Care of the Elderly (2013)
4. Doi, T., Kuwahara, N., Morimoto, K.: Effective Design of Recreation Activities in the Group Home for the Elderly with Dementia (2014)
5. Watanabe, Y., Takayama, S.: The Effects of Nursing Intervention which Provides Opportunities for Elderly People Living in Facilities that Suffer from Moderate to Severe Dementia to Make Decisions for Themselves (2010)
6. Wakashi, K., Kunitomo, T., Shimada, A., Tsuji, T.: Practical Research of Tasks that Effectively Prevent Dementia: A Comparative Investigation of Engagement in Music Therapy and Recreational Activities (2007)

Usability of Mobile Applications Supporting Training in Diagnostic Decision-Making by Radiologists

Min Soon Kim[1,2(✉)], Awatef A. Ben Ramadan[2], Martina A. Clarke[2],
Mia K. Markey[3], Kraig J. Lage[4], Michael R. Aro[4],
Kevin L. Ingalls[4], and Vivek Sindhwani[4]

[1] Department of Health Management and Informatics,
University of Missouri, Columbia, MO, USA
[2] University of Missouri Informatics Institute, University of Missouri, Columbia, MO, USA
[3] Department of Biomedical Engineering, University of Texas, Austin, TX, USA
[4] Department of Radiology, University of Missouri, Columbia, MO, USA
kimms@health.missouri.edu

Abstract. The objective of this study is to systematically review the usability of mobile applications currently available in radiology to support training in diagnostic decision-making. Two online stores with major market share (Google Play and iTunes) were searched. A multi-step review process was utilized by three usability investigators and five radiology experts to identify eligible applications and extract usability reviews. From 381 applications that were initially identified, user reviews of final 52 applications revealed 79 usability issues. Usability issues were categorized according to Nielsen's heuristic usability evaluation principles (HE). The top three most frequent types of usability issues were: Naturalness (43), Simplicity (43), and Efficient Interactions (21). Examples of the most frequent usability issues were: lack of information, lack of labeling, and details about images. This study demonstrates the urgent need of usability test to provide evidence-based guidelines to help choose mobile applications that will yield educational and clinical benefits.

Keywords: Education · Mobile application · Radiology · Training · Usability

1 Introduction

1.1 Mobile Applications in Improving Radiology Education

About 90 % of medical professionals have used mobile devices in medical practice to access their patients' electronic health records and medical information. Currently, there are four major application stores in the market: iTunes, Google Play, Windows, and Blackberry. iTunes and Google Play stores contain the majority of mobile applications. iTunes' application store consist of approximately 20,000 medical mobile applications while Google Play's application store has about 9,000 medical applications [1].

Radiology is a specialty that requires extensive training in image analysis for decision making. Radiology residents are physicians who are being trained in the specialty,

© Springer International Publishing Switzerland 2015
V.G. Duffy (Ed.): DHM 2015, Part II, LNCS 9185, pp. 448–454, 2015.
DOI: 10.1007/978-3-319-21070-4_45

and are increasingly using mobile devices. It is estimated that in professional settings, 78 % of physicians use smartphones for work-related purposes [2]. Smartphone usage has spread to healthcare settings with numerous potential and realized benefits. Mobile applications that are installed on smartphones have provided clinicians with readily available evidence-based decisional tools [3]. Medical applications fall under many different categories, including but not limited to, reference applications, such as the Physician's Desk Reference (PDR®) or WebMD®, medical calculators, and applications designed to access electronic health records (EHR) or personal health information (PHI) [4].

1.2 Poorly Designed Mobile Application Hinders User Acceptance

Recently, the functionality of mobile applications has increased greatly. This increase in functionality has come at the expense of the usability of these applications. The international standard, ISO 9241-11:1998 Guidance on Usability defines *usability* as:

> "The extent to which a product can be used by specified users to achieve specified goals with effectiveness, efficiency and satisfaction, in a specified context of use of the system" [5].

While technical evaluations of mobile applications receive much attention, few usability evaluation studies have been conducted, especially, for healthcare mobile applications. As such, there have been few studies that investigated the efficacy of using mobile applications that are used in hopes of assisting in training [4, 6].

Consequently, it is estimated that 95 % of downloaded mobile applications are abandoned within a month [7] and 26 % of applications are only used once, possibly because of the lack of attention to usability [8]. Poor healthcare system design may lower effectiveness [9, 10], decrease efficiency [11], and decrease team collaboration [12]. This, in turn, may lead to high cognitive load [13], medical errors [14], and decreased quality of patient care [15]. These issues are correlated within the scope of usability.

The objective of this study is to review and measure the usability of mobile applications currently available in radiology to support training in diagnostic decision-making.

2 Method

2.1 Setting

The University of Missouri Health Care (UMHC) is a tertiary care academic medical center located in Columbia, Missouri, with a total of 564 beds. With 626 medical staff at clinics throughout mid-Missouri, UMHC had an estimated 553,300 visits in 2012 [16]. Department of Radiology includes a full complement of 28 + highly trained clinicians and researchers, and successful training programs of 25 + resident physicians involving cutting-edge technologies and specialized clinical experiences. The department also operates Missouri Radiology Imaging Center, one of the most advanced resonance imaging facilities in the state.

2.2 Systematic Review of the Mobile Application

To determine usability issues of mobile applications in radiology, systematic review process was conducted. Two online stores with major market share (Google Play and iTunes) were searched on July 10, 2014 for mobile radiology applications that assist in training.

A multi-step review process was utilized by three usability investigators and five radiology experts to identify eligible applications and extract usability reviews. Distinct and broad search terms were used to capture a wide range of radiological applications: radiology, X-ray, ultrasound, MRI, CT, radiography, nuclear medicine, mammogram, mammography, and fluoroscopy.

Through screening of the titles and descriptions, applications were selected if they supported education and training of radiological diagnostic decision-making processes. They were excluded if they:

1. only provided access to journals, books, encyclopedias, or other reference material;
2. were designed solely for trivial medical calculations;
3. were designed solely for specific commercial vendor products;
4. were designed for use by a specific hospital/clinic only; or
5. were written in a non-English language.

The investigators extracted the usability reviews to be analyzed and coded them according to validated Nielsen's heuristic usability evaluation principles (HE) [17, 18]. Two independent investigators (ABR, MAC) cross-examined the usability reviews of the counterpart to reach agreement. An experienced usability investigator (MSK) adjudicated any disagreement. Finally, the entire team collectively reviewed the findings for validity before analysis was carried out.

3   Results

From 381 applications that were initially identified, 52 applications of the total searched applications were eligible applications with user reviews. Using HE was instrumental in understanding areas in need of improvement. For the studied 52 radiology training applications, the usability-related reviews are 79 reviews. The types of usability issues with frequency by principles discovered were (some usability issues were cross-listed):

- Naturalness (43)
- Simplicity (43)
- Efficient Interactions (21)
- Consistency (16)
- Effective Information Presentation (11)
- Preservation of context (11)
- Minimize cognitive (10)
- Effective use of language (5)
- Forgiveness and feedback (1).

The example usability problems were: applications lacking in content (17 apps), requests for scientifically based information (5 apps), downloading and crashing systems problems (5 apps), more images (3 apps), and more labels (2 apps).

The usability issues were classified according to 3 point usability severity scale [19]. Examples of the catastrophic usability issues (level 3 severity) were: crashing/force closing, and inability to install application to the user's mobile devices. Level 3 usability issues prevent users from completing their task. Level 2 usability issues include: inadequate content, insufficient cases and quizzes, non-intuitive labels to the images, and inefficient interfacing problems. Level 2 usability issues delay users significantly but eventually allows them to complete the task. Minor usability issues (level 1) include: the small font size, lack of zoom option in on the image. Level 1 issues could only delay user briefly to complete the task.

4 Discussion

4.1 Mobile Applications in Radiology Need Further Usability Evaluation

Most existing mobile applications in radiology fall short in adequately engaging stakeholders and ensuring that the system designs are user-centered. This may be attributed to a number of reasons, for example, a system designers' lack of understanding of clinical workflow, unclear guidelines in how user-engaged technologies should be implemented and actively used. Of most important is an insufficient understanding of users' information needs, socio-demographic status, preferences, health and literacy, computer literacy, and values. Medical mobile applications that do not take account of these factors can impair the effectiveness of clinical management.

While the majority of mobile applications in radiology have been evaluated using tablet platforms [20–28], there are very few studies available that investigated the potential benefit of mobile applications on smartphone platforms, potentially because of the small display size [20, 29]. However, advancement of display technology and better mobility will allow increasing use of smartphones in the near future [30]. Thus, it is important to explore the feasibility of mobile applications on smaller mobile devices among physicians.

4.2 User-Centered Design Process in Mobile Application Development

Prior studies showed that mobile applications, including radiology, can be utilized to enhance education, with the potential to improve overall patient care [31, 32] but suffered from poor usability. User-Centered Design (UCD) is a process wherein the needs, wants, and limitations of end users of a product are given extensive attention at throughout the design process [33, 34].

The UCD process involves engagement of users throughout the processes:

1. user needs analysis,
2. algorithm development,
3. cyclical prototype design, and
4. development.

In user needs analysis, the design team collects users' information needs, wants, and motivations for using mobile applications to acquire an understanding of potential factors that may impact the intended goals. Information items include: basic education-related demographics, prior mobile application experiences, perceived mobile device skills, and expectations (contents, features and functionalities) on usage of the mobile application in their clinical management setting. In algorithm development stage, design team sketches several ideas for potential prototype design through an iterative review process. Collected users' needs are reviewed to ensure if they could be integrated within the application's limitations. The team should decide on whether or not to include certain educational contents, features, and functional elements. Once the optimal algorithm is established, the team begins to design and develop a few low-fidelity (Lo-Fi) prototypes (i.e., sketches on paper or slides). The Lo-Fi prototypes will then be evaluated utilizing formative evaluations, such as, heuristic evaluation [17, 18] and cognitive walkthrough [35, 36]. When the final prototype has been selected, the team work to develop the high-fidelity (Hi-Fi) prototype with partial to complete functions. The Hi-Fi prototype are evaluated using summative lab-based usability testing [37].

After implementation, continuous data collection on usability should be warranted to measure usability [5, 38, 39] and acceptance [40] of the mobile application. This continuous evaluation will allow the team to adjust the design of the application for improving user acceptance and maintaining maximal educational effectiveness. Following the UCD process, mobile applications in radiology education and training may ultimately increase usability and therefore decrease cognitive overload, and may increase the quality of healthcare services.

4.3 Weakness to the Study

As with all study designs, there are limitations. First, due to this study's exploratory nature, this study involved mobile applications in two mobile application stores. Selection of iOS (iTunes) and Android (Google Play) platforms for this study was made based on current trend and it may change in the future considering the fast-changing IT market. As such, evaluation of mobile applications in other platforms, such as, Windows or BlackBerry, should be warranted. Second, while Nielsen's heuristic usability evaluation principles (HE) is an exemplary evaluation method, summative usability testing [37, 41] comparing multiple representative mobile applications could provide evidence-based guidelines to help choose mobile applications that will yield maximal educational and clinical benefits.

5 Conclusion

This study demonstrates the urgent need for usability evaluation in the development of radiology mobile applications. Investigators suggest that the approval process of any medical mobile applications should undergo a more systematic and rigorous process to improve the applications that will satisfy the users' experience and meet clinical training goals. In addition, the investigators suggest an institution of systematic and standardized guidelines regarding design and test of healthcare mobile applications to achieve maximal adoption.

References

1. Aungst, T.D., Clauson, K.A., Misra, S., et al.: How to identify, assess and utilise mobile medical applications in clinical practice. Int. J. Clin. Pract. **68**(2), 155–162 (2014)
2. Sources & Interactions Study, September 2013: Medical/Surgical Edition. [electronic article] (2013)
3. Prgomet, M., Georgiou, A., Westbrook, J.I.: The impact of mobile handheld technology on hospital physicians' work practices and patient care: a systematic review. J. Am. Med. Inform. Assoc. **16**(6), 792–801 (2009)
4. Szekely, A., Talanow, R., Bagyi, P.: Smartphones, tablets and mobile applications for radiology. Eur. J. Radiol. **82**(5), 829–836 (2013)
5. Standard ISO 9241: Ergonomic requirements for office work with visual display terminals (VDTs), part 11: Guidance on usability (1998)
6. Harrison, F., Duce, D.: Usability of mobile applications: literature review and rationale for a new usability model. J. Interact. Sci. **1**(1), 12 (2013)
7. Mocherman, A.: Why 95 % of apps are quickely abandoned - and how to avoid becoming a statistic [ectronic article] (2011)
8. First Impressions Matter! 26 % of Apps Downloaded in 2010 Were Used Just Once: Localytics [electronic article] (2011)
9. Koppel, R., Metlay, J.P., Cohen, A., et al.: Role of computerized physician order entry systems in facilitating medication errors. JAMA **293**(10), 1197–1203 (2005)
10. Steele, E.: EHR implementation: who benefits, who pays? Health Manag. Technol. **27**(7), 43–44 (2006)
11. Crabtree, B.F., Miller, W.L., Tallia, A.F., et al.: Delivery of clinical preventive services in family medicine offices. Ann. Fam. Med. **3**(5), 430–435 (2005)
12. Han, Y.Y., Carcillo, J.A., Venkataraman, S.T., et al.: Unexpected increased mortality after implementation of a commercially sold computerized physician order entry system. Pediatrics **116**(6), 1506–1512 (2005)
13. Tang, P.C., Patel, V.L.: Major issues in user interface design for health professional workstations: summary and recommendations. Int. J. Biomed. Comput. **34**(1–4), 139–148 (1994)
14. Ash, J.S., Berg, M., Coiera, E.: Some unintended consequences of information technology in health care the nature of patient care: information system-related errors. J. Am. Med. Inf. Assoc. **11**(2), 104–112 (2004)
15. Beuscart-Zéphir, M.C., Elkin, P., Pelayo, S., et al.: The human factors engineering approach to biomedical informatics projects: state of the art, results, benefits and challenges. Yearb. Med. Inform. 109–127 (2007)
16. MO: University of Missouri Health Care. Annual Report, Columbia
17. Selecting a mobile app: evaluating the usability of medical applications (2012)
18. Nielsen, J., Hackos, J.T.: Usability Engineering. Academic press, Boston (1993)
19. Sauro, J.: Rating The Severity Of Usability Problems, [News article] (2013)
20. Ridley, E.L.: Size Matters: IPad Tops IPhone for Evaluating Acute Stroke. AuntMinnie.com (2011). http://www.auntminnie.com/index.aspx?sec=ser&sub=def&pag=dis&ItemID=97731
21. Ridley, E.L.: Despite Speed Bump, IPad Up for Task of Assessing Tuberculosis. AuntMinnie.com (2012). http://www.auntminnie.com/index.aspx?sec=ser&sub=def&pag=dis&ItemID=98084

22. McNulty, J.P., Ryan, J.T., Evanoff, M.G., et al.: Flexible image evaluation. iPad versus secondary-class monitors for review of mr spinal emergency cases, a comparative study. Acad. Radiol. **19**(8), 1023–1028 (2012)
23. Johnson, P.T., Zimmerman, S.L., Heath, D., et al.: The iPad as a mobile device for CT display and interpretation: diagnostic accuracy for identification of pulmonary embolism. Emerg. Radiol. **19**(4), 323–327 (2012)
24. Ridley, E.L.: IPad Up for Challenge of Plain Radiographs. AuntMinnie.com http://www.auntminnie.com/index.aspx?sec=sup_n&sub=pac&pag=dis&itemId=97736 (2011)
25. Ridley, E.L.: IPad Up for Task of Assessing Pulmonary Nodules. AuntMinnie.com http://www.auntminnie.com/index.aspx?sec=rca&sub=rsna_2011&pag=dis&itemId=97565 (2011)
26. Ward, P.: IPads Are OK for VC Reviews, but Take Longer. AuntMinnie.com (2011). http://www.auntminnie.com/index.aspx?sec=rca_n&sub=rsna_2011&pag=dis&ItemID=97597. Accessed 22 Jan 2014
27. Hammon, M., Schlechtweg, P.M., Schulz-Wendtland, R., et al.: iPads in breast imaging - a phantom study. Geburtshilfe Frauenheilkd. **74**(2), 152–156 (2014)
28. iPads show the way forward for medical imaging, [online article] (2012)
29. Wolf, J.A., Moreau, J.F., Akilov, O., et al.: Diagnostic inaccuracy of smartphone applications for melanoma detection. JAMA Dermatol. **149**(4), 422–426 (2013)
30. Qiao, J., Liu, Z., Xu, L., et al.: Reliability analysis of a smartphone-aided measurement method for the Cobb angle of scoliosis. J Spinal Disord. Tech. **25**(4), E88–E92 (2012)
31. Trelease, R.B.: Diffusion of innovations: smartphones and wireless anatomy learning resources. Anat. Sci. Educ. **1**(6), 233–239 (2008)
32. Torre, D.M., Treat, R., Durning, S., et al.: Comparing PDA- and paper-based evaluation of the clinical skills of third-year students. WMJ **110**(1), 9–13 (2011)
33. Johnson, C.M., Johnson, T.R., Zhang, J.: A user-centered framework for redesigning health care interfaces. J. Biomed. Inform. **38**(1), 75–87 (2005)
34. Da Silva, T.S., Martin, A., Maurer, F., et al. (eds.): User-centered design and agile methods: a systematic review. *AGILE* (2011)
35. Polson, P.G., Lewis, C., Rieman, J., et al.: Cognitive walkthroughs: a method for theory-based evaluation of user interfaces. Int. J. Man Mach. Stud. **36**(5), 741–773 (1992)
36. Partala, T.: The combined walkthrough: measuring behavioral, affective, and cognitive information in usability testing. J. Usability Stud. **5**(1), 21–33 (2009)
37. Bastien, J.M.: Usability testing: a review of some methodological and technical aspects of the method. Int. J. Med. Inform. **79**(4), e18–e23 (2010)
38. Brooke, J.: SUS - a quick and dirty usability scale. In: Jordan, P.W., Thomas, B., Weerdmeester, B.A., McClelland, I.L. (eds.) Usability Evaluation in Industry. Taylor & Francis, London (1996)
39. Bangor, A., Kortum, P.T., Miller, J.T.: An empirical evaluation of the system usability scale. Int. J. Hum. Comput. Interact. **24**(6), 574–594 (2008)
40. Renaud, K., Biljon, J.V.: Predicting technology acceptance and adoption by the elderly: a qualitative study. In: Proceedings of the 2008 Annual Research Conference of the South African Institute of Computer Scientists and Information Technologists on IT research in Developing Countries: Riding the Wave of Technology, Wilderness, South Africa, 1456684, pp. 210–219. ACM (2008)
41. Faulkner, L.: Beyond the five-user assumption: benefits of increased sample sizes in usability testing. Behav. Res. Methods Instrum. Comput. **35**(3), 379–383 (2003)

An Investigation of Caregiver's Fatigue During Nursing Work in China

Mengyuan Liao[1(✉)], Yuqiu Yang[2], Yuka Takai[3], Takashi Yoshikawa[4], Akihiko Goto[3], Ting Yang[1], Tomoko Ota[5], and Hiroyuki Hamada[1]

[1] Advanced Fibro-Science, Kyoto Institute of Technology, Kyoto, Japan
ada.mengyuanliao@gmail.com
[2] College of Textile, Donghua University, Shanghai, China
amy_yuqiu_yang@dhu.edu.cn
[3] Department of Information Systems Engineering, Osaka Sangyo University, Osaka, Japan
gotoh@ise.osaka-sandai.ac.jp
[4] National Institute of Technology, Niihama College, Niihama, Japan
yosikawa@mec.niihama-nct.ac.jp
[5] Chuo Business Group, Osaka, Japan
tomoko.ota@k.vodafone.ne.jp

Abstract. In order to evaluate caregiver's fatigue during daily care work, an investigation was carried out in Chinese nursing house. 100 employees from four different nursing houses including day and night working shift were selected in random for sampling survey. And the fatigue situation was evaluated applying Japanese "subjective fatigue symptoms" (new edition of 2002) and "Tired body parts" questionnaires in field question-answer form. Collecting "subjective fatigue symptoms" questionnaire results were analyzed, which showed that caregiver's fatigue degree at the end of working day is more serious with larger scores than that of the beginning, especially caregiver in night shift displayed more fatigue in blurry vision and languidness. The aim of this work is to get a good knowledge of caregiver's fatigue situation basically and put forward some effective measures and necessary assisted device to adjust to Chinese nursing house development.

Keywords: Caregiver · Fatigue investigation · Nursing work

1 Introduction

Accompanying with economic and technology improvement, in recent years, ageing society rapid development has became a global trend issue, especially for large dementia and bedridden elderly population growth, the extended care period. Elderly dependency ratio and nursing care career have obtained increasing attention, and increasing elderly nursing demand also bring out huge promising market opportunity and challenge. Comparing with previous elderly nursing care mode and care service focus (basic life care), nowadays and future elderly nursing care is paying more attention to long-term period, diversity and personal care service items owing to living quality improvement.

© Springer International Publishing Switzerland 2015
V.G. Duffy (Ed.): DHM 2015, Part II, LNCS 9185, pp. 455–464, 2015.
DOI: 10.1007/978-3-319-21070-4_46

In other words, long-term care and diversified care service supply for elder population become more and more important mainstream development direction, which could help nursing industry to go across current development bottleneck.

According to the international standard, China has stepped into Aging Society from 1999 with 126 million elder people over 60 years old (accounting for 10 % of total population). By the end of 2014, ministry of civil affairs of the People's Republic of China reported that elderly population over 60 years old in China has been more than 200millions, 14.9 % of total population. China entered the Aged Society under the condition of weak pension consciousness and undeveloped economical reality, so in current social nursing facilities a large proportion of elders are disabled, semidisabled with high average nurse-care level or the elders need daily medical care for a long-term period. All those disabled and semi-disabled elders need professional care by caregivers. So according to the elderly to caregiver ratio 3:1, the national needs 10 million caregivers in minimum. Hard and long time care works usually make some great effects on caregiver's physical body situation or mental burder [1, 2, 3]. Due to high extensive work load but low salary and despise view for caregiver occupation, caregivers' shortage reality become more and more serious for urban and rural nursing institutions. For this reason, it is very urgent to increase caregiver's care work efficiency by skill training, more importantly is to get a good knowledge of caregiver's body fatigue situation and mental burden during daily care work period and then develop corresponding feasible solutions.

As well know that fatigue situation produced by work process is a serious issue if it could not be recovered timely, which not only lead to working efficiency decrease, but also affect worker's physical and psychological health, induce safety accident and even suicide and overwork death. Until now, some developed countries such as Europe, America and Japan are paying increasing attention to industrial fatigue investigation and study for ensuring worker's occupational circumstance. However such conscious in China is very weak, therefore this work is aim to get a good knowledge of caregiver's fatigue situation basically and put forward some effective measures and necessary assisted device as feedback to adjust to Chinese nursing house development. In this paper, 100 employees from four different nursing houses including day and night working shift were selected in random for sampling survey. And the fatigue situation was evaluated applying Japanese "subjective fatigue symptoms" (new edition of 2002) and "Tired body parts" questionnaires in field question-answer form. Collecting "subjective fatigue symptoms" questionnaire results were compared and analyzed before and after work, which showed that caregiver's fatigue degree at the end of working day is more serious with larger scores than that of the beginning, especially caregiver in night shift displayed more fatigue in blurry vision and languidness. Along with longer care-work time, "waist" and "shoulders" were most complained tired body parts among all subjects. For quantifying caregiver's body and mental fatigue by different care work contents during daily working period, "saliva test" was also conducted on 3 caregivers for continuous three days. It is found that different care content, work-shifts, caregiver's experience years make different type of body and mental fatigue effects on caregivers to varying degrees. Consequently, we proposed some fatigue countermeasures and optimized work schedules after statistics analyzing fatigue characteristics correlation with care work schedule and caregiver's experience years.

2   Methods

2.1   Investigation Subjects

100 caregivers from four different nursing houses including day and night working shift were selected as investigation subjects in random for sampling survey, and the subjects' characteristic was summarized in Table 1. Six caregivers from the same nursing house were also employed to carry out continuous three days tracking studies of saliva test.

Table 1. Characteristic of investigated subjects

	Women	Subject (people)	Average age (year)	Average work experience (year)
	No.1 (SD)	28 ·	44 (3.9)	5 (3.19)
	No.2 (SD)	11 ·	45 (3.3)	4 (1.55)
Day shift	No.3 (SD)	17 ·	52 (6.5)	4 (2.57)
	No.4 (SD)	16 ·	50 (6.8)	4 (2.97)
	合計 (SD)	72 ·	42.0 (12.9)	4.18 (4.83)
Night shift	No.1 (SD)	28 ·	24.8 (4.2)	3.61 (2.07)
	Total sum (SD)	100 ·	41.1 (11.7)	4.1 (2.64)

2.2   Fatigue Evaluation Items and Form

Caregivers' daily work fatigue situation was evaluated by applying Japanese "subjective fatigue symptoms" (new modified edition of 2002) and "Tired body parts" questionnaires in field survey. 25 question items were included in "subjective fatigue symptoms" and divided into five groups indicating five different type of fatigue characteristics/factors: (1) Drowsiness and dullness; (2) Uneasy feeling; (3) Illness situation; (4) Physical impairment/pain; (5) Fuzzy feeling, which listed in Table 1. And each item was given a mark/score by caregiver among five grade levels of "definitely no (1 point)", "hardly no (2 point)", "a little bit (3 point)", "exactly yes (4 point)" and "strongly agree (5 point)" through question-answer form before and after working (total in two times for each subject). "Tired body parts investigation" questionnaire was comprised of 17 body parts (head, shoulders, back, arms, front arms, hands, thighs, knees and leg, feet) for evaluating accumulated body loading after care working, so caregiver only required to record the pain feeling body part with "Yes" (Table 2).

2.3   Data Collation and Disposal

All the questionnaire data was collected and disposed with IBM SPSS Statics 20 software. Firstly of all, each evaluation item of "subjective fatigue symptoms" questionnaire

Table 2. Check-list of subjective symptoms of fatigue

Type 1	Type 2	Type 3	Type 4	Type 5
10. Give a yawn	2. Anxious about things	1. Feel heavy in the head	8. Feel stiffness in the shoulders	3. Feel dried in eyes
13. Become drowsy	5. Feel unsteady in standing	4. Feel ill	11. Feel a pain in hands or fingers	7. Feel a pain in eyes
14. Do not want to move	15. Feel uneasy	6. Have a headache	19. Get tired in wrist	
17. Get tired over the body	18. Feel sad or depressed	9. Feel the brain hot or muddled	23. Feel a pain in the back	
21. Want to lie down	20. Feel difficulty to thinking	12. Feel dizzy	25. Get tired in the legs	

was calculated and indicated by mean and SD value in the group of 4 nursing facilities. Afterwards, fiver fatigue factors were summarized with sum scores of items included in each type (1*5 = 5 lowest mark; 5*5 = 25 full mark). Fatigue location evaluated by subjective "Tired body parts" sheets was also counted and sort in to a rank. In order to investigate fatigue condition difference of before/after care work and day/night work shift, average value of each item and factor type in "subjective fatigue symptoms" questionnaire were compared applying Wilcoxon (paired test). Furthermore, relationship between subject's age or working experience and fatigue evaluation was also clarified by "Pearson correlation" analysis.

3   Results and Discussions

3.1   General Characteristics of "Subjective Fatigue Symptoms"

Table 3 listed 25 items of subjective fatigue symptoms (mean and SD values) for subjects' before and after care work process. It is found that "Feel a pain in the back" complaint item and other physical impairment items included in Type4 (IV) showed a comparative high score before work shift among 4 nursing house facilities. Fatigue condition before work shift is deemed as fatigue accumulation state in subject's body accompanied with long-term care-work occupation. Based on the subjective fatigue symptom investigation in current study, back pain was clarified as a serious puzzling issue for caregiver due to it was hardly recovered. Correspondingly, in the case of after work period, subjects' complained about items of "Want to lie down", "Feel stiffness in shoulder" and "Get tired in the legs" increased significantly except for "Feel a pain in the back" belonged to Type1 (I) and Type4 (IV). Fatigue factor types calculated by sum scores in respective type group were summarized in Table 4. It is obvious to note subject's fatigue complaints after care work were mainly concentrated in "Physical impairment" and "Drowsiness/dullness" factors in those 4 nursing house facilities, following by "Fuzzy feeling", "Illness condition" and "Uneasy feeling" factors.

In Fig. 1, fatigue condition change evaluation were illustrated by respective item and type group. Care work loading on investigated subjects was clearly reflected by all positive score change among 25 complaint items respectively. Especially, complaint items of "Want to lie down", "Get tied in the legs", "Feel a pain in the back", "Get tired in the wrist" and "Feel stiffness in shoulder" displayed obvious fatigue condition change

Table 3. Facility comparison of fatigue level for 25 items between before and after work

	No.1 before		No.1 after		No.2 before		No.2 after		No.3 before		No.3 after		No.4 before		No.4 after	
	mean	SD	mean	SD	mean	SD	mean	SD	mean	SD	mean	SD	mean	SD	mean	SD
16 Give a yawn	1.00	0.00	1.50***	0.69	1.27	0.47	1.82**	0.40	1.29	0.47	1.71**	0.69	1.63	0.50	2.81***	1.42
13 Become drowsy	1.07	0.26	2.61***	1.29	1.00	0.00	1.64***	0.50	1.12	0.33	2.00***	0.79	1.13	0.34	2.31***	0.70
I 14 Do not want to move	1.00	0.00	1.25**	0.52	1.00	0.00	1.00	0.00	1.00	0.00	1.00	0.00	1.00	0.00	1.06	0.25
17 Get tired over day	1.11	0.31	2.82***	1.33	1.00	0.00	1.00	0.00	1.18	0.39	1.94***	0.97	1.00	0.00	2.25***	0.93
21 Want to lie down	1.00	0.00	3.39***	1.69	1.09	0.30	2.09***	0.54	1.24	0.44	3.12***	1.11	1.06	0.25	2.63***	1.31
2 Anxious about things	1.00	0.00	1.54***	0.58	1.00	0.00	1.00	0.00	1.06	0.24	1.47**	0.80	1.19	0.40	1.38*	0.50
5 Feel unsteady in standing	1.07	0.26	1.46***	0.84	1.00	0.00	1.00	0.00	1.00	0.00	1.06	0.24	1.00	0.00	1.00	0.00
II 15 Feel uneasy	1.04	0.19	1.50***	0.88	1.00	0.00	1.00	0.00	1.00	0.00	1.06	0.24	1.00	0.00	1.00	0.00
18 Feel sad or depressed	1.00	0.00	1.25***	0.44	1.00	0.00	1.00	0.00	1.00	0.00	1.24	0.56	1.00	0.00	1.00	0.00
20 Feel difficult to thinking	1.00	0.00	1.32***	0.55	1.00	0.00	1.00	0.00	1.00	0.00	1.00	0.00	1.00	0.00	1.06	0.25
1 Feel heavy in the head	1.04	0.19	1.25*	0.65	1.00	0.00	1.09	0.30	1.12	0.33	1.65***	0.70	1.06	0.25	1.56	1.03
4 Feel ill	1.00	0.00	1.11*	0.31	1.00	0.00	1.00	0.00	1.06	0.24	1.24*	0.44	1.00	0.00	1.06	0.25
III 6 Have a headache	1.00	0.00	1.29***	0.46	1.00	0.00	1.00	0.00	1.00	0.00	1.24	0.56	1.06	0.25	1.25	0.58
9 Feel brain muddled	1.04	0.19	1.75***	1.14	1.00	0.00	1.00	0.00	1.24	0.44	1.76*	1.09	1.00	0.00	1.25	0.45
12 Feel dizzy	1.11	0.42	1.29*	0.85	1.00	0.00	1.00	0.00	1.06	0.24	1.71*	1.10	1.00	0.00	1.31	0.48
8 Feel stiffness in shoulder	1.21	0.42	3.00***	1.52	1.27	0.47	2.91***	0.94	1.71	0.59	3.12***	1.54	1.38	0.62	2.25***	1.13
11 Feel pain in hand/finger	1.21	0.42	2.82***	1.52	1.73	0.65	3.45***	0.69	1.06	0.24	1.59**	0.94	1.13	0.34	1.56**	0.73
IV 19 Get tired in the wrist	1.25	0.44	3.43***	1.48	1.18	0.40	3.09***	0.83	1.35	0.49	2.88***	1.17	1.13	0.34	2.06***	0.93
23 Feel a pain in the back	1.96	0.69	3.86***	1.27	1.73	0.90	3.36***	0.81	1.94	0.66	4.00***	1.17	1.56	0.51	2.88***	1.20
25 Get tired in the legs	1.14	0.36	3.11***	1.45	1.36	0.50	3.36***	0.81	1.12	0.33	3.06***	1.03	1.19	0.40	1.75**	1.06
3 Feel dried in eyes	1.07	0.26	1.36*	0.83	1.00	0.00	1.00	0.00	1.24	0.44	1.76**	1.09	1.56	0.63	2.00*	1.26
7 Feel a pain in eyes	1.00	0.00	1.25*	0.59	1.00	0.00	1.09	0.30	1.12	0.33	1.35	0.70	1.19	0.40	1.63***	0.81
V 16 Feel tired of things	1.11	0.31	1.32	0.72	1.00	0.00	1.00	0.00	1.12	0.33	1.88***	1.17	1.06	0.25	1.69***	0.60
22 Get tired in eyes	1.07	0.26	1.79***	1.07	1.09	0.30	1.18	0.40	1.06	0.24	2.06***	0.97	1.00	0.00	1.75***	0.86
24 Feel strained in the eyes	1.00	0.00	1.21	0.69	1.00	0.00	1.00	0.00	1.00	0.00	1.47**	0.62	1.06	0.25	1.81***	0.98

Table 4. Facility comparison of fatigue level in 5 factors between before and after work

	No.1 before		No.1 after		No.2 before		No.2 after		No.3 before		No.3 after		No.4 before		No.4 after	
	mean	SD	mean	SD	mean	SD	mean	SD	mean	SD	mean	SD	mean	SD	mean	SD
I (Drowsiness/dullness)	5.18	0.48	11.57***	3.38	5.36	0.67	7.55***	0.93	5.82	1.19	9.76***	2.91	5.81	0.66	11.06***	3.17
II (Uneasy feeling)	5.11	0.31	7.07***	2.32	5.00	0.00	5.00	0.00	5.06	0.24	5.82**	1.13	5.19	0.40	5.44*	0.51
III (Illness situation)	5.18	0.48	6.68***	2.34	5.00	0.00	5.09	0.30	5.47	0.80	7.59***	2.21	5.13	0.34	6.44***	1.41
IV (Physical impairment)	6.79	1.10	16.21***	4.81	7.27	0.79	16.18***	3.40	7.18	0.88	14.65***	3.44	6.38	1.26	10.50***	3.37
V (Fuzzy feeling)	5.25	0.70	6.93***	2.61	5.09	0.30	5.27	0.47	5.53	0.62	8.53***	2.79	5.88	1.02	8.88***	3.48

during work. Through on-scene interview and observation for investigated caregivers' care work process among four nursing house facilities, caregiver with big age and large numbers of turn-over care in wide work distribution were considered to be important reasons for complained items.

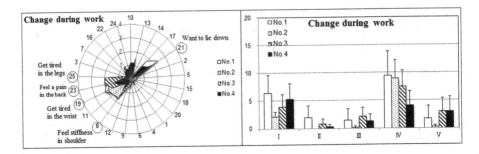

Fig. 1. The evaluation of fatigue condition change during care work

3.2 Discussion of Work Shift Effect on "Subjective Fatigue Symptoms"

In Tables 5 and 6, day and night work shift fatigue level along with care work were compared by each complaint item and type factor respectively. All the subjects employed for work shift effect discussion on fatigue symptom were originated from No. 1 facility with the same sample numbers. Comparing with day-work shift, night-work shift subjects showed more fatigue symptom such as "Give a yaw", "Become drowsy" and "Want to lie down" in addition to "Feel a pain in the back" item before work. In general, fatigue symptoms included in Type1 (I)-"Drowsiness/dullness" displayed an obvious complaint total-points. Predetermined night shift working schedule for subjects was required to charge from 9:00 pm to 7:00am (+1day) in No.1 facility. Because night shift caregiver's working period is just as the same with normal people's regular bedtime, so as you can imagine, most of night shift subjects may presented a dullness state before work. According to subjects' fatigue complaint items after care work, it is clearly to find that night shift caregiver suffered from a painful work period of physical (care work loading) and mental (sleep breaking) torture with a higher score in Type1 (I), Type3 (III) and Type5 (V) factors than day shift subjects except fatigue symptom score of Type4 (IV)-"Physical impairment". Based on site survey results, it is found that most elders fall into sleep with sharp activities reduce during night period, and for caregiver their main work was to assist bedridden elder to turn-over and check sick elder's body condition every 2 h. In other words, night shift subjects burdened less amount of care work than day shift, but they suffered from larger mental challenge as sleep broken, fear, loneliness and so on.

The comparison of subjects' fatigue condition change during work between day and night shift was clarified in Fig. 2 combining detailed items change painting in Radar map and type factor summary bar. It is worthwhile to note that both day and night work shift subjects displayed the obvious fatigue symptom change in "Want to lie down" and "Feel stiffness in shoulder" items. Furthermore, work shift's characteristics were also reflected on subjects' different fatigue symptom factors, where day shift subjects' fatigue complaints concentrated in Type4 (IV) because of heavier workload but night shift subjects' fatigue mainly stated in Type1 (I) as the result of regular rest violation.

Table 5. Work shift comparison of fatigue level for 25 items before and after work

	Day shift before		Day shift after		Change of day shift		Night shift before		Night shift after		Change of night shift	
	mean	SD	mean	SD	mean	SD	mean	SD	mean	SD	mean	SD
I												
10 Give a yawn	1.00	0.00	1.50***	0.69	0.50	0.69	1.29	0.60	3.29***	1.21	2.00	1.22
13 Become drowsy	1.07	0.26	2.61***	1.29	1.54	1.23	1.29	0.46	3.46***	1.06	2.18	1.09
14 Do not want to move	1.00	0.00	1.25**	0.52	0.25	0.52	1.04	0.19	1.46***	0.74	0.43	0.69
17 Get tired over day	1.11	0.31	2.82***	1.33	1.71	1.24	1.04	0.19	2.43***	1.03	1.39	1.03
21 Want to lie down	1.00	0.00	3.39***	1.69	2.39	1.69	1.32	0.61	3.61***	1.42	2.29	1.38
II												
2 Anxious about things	1.00	0.00	1.54***	0.58	0.54	0.58	1.07	0.26	1.71***	0.76	0.64	0.68
5 Feel unsteady in standing	1.07	0.26	1.46***	0.84	0.39	0.74	1.04	0.19	1.11	0.31	0.07	0.26
15 Feel uneasy	1.04	0.19	1.50***	0.88	0.46	0.84	1.00	0.00	1.32**	0.61	0.32	0.61
18 Feel sad or depressed	1.00	0.00	1.25***	0.44	0.25	0.44	1.00	0.00	1.18*	0.39	0.18	0.39
20 Feel difficult to thinking	1.00	0.00	1.32***	0.55	0.32	0.55	1.00	0.00	1.21*	0.63	0.21	0.63
III												
1 Feel heavy in the head	1.04	0.19	1.25*	0.65	0.21	0.50	1.00	0.00	2.18***	0.94	1.18	0.94
4 Feel ill	1.00	0.00	1.11*	0.31	0.11	0.31	1.04	0.19	1.57***	1.00	0.54	0.96
6 Have a headache	1.00	0.00	1.29***	0.46	0.29	0.46	1.00	0.00	1.50***	0.75	0.50	0.75
9 Feel brain muddled	1.04	0.19	1.75***	1.14	0.71	1.08	1.00	0.00	1.39***	0.57	0.39	0.57
12 Feel dizzy	1.11	0.42	1.29*	0.85	0.18	0.48	1.00	0.00	1.29***	0.46	0.29	0.46
IV												
8 Feel stiffness in shoulder	1.21	0.42	3.00***	1.52	1.79	1.32	1.07	0.26	2.71***	1.24	1.64	1.19
11 Feel pain in hand/finger	1.21	0.42	2.82***	1.52	1.61	1.34	1.00	0.00	1.54***	0.69	0.54	0.69
19 Get tired in the wrist	1.25	0.44	3.43***	1.48	2.18	1.36	1.04	0.19	2.46***	1.04	1.43	1.00
23 Feel a pain in the back	1.96	0.69	3.86***	1.27	1.89	0.99	1.29	0.53	2.89***	1.17	1.61	0.96
25 Get tired in the legs	1.14	0.36	3.11***	1.45	1.96	1.35	1.04	0.19	2.43***	0.96	1.39	0.96
V												
3 Feel dried in eyes	1.07	0.26	1.36*	0.83	0.29	0.76	1.11	0.31	2.61***	1.20	1.50	1.14
7 Feel a pain in eyes	1.00	0.00	1.25*	0.59	0.25	0.59	1.07	0.26	2.18***	1.31	1.11	1.20
16 Feel fuzzy of things	1.11	0.31	1.32	0.72	0.21	0.69	1.00	0.00	1.25*	0.59	0.25	0.59
22 Get tired in eyes	1.07	0.26	1.79***	1.07	0.71	1.01	1.11	0.31	2.89***	1.20	1.79	1.03
24 Feel strained in the eyes	1.00	0.00	1.21	0.69	0.21	0.69	1.00	0.00	1.82***	1.33	0.82	1.33

Table 6. Work shift comparison of fatigue level in 5 factors between before and after work

	Day shift before		Day shift after		Change of day shift		Night shift before		Night shift after		Change of night shift	
	mean	SD	mean	SD	mean	SD	mean	SD	mean	SD	mean	SD
I (Drowsiness/dullness)	5.18	0.48	11.57***	3.38	6.39	3.22	5.96	1.50	14.25***	3.12	8.29	3.29
II (Uneasy feeling)	5.11	0.31	7.07***	2.32	1.96	2.17	5.11	0.31	6.54***	1.32	1.43	1.29
III (Illness situation)	5.18	0.48	6.68***	2.34	1.50	2.01	5.04	0.19	7.93***	2.11	2.89	2.06
IV (Physical impairment)	6.79	1.10	16.21***	4.81	9.43	4.36	5.43	0.69	12.04***	2.60	6.61	2.41
V (Fuzzy feeling)	5.25	0.70	6.93***	2.61	1.68	2.39	5.29	0.71	10.75***	4.48	5.46	4.11

3.3 Fatigue Location Discussion by "Tired Body Part" Questionnaire

Figure 3(a) and (b) indicated the fatigue location rank of day work and work shift comparison respectively. It is obvious to obtain a general tired body part rank for 4 nursing house facilities (day shift) in total counting as: waist > shoulder > knee > arm > foot > head > back = hand/finger = thigh. Extraordinary, "waist pain" accounted for 80 % of subjects through one day-shift care

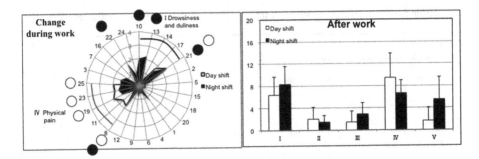

Fig. 2. Fatigue condition change during care work comparison between day and night shift

work, which confirmed that accumulated fatigue of waist part was serious and urgent issue. When we took the same fatigue location rank to sort corresponding day/night shift complaint feedback from No.1 facility, similar rank trend in night shift subjective reply was also demonstrated. However, night shift subjects showed a general lower percentage of fatigue complaints on body parts than day shift one.

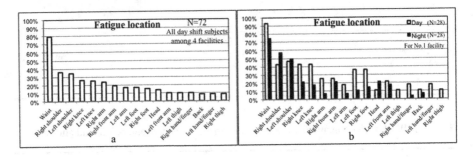

Fig. 3. Tired body part rank summary

3.4 Relationship Between Subjects' Characteristic and Fatigue Symptom

The correlation between subjects' fatigue symptom change and age or experience years was carried out by SPSS Pearson tests. The results did not showed correlation between subjects' fatigue symptom change and age based on limited data collection from current study. On the other hand, experience year indicated low negative linear correlation (-0.402) with fatigue symptom of Type4 (IV) under the significance interval $P < 0.05$, which means that expert caregiver with longer occupational years could master better skill of care work with less body loading.

3.5 Saliva α-Amylase Assay Test Results

The information of two groups subjects employed in saliva α-Amylase assay were recorded in Table 7, in which yellow group charged with shower care job during 9:30am to 10:30am. As the talk interview with subjects, we found that most of caregivers complained of physical fatigue and high stress during shower care job. As well known that larger numbers of elders were not cooperative or move around during shower process, which may result in increased elder fell-down risk and requirement of physical power for caregiver. Saliva α-Amylase is a kind of indicator of subject's fatigue and mental stress reflection. Figure 4 illustrated the average value of saliva tests for both two groups among three continuous observation days. It was found that either with or without shower care job both two groups subjects showed increased saliva α value along with increasing work duration time compared with first time measurement. Especially, saliva α value measured at 10:30am for the group charged with shower job manifested a large increase peak, which quantified shower care work loading on subject's body. However, after the day rest period from 13:00 to 15:00, both two groups kept the similar saliva α value for the third saliva test (tested at 16:30) as 2 times of first test measurement value. In other words, shower care job fatigue loading could be recovered effectively by lunch rest period.

Table 7. Subjects' information for saliva α-Amylase assay

Name code	Age (year)	Working experience (year)	Height (cm)	Weight (Kg)
Liu...	47	3.5	159	49
Wang...	41	4	150	47
Wu...	44	10	156	53
Zai...	45	4	150	50
Yang...	40	5	156	45
Li	41	10	160	57

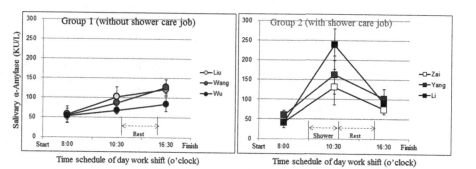

Fig. 4. Saliva α-Amylase assay results of two groups' subjects during work shift

4 Conclusions

In this research, Japanese "subjective fatigue symptoms" and "Tired body parts" questionnaire were employed to investigate caregiver's fatigue situation in Chinese nursing house facility. As a conclusion, fatigue pattern characteristics of Type4-"Physical impairment" and Type1-"Drowness/dullness" were clarified for day shift and night shift caregiver respectively. Furthermore, fatigue body location rank was also demonstrated according to complaint counting from "tired body parts" with "waist pain" as top spot. Finally, physical body loading and mental stress caused by shower care job was quantitatively confirmed by salivaα-Amylase assay.

Combined caregivers' nursing work interview and fatigue investigation feedback, some measures were proposed for improving the fatigue condition of Chinese elder nursing occupation as: (1) shower-assisted device application; (2) effective arrange of rest period during day shift; (3) optimize night shift work schedule by shift system with shorter work duration; (4) specific body exercise for tired body part recovery.

References

1. Marras, W.S., Davis, K.G., Kirking, B.C., Bertsche, P.K.: A comprehensive analysis of low-back disorder risk and spinal loading during the transferring and repositioning of patients using different techniques. Ergonomics 42(7), 904–926 (1999)
2. Coenen, P., Kingma, I., Boot, C.R., Bongers, P.M., van Dieën, J.H.: Cumulative mechanical low-back load at work is a determinant of low-back pain. Occup. Environ. Med. 71(5), 332–337 (2014). doi:10.1136/oemed-2013-101862. Epub 27 March 2014
3. Ito, M., Endo, A., Takai, Y., Yoshikawa, T., Goto, A., Kuwahara, N.: Study on kind transfer assistance between wheelchair and bed in the case of eye movement analysis. In: Proceedings of 5th International conference on Applied Human Factors and Ergonomics, AHFE (2014)

Mobile Application to Aid in the Prevention of Pressure Ulcers

Alvaro G. Lima[1]([⊠]), Lara Araújo[2], Isabel Italiano[1],
and Luciano V. Araujo[1]

[1] School of Arts Science and Humanity, University of Sao Paulo - USP,
Sao Paulo, Brazil
{alvarogulliver,isabel.italiano,lvaraujo}@usp.br
[2] Federal University of Sao Paulo - UNIFESP, Sao Paulo, Brazil
lara.araujo@unifesp.br

Abstract. Pressure Ulcer (PU) is a wound in the skin and underlying tissues caused by the lack of patient's movement leading to prolonged pressure exposure on certain body part. The PU's may cause complications to the patient's treatment, since it becomes a route of infection. Consequently, it can extend the length of hospital stay and treatment costs. This paper presents the development of a smartphone app to assist healthcare professionals in the prevention of Pus in bedridden patients. The developed app aims to collect and analyze data for estimating the severity of a health episode regarding suffering from patients. In addition, a prototype was developed for testing using the Wearable platform, based on temperature and humidity sensors together with ZigBee modules for data acquisition and communication between architecture components. This approach simplifies the interaction between sensors, applications, and medical staff with a focus on improved patient care.

Keywords: Pressure ulcer · Temperature sensor · Humidity sensor · Bedridden patient monitoring · Pressure ulcer prevention · M-Health application

1 Introduction

Reports of the NPUAP (National Pressure Ulcer Advisory Panel) in 2014, show that spending on treatment of pressure ulcers (PUs) in the United States are estimated about $11 billion (USD) annually. There is an economic impact of PU, because it may cause increased hospital stay and consequently generates an increase in spending with its treatment. The increase in the cost of hospitalization can reach up $70,000.00 (USD) per patient. Beyond the economic impact, the PU also affects the quality of life for patients, as they are painful and difficult to heal and can even lead to death [3].

The PUs are lesions on the skin, usually over a bony prominence, which affects the underlying tissues in bedridden, or that have any trouble changing the body position. With the emergence of PUs, the patient is at risk of getting infections. The variation of temperature and moisture of the body are important factors that contribute to increase the vulnerability, skin damage and avoid the recovery process. The automated and

V.G. Duffy (Ed.): DHM 2015, Part II, LNCS 9185, pp. 465–473, 2015.
DOI: 10.1007/978-3-319-21070-4_47

continuous monitoring of bedridden patients can collect detailed data about the patient. Such data can be used to assess the risk of developing ulcers and inference level of consciousness of the patient. The transformation of these data into indicators is a way to produce information to assist in monitoring the progress of PUs and deciding on the best treatment for the patient. The Human-Computer Interaction (HCI) area has made several contributions to the development of technologies that assist in disease prevention in healthcare, such as the miniaturization of hardware, network communications and distributed computing. Furthermore, with the popularization of electronic devices, such sensors and processors are increasingly available at affordable prices and can be used for software development and functionality for performing tasks related to prevention of PUs.

The risk factors of PUs include pressure shearing forces, frictions and so on. Pressure applied on the skin that is higher than arteriolar pressure (32 mmHg) causes and insufficiency of oxygen and nutrients in tissue, which results in tissue damage [2]. Damage can occur with as little as 2 h immobility. Other factors may not cause the PUs, but it could have additive effects during the development of PUs or more severe tissue damage [2]. Although some recommendations contained on this research are recognized, and are apparently simple, actually the logistics involved for replacement position demands a need for more specialized monitoring, and this work presents an alternative to contribute to the monitoring of bedridden patients as a way to increase the prevention of PUs.

2　Materials and Methods

This project presents integration between hardware and software, because we developed a wearable prototype with sensors and a mobile application to monitor the health status of the bedridden patients. The clothes developed and used in the test with temperature and moisture sensors are connected to an electronic board with microcontroller Atmel ATMEGA328P and uses Xbee Shield modules for data transmission to PC. We created a prototype with SHT15 sensor, since it is one of the smallest sensors found and according to the manufacturer [1] is one of the few sensors available on the market suitable for medicine purposes.

We developed an application for the Android platform using the SDK API 19. We tested it with Samsung Galaxy S4 smartphones with Android 4.2 and Sony Xperia with android 4.3. It was developed by using Android Studio, whose function is to monitor the variation of temperature and moisture where are the two main factors responsible for the emergence of PUs.

Furthermore, for connection between the modules, we used the XBee module technology, where is an embedded solution providing wireless end-point connectivity to devices. These modules were used with the same Zigbee networking protocol for fast peer-to-peer networking. Furthermore, the XBee Explorer Dongle is an extension used to connect directly to PC USB port.

2.1   Global System Architecture

The project was structured and divided into components to further specify your goals. There are four components that consisting on the Global System Architecture (GSA); each one is responsible for a specific function, and the Core Component, as shown on Fig. 1, orchestrates all these.

The Graphical User Interface (GUI) is responsible for the graphical display of indicators and alerts generated by the system. It also responsible for input data.

The Core Component is responsible for storing and processing the data over the Internet by using cloud computing providers (e.g.: Elastic Compute Cloud - AWS). Additionally, it manages the system operation and communication between GSA components, as shown in Fig. 2.

The next component of the GSA is called Wireless modules, collects the information reading of temperature and moisture sensors and transmits the data to a Core Component.

The last GSA component is called Wearable modules that collects temperature and moisture data from bedridden patients.

3   The Skin Health Advisor

In our work, we developed an app called Skin Health Advisor (SHA) that belongs to User Interface component. According to Fig. 3, we present some features used in the experiment. The collected data is retrieved through the functionality Capture Date and transmitted to the application with processed data on the clinical situation of each patient. The application accesses the data already collected and uses for alerting nursing staff to perform procedures for prevention and treatment (Capture Data functionality). It works as alert for medical decision making, once, with a profile of temperature and

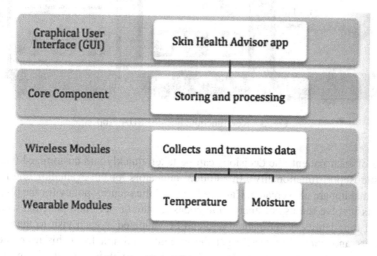

Fig. 1. Global System Architecture

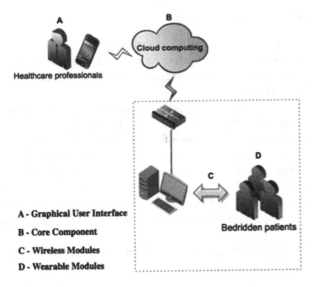

Fig. 2. Network diagram of each GSA component

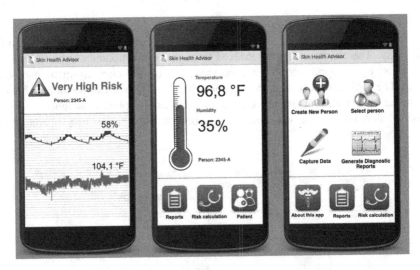

Fig. 3. Key functionalities of SHA App

moisture of each patient, the decisions can be taken quickly and customized (Generate Diagnostic Report functionality). In addition, indicators for the evaluation and medical decision-making are also created. Capture Data and the security policy for the protection of patients involve the use of encryption codes for the devices and patients, which did not reveal the identity of the patient and can be validated at each visit to the bed.

Doctors and nurses can easily get the current condition from this user interface. They can see if the current condition of the patient`s health is normal through a green color. If the patient's condition is dangerous, then the color will be red. In addition, other diagnostic reports may provide in advance if the bedridden patients at risk of developing the PUs over time.

3.1 Data Storage

Our system was developed to use a database management class that supports distributed processing by sharing data across multiple servers to balance the load because the amount of data collected by sensors was very huge, what every 10 s is collected samples of temperature and humidity over a patient and a day increases the size of the data very fast way [4]. To plan its scalability in the future, we opted for NoSQL database to meet these performance requirements.

3.2 Wearable Clothing with Sensors

The clothing of bedridden patients uses textile to connect with the electronic board and sensors, as shown on Fig. 4. The prototype integrated in the patient's clothing is adapted for removal from the sensors, since the sensors are removable and do not constitute a point of friction with the skin because the material has a soft encapsulation.

This sensor works stable within recommended normal range because it operates under conditions of temperature between −4°F and 176°F. Long period exposures to conditions outside normal range may temporarily offset the relative humidity signal (+3 %RH). After return to a normal range it will slowly return towards calibration state by itself [1].

3.3 Data Transmission Network

The ZigBee mesh networks are designed with the inverse square law in mind. Rather than using big batteries to generate the large amount of power needed to send a signal

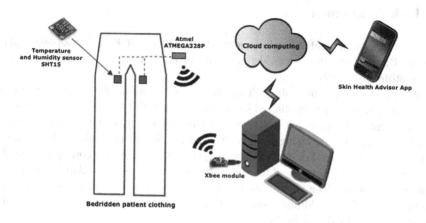

Fig. 4. The infrastructure integrated with the wearable clothing

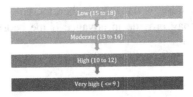

Fig. 5. Risk calculation given the Braden scale

over a great distance, each radio needs only small amounts of power to go a short distance to its nearest neighbor in the network [5]. By adding nodes to the network, great distances can be traversed without any node needing access to large amounts of energy.

The network layer below ZigBee that supports its advanced features is known as IEEE 802.15.4. This is a set of standards that define power management, addressing, error correction, message formats, and other point-to-point specifics necessary for proper communication to take place from one radio to another. XBee-brand radios can be used with or without ZigBee [5].

3.4 Non-invasive Method of Thermometry on Humans

The method is based on the body temperature and moisture measure, where is an influential indicator that reflects overall physiological health states [6]. The two critical factors and prolonged exposure to pressure compromise blood supply of nutrients and oxygen to the cells, causing tissue death and consequently leads to injury.

The sensors connected to the patient's clothing transmit the data to be processed and generated information to the SHA application. The module sensor used to collect thermometry data is soft and does not constitute a point of friction to increase the risk of emergence of new PU.

4 Risk Assessment

To assist healthcare professionals in identifying the risk of PUs development, SHA uses the Braden Scale that is considered the most comprehensive and widely utilized by health professionals [8].

We asked four questions through the SHA app, that assess the patient's condition considering: sensory perception, which is the patient's ability to react to discomfort; skin moisture; activity, which is the level of physical activity of the patient; mobility, which is the capacity to change and control the position of the body itself; nutrition; and body temperature. For each answer is given a score, which corresponds to the column number. For example, if for "moisture" the answer is "very clammy skin," are awarded two points. The sum of the points indicates the risk of PUs development as shown in Fig. 7. In addition, some additional information is needed to trace the patient's profile, as shown in Table 1.

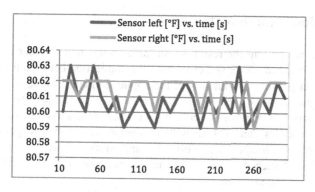

Fig. 6. First test period with dry cloth

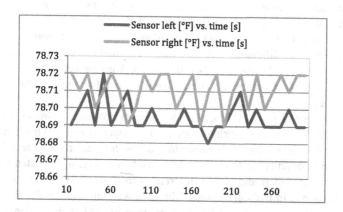

Fig. 7. Second test period with wet cloth

Table 1. Key attibutes used by the system

Attribute	Data type	Source
Ambient Temperature	Numeric	Relative Temperature Sensor
Age	Numeric	GUI
Body temperature	Numeric	Temperature sensor
Body moisture	Numeric	Moisture sensor
Weight	Numeric	GUI
Gender	Char	GUI
Day period	Date	Computed
Activity	Numeric	GUI
Humidity Relative	Numeric	Relative Humidity Sensor
Nutrition	Number	GUI

5 Simulation Experiments

In this section, we present the results of an initial simulation in order to evaluate the infrastructure described above and evaluating the connection between the modules, on this way we can perform a validation of the application and its connectivity.

For this simulation we used a prototype, not human to validate the exact position where the sensors will be placed to collect data. These tests served to validate how far up the XBee modules can achieve without compromising system performance. In addition, we collected temperature information and humidity every 10 s to also validate the transmission of such data for storage in the database. The test used two fabrics, a dry, another controlled moist.

During the first test, to measure the temperature and humidity, we used a sensor of doll panties, on each side of the legs, more precisely in the region above the pectineus muscle on humans. To measure it in different positions of these prototype, we simulated the situation where a patient is in the supine position for 10 min. Every 10 s, the temperature was collected through the body sensor. In this simulation we use a dry cloth to measure and collect the two vital signs at a distance of 2 m from the base where is the central computer where the data collected and transmitted is stored. According to Fig. 5, the temperature difference collected was very small and the tests were successful as the performance of the module, because we had no packet loss or drop in data transmission to the host computer. The ambient temperature was 82,40°F during the first experiment.

During the second test, we repeated the same experiment, however with slightly moistened cloth. We use a measuring instrument, dropper, in order to transfer the liquid into an exact amount of 20 ml of water in panties doll and repeat the collection of temperature and humidity for five minutes. According to Fig. 6, the listed temperature difference was very small and obtain differences from the first simulation performed due to the difference in moisture tissues. The tests were also successful as the module performance, as there was no packet loss or drop in data transmission to the host computer. The ambient temperature was 82.40° F during the second experiment.

6 Results

The SHA application presents an alternative for monitoring bedridden patients as a way to support the prevention and treatment of pressure. With it, the health care team receives alerts and indicators that support and enable an agile action in patient care. Through the split system architecture in well-defined layers, it was possible to complete the application development and deliver results that met the initial expectations of the project. Automated monitoring and continuous of bedridden patients can collect detailed data on their clinical status. The data collection made in the simulation was used as an initial test to validate the communication between components. As future work, tests will be performed to verify some limits, such as stress test to assess the ability of collecting temperature and humidity data. After these step, we will begin testing in humans.

References

1. SHT1x – Digital Humidity & Temperature Sensor (RH/T). http://www.sensirion.com/en/products/humidity-temperature/humidity-temperature-sensor-sht1x/. Accessed 17 November 2014
2. Bellos, C.C., Papadopoulos, A., Rosso, R., Fotiadis, D.I.: Extraction and Analysis of features acquired by wearable sensors network. In: 2010 10th IEEE International Conference on Information Technology and Applications in Biomedicine (ITAB), pp. 1, 4. 3–5 November 2010
3. National Pressure Ulcer Advisory Panel (NPUAP): 2014 World Wide Pressure Ulcer Prevention Day. http://www.npuap.org/2014-world-wide-pressure-ulcer-prevention-day-press-release/. Accessed 20 October 2014
4. Khadka, S.: Privacy, security and storage issues in medical data management. In: 2012 Third Asian Himalayas International Conference on Internet (AH-ICI), pp. 1, 5. 23–25 November 2012
5. Niswar, M., Ilham, A.A., Palantei, E., Sadjad, R.S., Ahmad, A., Suyuti, A., Indrabayu Muslimin, Z., Waris, T., Adi, P.D.P.: Performance evaluation of ZigBee-based wireless sensor network for monitoring patients' pulse status. In: 2013 International Conference on Information Technology and Electrical Engineering (ICITEE), pp. 291, 294. 7–8 October 2013
6. Sim, S.Y., Lee, W.K., Baek, H.J., Park, K.S., A nonintrusive temperature measuring system for estimating deep body temperature in bed. In: 2012 Annual International Conference of the IEEE Engineering in Medicine and Biology Society (EMBC), pp. 3460–3463, 28 August 2012–1 September 2012
7. Fard, F.D., Moghimi, S., Lotfi, R.: Pressure ulcer risk assessment by monitoring interface pressure and temperature. In: 2013 21st Iranian Conference on Electrical Engineering (ICEE), pp. 1, 5. 14–16 May 2013
8. Hyun, S., Li, X., Vermillion, B., Newton, C., Fall, M., Kaewprag, P., Moffatt-Bruce, S., Lenz, E.R.: Body mass index and pressure ulcers: improved predictability of pressure ulcers in intensive care patients. Am. J. Crit. Care 23(6), 494–501 (2014). American Association of Critical-Care Nurses
9. Raju, D., Su, X., Patrician, P.A., Loan, L.A., McCarthy, M.S.: Exploring factors associated with pressure ulcers: a data mining approach. Int. J. Nurs. Stud. 52, 102–111 (2015)

Development of a Self-learning System
for Chest Auscultation Skills Using an RFID
Reader for Nursing Students

Mitsuhiro Nakamura[1]([✉]), Kyohei Koyama[2], Yasuko Kitajima[1],
Jukai Maeda[1], and Masako Kanai-Pak[1]

[1] Faculty of Nursing, Tokyo Ariake University of Medical and Health Sciences,
2-9-1 Ariake, Koto-Ku, Tokyo 135-0063, Japan
{m-nakamura,kitajima,jukai,p-kanai}@tau.ac.jp
[2] GOV Co. Ltd., Bldg.#1 134 Chudoji Minamimachi, Shimogyo-Ku,
Kyoto-Shi, Kyoto 600-8813, Japan
koyama@go-v.co.jp

Abstract. The purposes of this study are (1) To develop a chest auscultation
self-learning system for nursing students with which both a self-learning tool
and an evaluation tool are integrated, and (2) To evaluate the system whether
nursing students are able to acquire the chest ausculation skills. We have
developed a system using RFID tags and RFID reader (TECCO). Six nursing
students used this system for 15 min, and received feedback after each performance from this system. The students' performance was evaluated. The highest
score was 85, and the lowest score was 10. The range of practice time was
between 5 and 13. The differences between highest score and lowest score for
each examinee ranged from 63 to 25. The results indicated that nursing students
can learn the chest auscultation skills using this system even they spend a
limited time for practice if they use repeatedly.

Keywords: Chest auscultation skill · Nursing education · Nursing skill ·
Nursing student · RFID reader · Simulation

1 Background

In Japan, a shortage of nurses due to increased demand from a super aging society and
decreased supply from declining birth rates has been pointed out, and ensuring the
number of nurses is an urgent issue [1]. The Japanese government is taking measures
relating to the supply of nurses, and it increased the enrollment capacity of registered
nurse education from 40,865 to 61,629, in 1991 to 2013, respectively [2, 3].

On the other hand, according to a survey conducted by the Japan Nursing Association in 2002, of 103 "skills you could perform on your own when you started
working," more than 70 percent could only name four: bed-making, changing linens,
taking vital signs and measuring height and weight. It is a serious issue that new
graduates do not acquire competent nursing skills upon their graduation [4].

Nursing students have to learn nursing skills in nursing skill lab rooms. Usually,
teaching nursing skills are structured as lectures and practice in lab with mock patients.

© Springer International Publishing Switzerland 2015
V.G. Duffy (Ed.): DHM 2015, Part II, LNCS 9185, pp. 474–481, 2015.
DOI: 10.1007/978-3-319-21070-4_48

They receive technical instructions from the teachers. However, there is severe nursing faculty shortage due to recent rapid increase of nursing colleges in Japan. In the nursing program where the researchers work, for example, there are four faculty giving skill instructions to 60 students. It is obvious that the students do not receive sufficient skill instructions.

Also, previous research results indicated that the average time faculty can give direct instructions to a student in nursing skill lab rooms was 9.4 min [5], in order for students to acquire nursing skills, more effective teaching methods is required to develop. In such a situation, self-learning on the part of the nursing education is essential for acquiring nursing skills. Students work hard to acquire through self-learning nursing skills which were taught once during in-school practice by teachers, however when teachers evaluate the students' nursing skills after self-learning, they often find the students have learned a skill incorrectly. This is thought to be attributable to the fact that students cannot objectively observe their own skill and correct incorrect performance [6]. In other words, for nursing students to acquire nursing skills through self-learning, it is essential to have a third party who can provide correct feedback. However, as mentioned earlier, teachers who have expert knowledge and have skills to give accurate feedback to students cannot find enough time to be involved with self-learning until all students acquire nursing skills.

In order to support nursing students' self-learning, various tools are available. Audiovisual educational materials such as videos and DVDs (Fig. 1), e-learning systems that can be used not just with computers but also with mobile devices that can connect to the Internet (Fig. 2), and various tools such as those that use anatomical models of the human body (Fig. 3) are available in market. However, these are only one-way tools for showing correct skills and they have no skill evaluation functions. That is why students cannot learn correct skill even when they use such learning materials.

In order to solve this problem, it is necessary to provide an environment in which students can receive precise instructions and evaluation of their performance.

If there were an automated system that seamlessly linked a nursing skill self-learning tool with an evaluation tool, rapid improvement could be made in

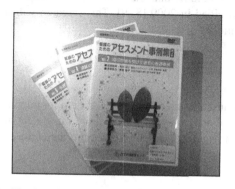

Fig. 1. Learning DVD (The Nursing Education Series by Institute of Audio-Visual Medical Education)

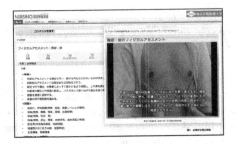

Fig. 2. E-learning systems (Nursing Skills by Elsevier Japan)

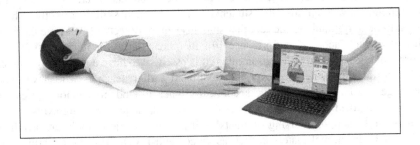

Fig. 3. Physical Assessment Simulator (Physiko by Kyoto Kagaku Co., Ltd.)

effective and efficient acquisition of nursing skill through self-learning. This is why this research team developed a system that can be used when nursing students study nursing skills on their own.

Although nursing students have to learn numerous nursing skills, this system focuses on chest auscultation skills. The chest auscultation skills are one of the physical assessment which assesses the body conditions non-invasively. The previous research indicated that chest auscultation is one of the most frequently performed physical assessment skills during the clinical practicum [7]. Physical assessment is a required skill in many nursing programs that the Ministry of Health, Labour and Welfare, a license issue body, specified in 2009 [8, 9]. This research will fit for the issue of the current nursing education.

2 Purposes

1. To develop a chest auscultation self-learning system for nursing students with which both a self-learning tool and an evaluation tool are integrated, and 2. To evaluate the system whether nursing students are able to acquire the chest auscultation skills.

3 Methods

3.1 System Development

In order to develop the system, the researchers sought opinions of several nursing faculty members who teach nursing skills at universities about what kinds of functions are essential for the system. Based on their comments, the specifications of the system were developed. The specifications are as follows:

- The system will recreate three-dimensionally of the upper body of an adult male.
- It is desirable for nurses to confirm the accurate point of the breathing auscultation part by touching the clavicles and ribs of the patient, so the lay figure of the upper body was created that the nursing students are able to touch clavicles and ribs from the surface of the chest.
- Because auscultation skill is performed using a stethoscope, the system will have a stethoscope-type device.
- When the stethoscope-type device is touched to the chest area, the nursing student will be able to listen to the breathing sound in the area being auscultated.
- The system will be able to record the location being touched with the stethoscope-type device and to record the length being touched.
- The nursing student will be able to use the system on his own without any instructions and teachers for a system operator.
- The system will be able to provide feedback by converting an evaluation to a score.
- The system will be able to provide feedback by presenting an evaluation visually.
- The system will be able to record scores.

3.2 Built a System that Fulfills the Above Requirements

For the stethoscope-type device, we used TECCO by GOV Co., Ltd. TECCO is a RFID reader (13.56 Hz band) in the form of a covering for the back of the hand and wrist that is worn on the wrist and can be used wirelessly. The reading part of the reader was refashioned to be small like the chest piece of a stethoscope to create a stethoscope-type device (Fig. 4).

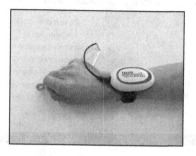

Fig. 4. A stethoscope-type device

To recreate the upper body of an adult male, the upper body of a simulation mannequin was used. The chest area surface is made of sponge material and the inside is a faithful recreation of the rib cage of a person, so by touching the skin one can feel the ribcage. Round, thin, 15 mm diameter REID tags are placed in a mesh pattern at roughly 20 mm intervals the reverse side of the sponge material.

For the system's operation and feedback display device, an Android operating system tablet (Toshiba's REGZA Tablet AT703 28 J) was used.

On the tablet, a chest auscultation evaluation application which we developed was installed. This has the functions of recording the time when the TECCO device contacts with an RFID tag and the tag's ID by comparing it with chest auscultation evaluation criteria developed in advance by the researchers (Table 1), assigning a score, recording it and displaying it as feedback (Fig. 5).

Table 1. Evaluation criteria

	Evaluation Criterion	Basis for Evaluation Criterion
1	Listening at an intercostal space	Because it is difficult to hear breath sounds just above the rib
2	Listening at the central part of the lung	Because it is difficult to hear breath sounds on either end of the lung
3	The order of auscultation is correct	Because auscultation is performed listening symmetrically from left to right and the top to bottom by comparing the sounds
4	The nursing student can move the stethoscope smoothly and in a short time	Because a long period of time for auscultation will be a physical burden on the patient
5	The nursing student listens to inhale and exhale of breathing as one cycle	Because chest auscultation requires listening to both inhale and exhale of breathing sounds

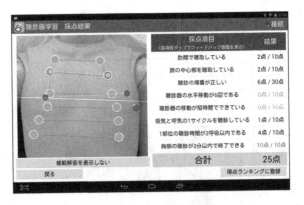

Fig. 5. Screen of tablet

3.3   The Learning Process with the Self-learning System

The learning process with the self-learning system is as follows:

1. Start up the tablet and stethoscope-type device and establish a bluetooth connection.
2. Activate the chest auscultation evaluation application.
3. Perform chest auscultation on the upper-body model.
4. When the "Finish" button is tapped, the scores for each evaluation criterion are displayed. Detailed explanation of each criterion is also displayed by tapping the criteria.
5. If the examinee desires, the scores can be registered in the ranking order.

3.4   Evaluation of the System

Six nursing students participated in the evaluation of the self-learning system of chest auscultation. They were four freshman and two sophomore nursing students. They engaged in self-learning using the system repeatedly for 15 min.

4   Results

The results are shown in Table 2. The top score was 85 for Examinee 1, and the lowest score was 10 for Examinee 4. The lowest number of times practicing was 5 for Examinee 5, and the highest number of practice was 13 for Examinee 4. The differences between highest score and lowest score for each examinee ranged from 63 to 25.

Table 2. Scores of the Subjects

#	Grade	The Number of Self-learning													Difference*
		1	2	3	4	5	6	7	8	9	10	11	12	13	
1	2	80	39	69	63	**85**									46
2	2	37	47	**80**	52	48	54								43
3	1	21	17	36	39	21	33	39	**80**						63
4	1	13	12	10	12	12	24	24	23	27	23	29	**35**	31	25
5	1	18	40	30	**56**	42	55	55	43						38
6	1	25	51	49	47	47	**59**	57							34

* Difference between the highest and lowest points
Bold is the highest score

5 Discussion

The participants were told that they could practice as many times as they wish with in 15 min. As a result, the sophomore students practiced fewer times than that of freshman students. On the other hand, comparing the scores at the end of practice, the scores of the freshman students were lower than that of the sophomore students except one student. This could be a difference in their school year. At the time of this experiment, the sophomore students had already learned chest auscultation skills, but the freshman students had not. This could be the reason for this result. However, the scores increased as they practice regardless of the students' previous study. There is no doubt that repeated practice while receiving an unerring evaluation is a factor for students to acquire skills. There is also a surprising result that the freshman students were able to score a certain number of points ranging from 35 to 80 even though they had not learned chest auscultation skills.

Self-learning is usually introduced after gaining knowledge from the lecture and practice. It can be said that students who did not learn skills could gain certain skills using this kind of self-learning system. This self-learning system could be an effective teaching/learning method for nursing students to prepare for new subjects. For students who have already learned chest auscultation skills, this self-learning system could be used for reinforcing their skills. The scores at the end is higher than that of the beginning, however, the scores are not positively correlate with the number of practice. One of the reasons for this result could be that the students did not obtain correct skills even though they received feedback. Based on the feedback, the students tried to correct their performance and they may not pay attention to the skills that they performed correctly. As a result, during the following practice, they made mistake on the skills which they previously performed correctly. This is also due to the design of the system which focuses on how effectively the learners could correct their incorrect performance. There should be a system including how the learners are able to obtain steady skills. For example, the system gives an alert when the learners perform an incorrect skill which they performed correctly during their previous practice. Also, it is helpful that displaying the list of the correct and incorrect records of the skills could be incorporated.

Although the examinee 4 practiced many times, the scores are lower than those of other examinees. There are two reasons to be considered. First, the examinee 4 was not familiar with manipulating computers. Second, she chose the style of learning by exit after each skill not by finishing through performing all skills. The system aggregates the score of each skill upon the exit button is tapped. This could be a reason for the low scores of the examinee 4 who practiced 13 times in 15 min.

6 Conclusion

Based on this research, even in a limited amount of time, if a nursing student uses this system repeatedly for self-learning, she can learn chest auscultation skills.

In Japan, ensuring work-ready, new graduate nurses is an urgent issue, but under the current situation of a shortage of faculty, it is difficult to accomplish nursing skill acquisition for nursing students through only instruction from teachers. This research was successfully proceeded because of collaboration of not only nursing science with engineering. This kind of collaboration will not only solve various problems in nursing science but also to contribute the development of nursing science as profession. The researchers strongly believed that the collaborations between nursing science and engineering will be future approach to improve and contribute both professions.

References

1. Ministry of Health, Labour and Welfare.: The seventh report of committee on nursing staff supply and demand outlook (2010). (in Japanese)
2. Nursing division, Health policy bureau, Ministry of Health and Welfare.: Statistical data on nursing service in Japan 1995 (1995)
3. Japanese Nursing Association Publishing Company.: Statistical data on nursing service in Japan 2013 (2014)
4. Japanese Nursing Association.: Survey of basic nursing skills of freshman nurses (2002). (in Japanese)
5. Nakamura, M.: Building the foundation for a new nursing skill education system based on patient moving. Handout, Special Interest Group of Nonverbal Interface, Human Interface Society (2011). (in Japanese)
6. Kanai-Pak, M.: Innovation in collaborative research between nursing and engineering.: a new approach for skill acquisition. Japan. J. Nurs. Res. **44**(6), 554–558 (2011). (in Japanese)
7. Yokoyama, M. Sakyo, Y.: Practice of Physical Assessment Skills by Nurses.: Comparing the Frequency of Physical Examination Skills Performed by Nurses Who Took the Physical Assessment Course and Who did not Take That Course. Bulletin of St. Luke's College of Nursing, vol. 33, pp. 1–16 (2007). (in Japanese)
8. Ministry of Health, Labour and Welfare.: Curriculum guidelines for the operation of the nursing school (2012). (in Japanese)
9. Shinozaki, E., Yamauchi, T.: The physical assessment education in basic nursing education from nursing college survey 2005. Japan. J. Nurs. Educ. **47**(9), 810–813 (2006). (in Japanese)

The Digital Reminiscence Method: Effect on Dementia in Japanese Day Care Centers

Masayuki Nakamura[1], Takashi Yoshikawa[1(✉)], Kayo Tanaka[2], Mengyuan Liao[3], and Noriaki Kuwahara[3]

[1] National Institute of Technology, Niihama College, Niihama, Japan
nakamu1993@gmail.com, yosikawa@mec.niihama-nct.ac.jp
[2] Wagaya of the Dementia-Only Day Care Center, Niihama, Japan
k-tanaka@asokaen.jp
[3] Kyoto Institute of Technology, Kyoto, Japan
ada-guilin@live.com, nkuwahar@kit.ac.jp

Abstract. When considering working with dementia patients in communities or welfare facilities, manpower problems and the existing caregiver's support system must be considered. It is a modern reality that many facilities often struggle while coping with dementia patients. However, as recent studies have reported, depending on the way dementia patients are cared for, it is possible to suppress problematic behavior such as violence, screeching, and/or wandering.

In order to assist dementia patients while using the "digital reminiscence" method, students, facility staff members, dementia patients and their families worked together in this study.

Keywords: Effects on one's lifestyle · Movie production · Good staff coordination · Families and students

1 Introduction

Current, low birthrate and longevity is in progress in Japan. With it, we are faced with a variety of problems in the field of the social welfare and social security. A problem about dementia has taken up as one of the pressing issue as a national problem. Actually, when considering working with dementia patients in communities or welfare facilities, manpower problems and the existing caregiver's support system must be considered. And, comprehensions and concerns that youths hold are not enough in this current situation. As the result, these problems have led to a reduction in population of caregiver in Japan.

So, in order to assist dementia patients while using the "digital reminiscence" method, we, facility caregivers, dementia patients and their families worked together in this study using ability of students.

The changes of the users' state and consciousness of caregivers and students were focused in this research. In addition, we aim to discuss the concept of movies that elicit a more effective response from dementia patients and report the results in the future.

© Springer International Publishing Switzerland 2015
V.G. Duffy (Ed.): DHM 2015, Part II, LNCS 9185, pp. 482–489, 2015.
DOI: 10.1007/978-3-319-21070-4_49

The day service, it is one of the care services in Japan. This kind of service is targeted to improve or recover the mental and physical functions of the users. Facilities supply this kind of service and only take care of the users in the daytime. After that, the facilities conduct exercises and recreations to recover and inhibit declines of requisite functions for the users live a daily life by themselves. Merits of this service are not only a recovery of the mental and physical functions of the users, but also a reduction of the mental and physical load of families who take care of them every day. In this paper, an experiment using the digital reminiscence method was conducted in a small facility which is supplying the day service for dementia patients.

2 Experiment Method

2.1 Digital Reminiscence Method

The "reminiscence method" proposed by Robert Butler is a kind of psychotherapy [1]. This method uses conversation to retrieve memories from events in an elderly patient's past. It is said that makes their brains accelerate revitalization or emotional stability and prevent dementia or delay progression of dementia.

However, it is a load for caregivers to converse to dementia users with one to one than other assistances. So, we convert memories pictures to digital data and edit them to as a movie. As this result, we consider we can obtain effect as same as reminiscence method without assistances with one to one.

We use slideshows of memories pictures and add user's favorite music and comments about each picture into them. We term what user enjoys these slideshows "digital reminiscence method".

2.2 Movie Production for Digital Reminiscence Method

Nine subjects with dementia with the age from 74 up to 102 years old. They who were cooperated as test subjects in this study were 3 males with average age: 83.7 years old and 6 females with average age: 94.7 years old. Two criterions were followed when we choose the subjects: (1) Subjects can speak with oral excepting nutation. (2) Subjects' families agree and cooperate on this study.

Five stages were needed during movie production. (1) Since the subjects had dementia, we explained the purpose of this study to their families and obtained their consent to use their photos in our films. (2) The dementia patients and their families, facility caregiver staff members, and engineering students then gathered together to exchange impressions and discuss the potential photos, then created comments for the images. (3) We digitized the photos that elicited responses from the patients, then organized them in the chronological order and included the comments. In an attempt to use complete comments, not only the dates and locations were listed, but words expressing the patients' feelings when viewing the images. (4) We prepared memorable music for the subjects, combining them with the images and comments to produce completed films. (5) Finally, the films were transferred to DVDs which could be viewed anytime at home or in care facilities.

On the other hand, we selected twenty-eight students participated in movie production (with the age from 16 to 20 years old) with various backgrounds; some had never been in contact with elderly people, while some had lived with grandparents who had dementia. The students formed eight groups (four people per one group). In addition, they attend a lecture about dementia and visit day care center as a part of movie production.

2.3 Assessment Method for Verification

We assessed subjects' actions in daily life using GBS scale quantitatively [2]. All subjects watched each movie every day for four weeks and we assessed their actions before they have watched the movie for the first time and at intervals of seven days after first assessment. In addition, we also assessed changes of their actions by descriptive form excepting GBS scale.

GBS scale is a quantitative method which assesses about four fields: physical functions, intelligent functions, emotion functions and other symptoms. It is composed by twenty-six questions in the total. But, we assess only six items in emotion functions and other symptoms: "dullness", "instability of emotion", "shortage of motivation", "anxiety", "depressed mood" and "restlessness" [3]. That is because we consider that physical functions and intelligent functions of subjects are difficult functions to improve.

3 Result

3.1 Change of Users' States

No specific improvement was observed in the GBS scale evaluation results. The reason is because we couldn't confirm improvements assessed by GBS scale from each subject in general daily life.

Assessments by descriptive form indicated some change of subjects in a part of daily life. First, all subjects smiled during watching each movie. Figure 1 shows a change of subject's expression. And, even if subjects watch other subject's movie, some subject was impressed with it. Therefore, it's effective for dementia patients to enjoy pictures and music in old days they were young even if they watch pictures which have no relation to them.

Furthermore, subjects could talk with other users and do some daily actions which they can't do well smoothly by repeating the number of times of the enjoying of the movie. Namely, digital reminiscence method makes dementia symptoms of subjects recover in a part of daily life. In this manner, we couldn't confirm quantitative assessments of digital reminiscence method by GBS scale. But, we could confirm many improvement effects as valuable as GBS scale. However, contents and features of improvement effect were different by each subject.

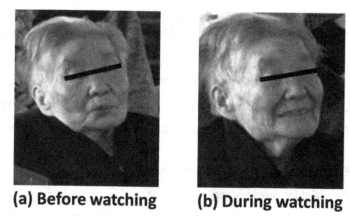

(a) Before watching   (b) During watching

Fig. 1. change of subject's expression

3.2 Change in the Consciousness of Caregiver Staffs and Students

The facility caregiver staff members answered about effect of digital reminiscence method, such as, "I can know about user's personal anew" and "I can see the users from a different angle in the context of care". Namely, staffs can understand and receive users' some actions because caregivers know about user's past. We consider that it's very important for facility staffs to understand users deeply because the quality of care improves.

Table 1 and Fig. 2 shows details of questionnaire about elderly facilities and change in the percentage of students' images about elderly facilities. Before they attend a lecture about dementia and visit day care center, 20 % of all students hold images, such as, "elderly facilities are places which users and caregiver staffs spend vividly and cheerfully". On the other hand, 20 % of all students also hold images, such as, "elderly facilities are places which users with a disability and sick spend" and "elderly facilities are gloomy and lonely facilities". And, 65 % of all students also hold images, such as, "care of elder people is very serious job". But, after they attend a lecture and visit, nobody hold the image. In addition, about 80 % of all students hold images, such as, "elderly facilities are places which users and caregiver staffs spend vividly and cheerfully".

Table 2 and Fig. 3 shows details of questionnaire about dementia and change in the percentage of students' images about dementia. Before they attend a lecture, 15 % of all students hold dementia images, such as, "dementia patients can't understand anything" and "to communicate with dementia patients is fearful". In addition, 35 % of all students hold images, such as, "dementia patients do strange and untoward actions", and 60 % of all students hold images, such as, "care of dementia patients is very serious job". On the other hand, about 20 % of all students hold images, such as, "if they be supported by suitable care, dementia patient can keep dignity and live" and "even if human fall dementia, he can find a new way to live". And, 10 % of all students hold images, such as, "dementia patients have liveliness and live very hard". But, nobody hold a variety of negative images about dementia. In addition, 50 % and over of all students hold images, such as, "if they be supported by suitable care, dementia patient can keep dignity and live".

Table 1. Details of questionnaire about elderly facilities

Q1	Elderly facilities are places which users with a disability and sick spend
Q2	Elderly facilities are places which elder people spend quietly as last where-abouts
Q3	Elderly facilities are gloomy and lonely places
Q4	Care of elder people is very serious job
Q5	Elderly facilities are places which users and caregiver staffs spend vividly and cheerfully
Q6	Elderly facilities are cheerful places

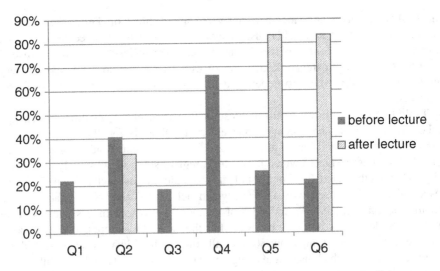

Fig. 2. Change in the percentage of students' images about elderly facilities

As the result, the number of student holds positive images about dementia and elder facilities increased through lecture as a part of movie production and communication with dementia users really. Care by youths is important in current Japanese society. Therefore, it's very important for Japanese youths to learn right knowledge about dementia and elder facilities. We consider that to concern students with movie production for digital reminiscence method is a suitable opportunity to learn them.

Table 2. Details of questionnaire about dementia

Q1	I can't imagine anything about dementia
Q2	Dementia patients can't understand anything
Q3	Care of dementia patients is very serious job
Q4	Dementia patients do strange and untoward actions
Q5	To communicate with dementia patients is fearful
Q6	If they be supported by suitable care, dementia patient can keep dignity and live.
Q7	Even if human fall dementia, he can find a new way to live
Q8	Dementia patients have liveliness and live very hard

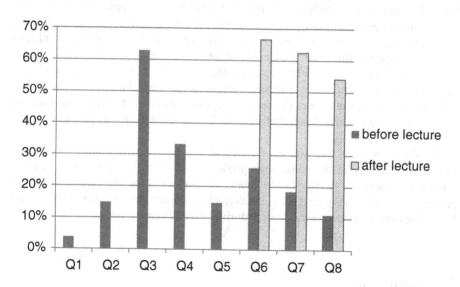

Fig. 3. Change in the percentage of students' images about dementia

4 Consideration

In previous discussion, some effect of dementia symptoms improvement was found, however it is pity that no results or influence was showed by check expression evaluation table.

Referring to GBS scale evaluation, it was said that check scheme was to be carried out in limited time. Furthermore, it was difficult to decide how many items should be focused, in other words, how to investigate elder subjects' daily life/activity, how to apply the monitor method individually and choose the proper/effective measures are very puzzling problems.

Namely, there is urgent desire should be considered, such as change the items individually to evaluate what you want as an effect of digital reminiscence method. However, it is very important to establish as a thesis, especially to clarify such effects. In reality, it is very meaningful to increase everyone's smile (including caregiver staffs), improve parts of dementia elder's life through applying digital reminiscence method. That is because, for both caregiver staffs and elder patient they have a win-win relationship, so in this direction it is able to aspire and achieve a better improvement in an aging society.

What's more, digital reminiscence's significant effect not only displayed during the movie watching period, but also showed a striking influence on caregiver staff's daily care activity. However, as the improvements, DVD method was lack of sustainability because of its indirect effects (for predetermined subjects' condition able to communicate).

In order to solve the problem of indirect effect, this research put more emphasis on the background music. Music has the magic effect of bringing people back into the past time memories and emotions, even after repeated viewing as well as person's favorite song is nostalgic memories of self-awareness and very good. Therefore, follow and align the music to specific time, match with photo content and story, such kind of music (slow tempo and up-tempo) could help to recovery the memories of the past. Moreover, alternative effect is also expected by listening to music for dementia elder without caregiver's daily support and mental care. Consequently, it is consider that users' strong mental fatigue of "uneasy feeling" suffered from daily life could be effectively release and eliminate.

On the other hand, four weeks daily repeat watching movie in multiple facilities showed a good basic of the future movie production. In a near future, movie production service will not only face to all elder users but also record the daily life/activity care process between caregiver and elder. Finally, it is considered to help everybody operate better lives and eliminate users' anxiety during dementia care process.

5   Conclusion

In this paper, digital reminiscence method was applied to investigate DVD movie effect on dementia lived in Japanese Day Care Centers. It could demonstrate the conclusions as following 5 key points;

1. Combining with past photos, background music and words, DVD movie could able to make everybody lived in center smile;
2. Corresponding to caregiver's uneasy feeling accumulated in previous dementia care process, DVD movie can recovery dementia elder's past memory, active their activity and finally staff's reduce anxiety;
3. As a side-effect, through photos showing, the relationship between caregiver staff and elder's family members become more familiar with each other deeply;

4. Continuing release of DVD movie in nursing facilities, a circle of communication among elder users was established and spread out;
5. Referring to students who make the DVD movie, they obtain some new value theory for elder nursing industry.

References

1. Butler, R.N.: The life review: an interpretation of reminiscence in the aged. Psychiatry **26**(1), 65–76 (1963)
2. Gottfries, C.G., Brane, G., Gullberg, B., et al.: A new rating scale for dementia syndromes. Arch Gerontol Geriatr **1**, 311 (1982)
3. Doi, T., Ikenobo, Y., Kuwahara, N.: The report on the utilization and effectiveness verification of the elderly care of traditional Japanese culture. In: 2013 fiscal Ergonomics Society Kansai Branch Conference Abstracts, pp. 89–92 (2013)

Verbal and Nonverbal Skills in Open Communication: Comparing Experienced and Inexperienced Radio Duos

Noriko Suzuki[1]([✉]), Yu Oshima[2], Haruka Shoda[2,3], Mamiko Sakata[2], and Noriko Ito[2]

[1] Faculty of Business Administration, Tezukayama University,
7-7-1 Tezukayama, Nara 631-8501, Japan
nsuzuki@tezukayama-u.ac.jp
[2] Department of Culture and Information Science, Doshisha University,
1-3 Tatara Miyakodani, Kyotanabe, Kyoto 610-0394, Japan
[3] Japan Society for the Promotion of Science, 5-3-1 Kojimatchi,
Chiyoda-ku, Tokyo 102-0083, Japan

Abstract. This paper examines how the difference in talk skill for open communication affects the orientation of the verbal and nonverbal behaviors of the talk partner or audience. An experiment was carried out using multiple radio duos having different levels of talk skill, i.e., experienced and inexperienced. The experiment's task was conducted in a pseudo-radio setting under three conditions: audience-present talk, audience-absent talk, and audience-absent/post-talk sessions. The speech and body gestures of all participants were video-recorded and analyzed. The results suggest that the different levels of experience in radio talk are expressed in different speech and gesture orientations. These findings seem applicable to the speech- and gesture-expression model for conversational robots, especially for nursing-care robots designed to talk with other robots or cohabitants.

Keywords: Open communication · Radio talk skill · Orientation of verbal and nonverbal behaviors · Experienced and inexperienced radio duos

1 Introduction

The development of domestic robots has progressed rapidly in recent years, targeting the needs of the coming aging society with fewer children. We will live at home with multiple robots for different purposes, i.e., nursing care, home care, and training, just like the movie droids "C-3PO and R2D2" in "Star wars" or the robotic boy "David" in "Artificial Intelligence: AI." What would you think about such robots interacting silently with each other via a network right in front of you? The response of many people might be a feeling of alienation or anxiety. To solve this perception problem, domestic robots should have a model

© Springer International Publishing Switzerland 2015
V.G. Duffy (Ed.): DHM 2015, Part II, LNCS 9185, pp. 490–499, 2015.
DOI: 10.1007/978-3-319-21070-4_50

of expressing explicit verbal and nonverbal behaviors to put users at ease [4]. The authors give attention to the mechanism of open communication as a key for expressing participant-oriented behaviors [2].

Open communication is a type of performer-to-audience communication in which the audience perceives indirect messages from direct conversation among performers [7]. Cooking shows and domestic comedies on TV program are typical examples of open communication. In particular, the authors focus on radio-duo shows as a distinct form of open communication. A radio-duo show is usually not watched directly by the audience. Nevertheless, the audience can perceive indirect messages from the conversation between the partners of a radio duo without any visual information. In other words, the radio duo can communicate to an invisible audience, although the duo partners seem to neglect the presence of the audience while talking to each other. The skill of radio talk in open communication might be a useful analog for increasing the ability of domestic robots to express participant-directed behaviors.

The authors conducted an experiment to explore radio talk skills by comparing experienced with inexperienced radio duos. A pseudo-radio session was selected as the task. Seven experienced and seven inexperienced radio duos took part in the experiment. In this paper, the partners in an experienced radio duo have at least one year of on-the-job experience on a university's radio show. The partners in an inexperienced radio duo have no experience in talking to each other on any radio show, although they may be acquaintances.

Conventional studies in multiparty interaction have shown that the presence or the absence of an audience affects the amount of speech or the speech orientation of the performer in a comic duo [9]. On the other hand, related works in gesture have shown that representational or beat gesture was produced more frequently in a face-to-face setting than in a separated setting [1,6]. However, few research works have taken into account the relationship between the difference in talk experience with an audience and the orientation of verbal and nonverbal behaviors.

A within-participants experimental design was used in three situations: audience-present talk, audience-absent talk, and audience-absent/post-talk sessions. Audience-absent/post-talk session was defined as closed communication, although both audience-present talk and audience-absent talk sessions are defined as open communication. The turn duration, speech intervals, frequency of back channels, duration of representational and beat gestures for each participant, and overlaps and gaps between the partners of the radio duo were annotated. The authors performed a two-way analysis of variance to examine the effects of skill (i.e., experienced versus inexperienced) and session (i.e., audience-present, audience-absent, post-talk) and to conduct a correlation analysis between a post-experiment questionnaire on attention given to the audience and the verbal/nonverbal behaviors of the performers.

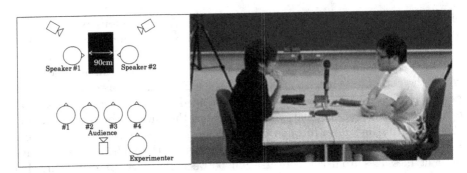

Fig. 1. Experimental setting: recording setup in audience-present talk session (left) and sample scene (right)

2   Method

2.1   Participants

A total of 28 graduate and undergraduate students (Mean age: 19.6 years, SD: 1.2) participated in the experiment, and they were assigned to either an "experienced radio duo" (n = 14, 7 pairs) or an "inexperienced radio duo" (n = 14, 7 pairs). In this paper, an experienced radio duo means that each partner has at least one year of on-the-job experience on a university radio show. The inexperienced radio duo means that the partners have no experience in talking to each other on any radio show, although they may be acquaintances.

2.2   Procedure

Each radio duo was instructed to sit down and face each other across the desk (Fig. 1). They participated in the pseudo-radio sessions: audience-present talk for 10 min, audience-absent talk for 10 min, and audience-absent/post-talk sessions for 10 min. In audience-present talk session, radio duo talked each other to four numbers of audience in front of the radio duo. It was a kind of open communication. In audience-absent talk session, radio duo talked each other to audience without physically being. They were instructed that audience listened their talk in a separate room. It was also a kind of open communication. Here, "post-talk" refers to a brief discussion after the simulated radio show in which the duo's partners evaluated their performance. It was a kind of closed communication as against open communication. The first two talk sessions were counter-balanced. All radio duos in both talk sessions discussed the same topic, i.e., the item they would take to a deserted island. We video-taped the upper body of each participant with three video cameras (HDR-XR550V, Sony) and four wireless microphones (ECM-AW3T, Sony). After three sessions, participants answered a questionnaire on such items as attention to the audience.

2.3   Parameters

For 3 min within the 10-min recording of each radio duo, we extracted verbal and nonverbal behaviors by using the annotation software ELAN (EUDICO Linguistic Annotator [3]). We measured the duration of each of the conversations and the gestures made according to the following criteria.

Turn Duration Per Minute (in sec.): We measured the turn duration per minute through a talk session. The turn duration means the length of speech turn while a partner talks until the other partner begins to talk. Back channels are not included in a speech turn.

Speech Interval Per Minute (in sec.): We measured the speech interval per minute between two participants through a talk session. The speech interval includes both response latency and speech overlap.

Frequency of Back Channels Per Speech: We measured the number of back channels per speech. The back channels are utterances such as "Yeah" or "Umm".

Frequency of Representational Gesture Per Speech: We extracted the number of each participant's representational gestures that express semantic content related to the speech by virtue of the hands' shape, placement, or motion (e.g., [8]).

Frequency of Beat Gesture Per Speech: We extracted the number of each participant's beat gestures that express simple, rhythmic gestures that do not convey semantic content (e.g., [5]).

2.4   Predictions

Verbal Behaviors: We predict that the difference in radio talk experience will affect the verbal behaviors of the radio duos as well as the presence of audience does (e.g., [9]).

Nonverbal Behaviors: We predict that the difference in radio talk experience will also affect the nonverbal behaviors of the radio duos as well as the presence of audience does (e.g., [1,6]).

3   Results

3.1   Verbal Behaviors

The authors performed two-way analysis of variance to examine the effects of skill (i.e., experienced versus inexperienced) and session (i.e., audience-present, audience-absent, post-talk).

For the turn duration, the main effect of skill and that of session were not significant, but the two-way interaction was significant: $F(1, 26) = 3.91, p = .04, \eta_p^2 = .13$ (skill $\times$ session) (Fig. 2). A post-hoc t-test with Bonferroni's correction showed that an inexperienced radio duo expressed longer turn duration per minute in the audience-present session than in the audience-absent session

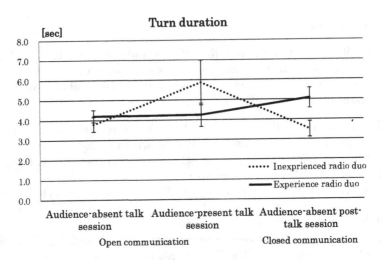

Fig. 2. Results of turn duration per minute

$(p = 0.09, d = 0.83)$, and in the audience-present session than in the audience-absent/post-talk session $(p = 0.07, d = 0.90)$.

For the speech interval, the two-way interaction was not significant, but the main effect of skill and that of session were significant: $F(1, 26) = 6.74, p = .02, \eta_p^2 = .21$ (skill) and $F(1, 26) = 41.40, p < .001, \eta_p^2 = .61$ (session) (Fig. 3). A post-hoc t-test with Bonferroni's correction showed that both inexperienced and experienced radio duos expressed a longer speech interval per minute in the audience-present session than in the audience-absent session $(p = 0.09, d = 0.82)$ and in the audience-absent/post-talk session than in the audience-present session $(p < 0.01, d = 2.51)$.

For the frequency of back channel, the main effect of skill and the two-way interaction were not significant, but the main effect of session was significant: $F(1, 26) = 9.09, p < .001, \eta_p^2 = .26$ (Fig. 4). A post-hoc t-test with Bonferroni's correction showed that both inexperienced and experienced radio duos expressed a larger number of back channels per speech in the audience-absent session than in the audience-absent/post-session $(p = 0.02, d = 1.08)$ and in the audience-present talk session than in the audience-absent/post-session $(p = 0.04, d = 1.24)$.

3.2 Nonverbal Behaviors

The authors performed two-way analysis of variance to examine the effects of skill (i.e., experienced versus inexperienced) and session (i.e., audience-present, audience-absent, post-talk).

For the frequency of beat gesture, the main effects of session and two-way interaction were significant: $F(1, 26) = 6.22, p = .007, \eta_p^2 = .19$ (session), and $F(1, 26) = 6.13, p = .004, \eta_p^2 = .19$ (skill $times$ session), respectively (Fig. 5).

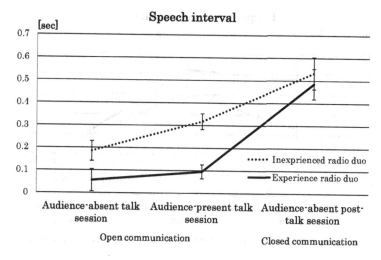

Fig. 3. Results of speech interval between radio duo partners per minute

In the results of the simple main effect, there was a significant difference in experienced radio duos through three sessions ($p = 0.03, d = 0.38$). A post-hoc t-test with Bonferroni's correction showed that experienced radio duos expressed longer frequency of beat gesture per speech in the audience-absent session than in the audience-absent/post-talk session ($p = 0.05, d = 1.16$) and in the audience-present talk session than in the audience-absent/post-talk session ($p = 0.02, d = 1.37$).

For the frequency of representational gesture, the main effect of skill was not significant but that of session and the two-way interaction did show a significant tendency: $F(1, 26) = 2.81, p = .07, \eta_p^2 = .10$ (session), and $F(1, 26) = 2.83, p = .06, \eta_p^2 = .10$ (skill $times$ session) (Fig. 6).

In the result of the simple main effect, there was a significant difference of experienced radio duo through three sessions ($p = 0.03, d = 0.24$). A post-hoc t-test with Bonferroni's correction showed that experienced radio duos expressed longer frequency of representational gesture per speech in the audience-absent session than in the audience-absent/post-talk session ($p = 0.03, d = 0.96$) and in the audience-present/post-talk session than in the audience-absent/post-talk session ($p = 0.08, d = 0.87$).

3.3   Post-experiment Questionnaire

Figure 7 shows the results of a post-experiment questionnaire on the attention of the performer to the audience.

The authors performed two-way analysis of variance to examine the effects of skill (i.e., experienced versus inexperienced) and session (i.e., audience-present, audience-absent).

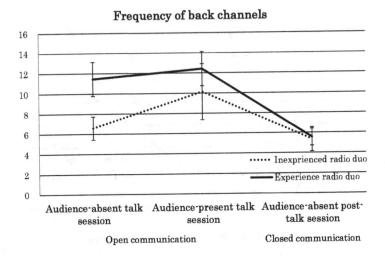

Frequency of back channels

Fig. 4. Results of frequency of back channels per speech

For the frequency of beat gesture, the main effect of session was significant: $F(1, 26) = 5.93, p = .02, \eta_p^2 = .16$). This result suggested that the partners in both experienced and inexperienced radio duos talked to each other while paying more attention to the audience in the audience-present talk session than in the audience-absent talk session.

3.4 Correlation Between Verbal/Nonverbal Behaviors and Attention to the Audience

The correlation analysis between the post-experiment questionnaire and verbal and nonverbal behaviors showed that there were both a negative correlation between the attention to the audience and the turn duration (r = −0.728, p < .01) and a positive correlation between the attention and the frequency of back channel (r = .560, p < .05) in the audience-absent session in inexperienced radio duos (Table 1). In other words, the more attentive the radio duo was, the shorter the turn duration in an inexperienced radio duo was, or the larger the back channel was.

On the other hand, there was a negative correlation between attention and the frequency of beat gesture (r = −0.659, p < .05) in the audience-present session in experienced radio duos. In other words, the more attentive the radio duo was in experienced radio duos, the smaller the frequency of beat gesture was.

4   Discussion

In the present study, we found differences in verbal and nonverbal behaviors between experienced and inexperienced radio-duo talk through three kinds of

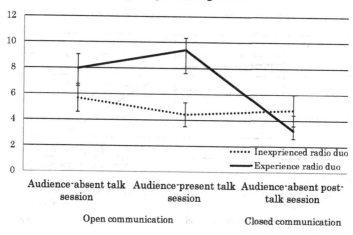

Fig. 5. Results of frequency of beat gesture

Table 1. Correlation between attention to the audience and verbal/nonverbal behaviors

	Attention to the audience			
	Experienced radio duo		Inexperienced radio duo	
	Audience-absent session	Audience-present session	Audience-absent session	Audience-present session
Turn duration	−.075	−.497	−.728 **	−.065
Speech interval	.109	−.028	−.318	.372
Back channel	.301	.140	.560*	.243
BG	−.253	−.659*	.234	.133
RG	.031	.029	−.079	.287

BG: Beat gesture, RG: Representational gesture
*: $p < 0.05$, **: $p < 0.01$.

sessions, i.e., audience-present, audience-absent as open communication and post-talk as closed communication, in terms of "turn duration," "speech interval," "frequency of back channel," "frequency of beat gesture," and "frequency of representational gesture." We also found correlations between the attention to the audience and the radio duo's behaviors.

In their verbal behavior, experienced radio duos did not change so much in turn duration. Inexperienced radio duos used a longer turn duration in the audience-present talk session than in the audience-absent sessions. On the other hand, both radio duos seemed to show the similar tendency on the speech interval or the frequency of back channels. Although the amount of speech with the audience present increased more than that without an audience in the case of

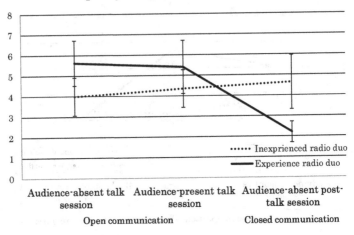

Fig. 6. Results of frequency of representational gesture

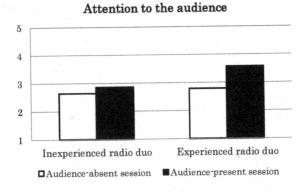

Fig. 7. Results of post questionnaire: attention to the audience

comic duos [9], our results suggested that the communication style, open or closed, affected the verbal behaviors. The difference in radio talk skill seemed not to affect the verbal behaviors so much except the speech interval. From the results of the correlation with attention to the audience, the turn duration has a negative correlation while the back channel has a positive correlation in inexperienced radio duos in the audience-absent session. The turn duration and the number of back channel might have a potential of participant-directed behaviors in inexperienced radio duos.

In the nonverbal behavior, inexperienced radio duos did not change so much their frequency of either beat or representational gestures. Experienced radio duos used a larger number of both beat and representational gestures in audience-absent and audience-present sessions than in the post-talk session. Although the presence of audience affects the frequency of both beat and representational gestures in the conventional studies in gesture production [1,6], our results suggest that both the communication style, open or closed, and the difference in radio talk skill seemed to affect the frequency of gesture production. From the results of the correlation with attention to the audience, the frequency of beat gestures has a negative correlation in experienced radio duos in the audience-present session. The frequency of beat gesture might have a potential of addressee-directed behaviors in experienced radio duos.

In conclusion, different levels of radio talk skills show different type of nonverbal expressions. The open commutation style also affects the radio duo's speech and gesture production. Besides, it might be possible that the verbal behaviors indicate participant-directed acts, although the nonverbal behaviors indicate addressee-directed acts. In our future work, we will search for explicit speech and gesture orientation by analyzing more detailed aspects of the verbal and nonverbal behaviors of radio duos based on Clark and Carlson, 1982 [2]. These results may lead to several implications for constructing a narrative-strategy model for communication robots that can alleviate the sense of alienation felt by the users.

Acknowledgment. The contents of this study are based on the second author's master thesis. We thank 28 students at Doshisha University for their participation in the experiment. We also thank Haru Nitta, Kana Shirai, Koshi Nishimoto, and Tomoki Yao for their fruitful discussions on this study.

References

1. Alibali, M.W., Heath, D.C., Myers, H.J.: Effects of visibility between speaker and listener on gesture production: some gestures are meant to be seen. J. Mem. Lang. **44**, 169–188 (2001)
2. Clark, H.H., Carlson, T.B.: Hearers and speech acts. Language **58**(2), 332–373 (1982)
3. ELAN. https://tla.mpi.nl/tools/tla-tools/elan/
4. Matsuyama, Y., Taniyama, H., Fujie, S. and Kobayashi, T.: Framework of communication activation robot participating in multiparty conversation. In: Proceedings of AAAI Fall Symposium, Dialog with Robots, pp. 68–73 (2010)
5. McNeill, D.: Hand and Mind: What Gestures Reveal about Thought. University of Chicago Press, Chicago (1992)
6. Mol, L., Krahmer, E., Maes, A., Swerts, M.: Seeing and being seen: the effects on gesture production. J. Comput.-Mediated Commun. **17**(1), 77–100 (2011)
7. Ohba, M., Okamoto, M., Enomoto, M., Iida, H.: Tittering and laughing: a case of manzai audience. In: Proceedings of LIBM 2008: First International Workshop on Laughter in Interaction and Body Movement, pp. 34–39 (2008)
8. Ozyurek, A.: The influence of addressee location on spatial language and representational gestures of direction. In: McNeill, D. (ed.) Language and Gesture: Window into Thought and Action, p. 6483. Cambridge University Press, Cambridge (2000)
9. Sakata, M., Tanno, M.: Multimodal interactions in duo-comic acts manzai. In: Proceedings of the 8th International Conference on Humanized Systems 2012 (ICHS 2012), pp. 63–66 (2012)

The Transfer of Expertise in Conducting a Participatory Music Therapy During a Combined Rehabilitation-Recreational Program in an Elderly Care Facility

Akiyoshi Yamamoto[1], Henry Cereno Barrameda Jr.[1(✉)],
Tatsunori Azuma[1], Hideaki Kasasaku[1], Kayoko Hirota[1],
Momo Jinno[1], Maki Sumiyama[1], Tomoko Ota[4], Akihiko Goto[3],
Noriyuki Kida[2], Noriaki Kuwahara[2], and Hiroyuki Hamada[2]

[1] Super Court Co. Ltd, Osaka, Japan
{yamamoto,henrybarramedajr,azuma,
kyo-shijyuoomiya}@supercourt.co.jp,
jiayuzi-5963@ezweb.ne.jp, zimal031@gmail.com
[2] Kyoto Institute of Technology, Kyoto, Japan
{kida,hhamada}@kit.ac.jp, organ0412@gmail.com
[3] Osaka Sangyo University, Osaka, Japan
gotoh@ise.osaka-sandai.ac.jp
[4] Chuo Business Group, Osaka, Japan
tomoko.ota@k.vodafone.ne.jp

Abstract. Not so long ago, in Japan, much emphasis were given to elderly`s basic life`s needs like eating, sleeping, excretion and bathing, however support for other problems of aging like mental and emotional health, muscle tone weakness, and life satisfaction are much left out. Just until recently, new concepts like QOL (Quality of Life) were seriously considered. This signaled the start of not just focusing on giving support on the material needs but also giving equal importance on issues pertaining to mental and emotional health, as well as life satisfaction of the residents in the elderly care facility. Recreation for improvement of mind and body functions of residents, as well as improvement of daily quality of life are now being carried out. Jurisprudence, administrative measures on recreational activities were also created. It has since been a standard for the elderly welfare care facilities of to provide recreational events appropriate to the number of residents. Different kinds of rehabilitation and recreational activities were introduced, one of them is Music Therapy. Activation of the brain, strengthening of the muscles for swallowing, and emotional and mental stability are just few of the most common beneficial effects of the said therapy. In this study, the setting for the music therapy is a paid elderly care facility.

Keywords: Caregiver · Paid elderly facility · Recreation · Participatory music therapy

© Springer International Publishing Switzerland 2015
V.G. Duffy (Ed.): DHM 2015, Part II, LNCS 9185, pp. 500–511, 2015.
DOI: 10.1007/978-3-319-21070-4_51

1 Research Background

1.1 Introduction

In Japan, music therapy has been introduced not so long ago as a new recreational and rehabilitation therapy. Activation of the brain, strengthening of the muscles for swallowing, and emotional and mental stability are just few of the most common beneficial effects improving the mind and body functions. It as well aim to improve of daily quality of life among the recipients. It has since been a standard for the elderly welfare care facilities of to provide recreational events, and recreation has also been the main in the life support provided by Day Service Institutions.

In a study, (Brotons, et al. 1997) stated that Music therapy is an effective intervention for decreasing behavioral problems of individuals with dementias and for maintaining and improving active involvement, social, emotional and cognitive skills.

The setting of our study is a paid nursing home facility in Japan. Providing music therapy in the said facility has yield positive results, and we have felt the need to expansion of the program to our other facility so that other residents could have access to music therapy. However, offering sustainable service has always been a challenge to currently the short-staffed and notoriously high turn-over rate caregiver work in Japan (Yamamoto 2015). So, in order to cope up and meet the increasing demand for the provision of higher quality nursing service to the residents in the elderly facilities, we believe that researches on transfer of certain nursing skills is indispensable. Many research works are being carried out to improve nursing services, however, studies related to sustainability of operation like research on skills transfer are not given much emphasis. In fact, our query on any research pertaining to transfer of expertise and skills in the nursing field in Japan yield us very limited result. In this particular experiment, we studied how to be able to transfer skills effectively by careful analysis of the technique used while performing.

We begin by analyzing the common techniques employed by expert performer, as characterized by her use of time, decisions and actions while performing a participatory music therapy in a paid nursing facility. We then present some background on music therapy and related work in the field of skills transfer, followed by the description and discussion of our research.

Our study shows that positive development can be achieved if the performance is well-arranged. This study also implies that the point of solving ingeniously while performing is the foundation that results to good performance. Finally, we believe that result of this study can be useful in producing the training video we wish to create. In the discussion section we present the analysis of the results and implications for future improvements.

1.2 Research Trends and Significance of the Study

Music therapy is an effective intervention for decreasing behavioral problems of individuals with dementias and for maintaining and improving active involvement, social, emotional and cognitive skills (Brotons, et al. 1997).

In Japan, in the paper, Effects of Music Therapy for Dementia: A systematic review (Watanabe 2005) suggested that after reviewing researches published within the past 20 years, they have found out that along with the findings of Koger, music therapy is an effective intervention for dementia.

In a separate study, Kuwahara (2001) stated that music has physiological and mental effects on human being. Their work that was conducted in a long term-care health facility, found significance on the activities, whether it is a music therapy or music recreational activity.

However, along with Japan's rapid aging society, experts on different fields are also growing old, remarkably low birth rate poses another challenge in transfer of these expertise to young generations later. Problems in skills transfer is not just being a business entity issue but becoming a Japan national issue as well (Gijutsu·Ginou Denshou no tame no Ginou Bunseki to Manyuaru Kousei no Houhou, Mori 2001).

This study will be a significant endeavor in the transfer of expertise in music therapy. Not only the expert and successor performers would benefit when they employ the learning from the training tool for transfer of expertise that will be created from this study, but if we are able to create more successor performers, it is the end-user of music therapy, who are residents in the paid nursing facility suffering from dementia would greatly benefit from this study. By understanding the important points to consider in order to be able to deliver an effective music therapy, smooth transfer of skills from expert and successor will be assured.

2 Design

2.1 Grounded Theory Methodology

Grounded theory method is a systematic generation of theory from data that contains both inductive and deductive thinking. One goal is to formulate hypotheses based on conceptual ideas. Generally speaking, grounded theory is an approach for looking systematically at (mostly) qualitative data (like transcripts of interviews or protocols of observations) aiming at the generation of theory. Sometimes, grounded theory is seen as a qualitative method, but grounded theory reaches farther: it combines a specific style of research (or a paradigm) with pragmatic theory of action and with some methodological guidelines.

Grounded theory method does not aim for the "truth" but to conceptualize what is going on by using empirical research. In a way, grounded theory method resembles what many researchers do when retrospectively formulating new hypotheses to fit data. However, when applying the grounded theory method, the researcher does not formulate the hypotheses in advance since preconceived hypotheses result in a theory that is ungrounded from the data (Glaser and Strauss 1967).

If the researcher's goal is accurate description, then another method should be chosen since grounded theory is not a descriptive method. Instead it has the goal of generating concepts that explain the way that people resolve their central concerns regardless of time and place. The use of description in a theory generated by the grounded theory method is mainly to illustrate concepts (Wikipedia 2015).

2.2   Subjects and Location of Study

In this study, there were two subjects: An expert music performer, (Female, 54 years old, with a total of 49 years of piano recital experience, 6 years of which is music therapy related, with averaging 2 performances a month) and a successor, (Female, 25 years old, with 19 years piano recital experience. Both subjects were working in the elderly nursing facility. The expert is a care manager with a total of 13 and half years of experience in the field of caregiving, and the successor is a caregiver with 1 year and 10 months experience in caregiving field. See Table 1.

Table 1. Data of the subjects

Subject	Age	No. of times performed music therapy	No. of years of years performing piano recital	No. of years of experience in caring for elderly suffering with dementia
Expert	54	72	49	13.5
Successor	24	2	20	1.8

The setting of our study is a paid nursing home facility in Japan. The facility houses 73 residents, with about 80 percent of them affected by dementia or having dementia symptoms. We have created the music therapy program to address dementia as well as to prevent it's onset on the residents.

2.3   Objective of Analysis

Our objective is to formulate hypotheses based on conceptual ideas presented by the expert performer. This study sought to analyze performance process and map core skill requirements, in order to create manuals for transfer of expertise in music therapy, employing the process analysis sheet format for SAT (Skills Analysis for Training) that was revised by Mori in 2000. Two types of manual will be created. (1) Text type manual in tutorial style for the general description of the performance process and (2) A video manual for the critical highlight parts of the performance process which needs to be carefully analyzed and explained by a fraction of a second. By using both text and video manual, the trainee is expected to have a better grasp of the learning material, and the transfer of expertise will be smoothly carried out.

2.4   Process Analysis Technique

In 2000, Mori, with the result of his studies, he revised the SAT (Skills Analysis for Training) and created manuals on technical skills namely, pencil sharpening, the use of knife, the use of hammer and cooking of the *Atsuyaki Tamago* (thick-sliced egg roll). We have employed identical process analysis technique with some revision on some parts in order to fit our goal and improvised through the addition a new element, the time usage analysis.

Video Recorded Participatory Music Therapy. Video footage of the actual performance served as an important medium that was used in analyzing the performance process, and profiling the core performance requirements. Camera Position. Figure 1 shows that, three video cameras were used, all were set on a tripod. One camera is positioned at the back of the Audience, capturing the entire general setting. This camera also is used for observing the performer in the direct view. The other two video cameras were position to the front left and to the right of the performer, aimed to capture the general movement of the performer, as well as some part of the audience. All of the video cameras were set to wide angle or zoomed-out to be able to capture wide area. The same camera set-up was used for both the expert and the successor performance analysis.

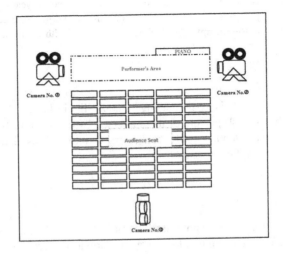

Fig. 1. Camera Position Diagram

Process Analysis I: Interview. To be able to map the core performance requirements and be able to arrange them in the Process Analysis Sheet, interview of the expert and successor were conducted. While watching the video footage of their own performances, the expert and successor were ask questions focusing on analyzing the performance protocol. Data gathered from these interviews were used in mapping the core performance requirements that were reflected in the process analysis sheet (Fig. 2).

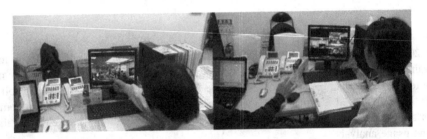

Fig. 2. Interview

Process Analysis II: Analysis of usage of time. Attention is a high-priced commodity especially in performances. In this experiment, we tried to analyze the difference in usage of time between the expert and successor. Rendition time of song and exercise as well as time used in between songs (Interval time) were analyzed.

3   Results and Consideration

3.1   Video Recorded Participatory Music Therapy

Figure 3 shows the flowchart we followed starting from video shoot of the actual music therapy until the performance process analysis.

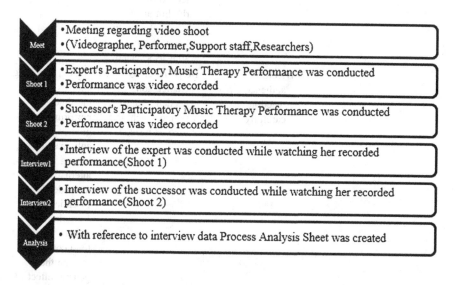

Fig. 3. Performance process analysis flowchart

3.2   Performance Process Analysis I (Interview)

As shown in Table 2, upon careful consideration of the collected data, it is suggested that as a requirement, every performance must have three stages, audience preparation stage, excite stage, and cool-down stages. (Stages were named after the main activity of each individual stage). Interview yield results that cooling down of the audience is proportionally important as preparation of the audience for the activity. It was known that the performer's knowledge of songs familiar to most of the audiences, ability to render songs related to hometown and season were essential components of the performance. Moreover, performer's ability to observe and make changes in tempo,

Table 2. Result of process analysis based on interview

Process	Main activity	Element /detailed action	Judgment standard	Core principle
Audience preparation stage	Rendition of familiar song This is essential on this stage but could be generally applied to other stages	Perform songs related to the audience time, hometown and current season	Find a song that is commonly liked by the audience. Reaction of the audience during performance like movement of their head, tapping hand and feet to the rhythm are essential cues to know if good song is selected	Familiarity helps to activate participation among audiences. Preparing also the audience for a performance is essential
		Watch the audience reaction carefully	Be prepared to change song as needed. Adjust tempo, pitch and tone as needed	Prepare a few song choices. Not all the time performances goes as anticipated, so having an alternative song to render is essential. Variation of tempo, pitch and tone could change the general effect of the song depending on situation
	Vocalization	Perform, simple, long and loud vocalization	This part will serve as their breathing exercise	Breathing exercise is essential prior to any strenuous activity
	Perform nature related song	Perform song related to moon and stars, etc.	Remind the audience the things they already know, but rarely seen or experienced, for being inside the facility. This will also facilitate their relaxation	A relaxed environment facilitates attention to performance

(Continued)

Table 2. (Continued)

Process	Main activity	Element /detailed action	Judgment standard	Core principle
Excite stage	Perform lively songs	Let the audience participate and experience music with their five senses •Grab the audience attention •Bring to climax •Compliment the audience	Create an emotionally pleasant atmosphere	Emotionally pleasant atmosphere lengthens the audience attention span
	Perform song combined with physical exercise	Use sticks, towels, newspapers as props	Use these things for maintenance and improvement of hand grip power, hand and eye coordination, etc.	Mobilization of muscles prevents muscle weakening especially for elderly residents
Cool down stage	Perform mellow songs	Let the audience cool down their emotions after a series of lively songs in order for them to have a complete totally satisfying experience	Not cooling down effectively could cause sleep cycle problems to audience.	Ending the music therapy abruptly without cooling down could leave the residents at aroused state.

rhythm, tone of the song is indispensable to be able to maintain the audience attention.

3.2.1 Performance Process Analysis II: Difference in Usage of Time

Figure 4 shows that the expert performance had used a total of 1637 s (27 min and 17 s) for rendition, 780 s (13 min) for Others (unspecified activity), and a total 1046 s (17 min and 26 s) for rendition interval. The performance timed a total of 3463 s (57 min and 43 s).

Figure 5 shows that the successor performance had used a total of 1252 s (20 min and 52 s) for rendition, 430 s (7 min and 10 s) for Others (unspecified activity), and a total 1669 s (27 min and 49 s) for rendition interval. The performance timed a total of 3351 s (55 min and 51 s).

On Figs. 6 and 7, the usage of time by the expert and successor were compared.

Performance Type	Song Name	Rendition Duration			Rendition Interval		
		s	m	s	s	m	s
Participatory Song	ドレミの歌	102	1	42	35	0	35
Participatory Song and Exercise	発声練習	107	1	47	14	0	14
Participatory Song and Exercise	パタカラ	150	2	30	57	0	57
Participatory Song	あのすばらしい愛をもう一度	168	2	48	47	0	47
Participatory Song	お座敷小唄(1回目)	71	1	11	63	1	3
Participatory Song	お座敷小唄(2回目)	64	1	4	48	0	48
Participatory Song	月がとっても青いから	92	1	32	65	1	5
Participatory Song	星影のワルツ	115	1	55	12	0	12
Participatory Song	指と手の運動	68	1	8	0	0	0
Participatory Song	2拍子・3拍子	112	1	52	86	1	26
Participatory Song	かかし(かなし)	37	0	37	12	0	12
Participatory Song	かかし(手を叩く)	34	0	34	82	1	22
Participatory Song	かかし(スタッフ伴奏)	35	0	35	90	1	30
Participatory Song	もしもしかめよかめさんよ(棒)	26	0	26	6	0	6
Participatory Song	もしもしかめよかめさんよ(棒)2回目	25	0	25	5	0	5
Participatory Song and Exercise	棒	292	4	52	55	0	55
Participatory Song	竹田の子守歌	121	2	1	63	1	3
Participatory Song	どんぐりころころ	75	1	15	37	0	37
Participatory Song	女ひとり	157	2	37	40	0	40
Participatory Song	もみじ	103	1	43	30	0	30
Participatory Song	旅愁	23	0	23			
		73	1	13	31	0	31
Participatory Song	里の秋	163	2	43	86	1	26
Participatory Song	夕焼け小焼け	95	1	35	82	1	22
Participatory Song	ふるさと	109	1	49			

Rendition Duration	1637	27	17
Others	780	13	0
Rendition Interval	1046	17	26
Total	3463	57	43

Fig. 4. Expert performance time data analysis (October 2014)

Attention was given to three variables, namely rendition duration, others and rendition interval. The expert's total rendition time was 6.41666667 min longer than the successor. On Others total (Unspecified activity, neither rendition nor rendition interval) the expert timed 5.83333333 min longer than the successor. While on the other hand, the rendition interval time for the successor is 10.3833333 min longer. This implies that the audiences waiting time for the next rendition was longer.

Performance Type	Song/Exercise Name	Rendition Duration			Rendition Interval		
		s	m	s	s	m	s
Participatory Song	まるたけえびす	35	0	35	13	0	13
Participatory Song and Exercise	発声練習(あいうべ)	115	1	55	62	1	2
Participatory Song	ふたりは若い	101	1	41	96	1	36
Participatory Song	富士の山	99	1	39	112	1	52
Participatory Song	津軽海峡冬景色	190	3	10	110	1	50
Participatory Song	おかあさん	93	1	33			
		19	0	19	83	1	23
Participatory Song	ジングルベル	107	1	47	40	0	40
Participatory Song	きよしこの夜	110	1	50	144	2	24
Participatory Song	もちつき	94	1	34	118	1	58
Participatory Song	じゃんけん	55	0	55	11	0	11
Participatory Song and Exercise	棒体操	240	4	0			
		20	0	20	61	1	1
Participatory Song	落ちた落ちた	44	0	44	95	1	35
Participatory Song	365歩のマーチ	64	1	4	286	4	46
Participatory Song	ふるさと	10	0	10	43	0	43
		12	0	12	37	0	37
		10	0	10	48	0	48
		9	0	9	14	0	14
Participatory Song	ふるさと全体	40	0	40	187	3	7
Participatory Song	雪	41	0	41			
		17	0	17	54	0	54
Participatory Song	たき火	69	1	9	55	0	55
Participatory Song	ふるさと	88	1	28			

Rendition Duration	1252	20	52
Others	430	7	10
Rendition Interval	1669	27	49
Total	3351	55	51

Fig. 5. Successor performance time data analysis (October 2014)

	Expert		Successor	
	m	s	m	s
Total Rendition Duration	27	17	20	52
Others	13	0	7	10
Rendition Interval	17	26	27	49
Total	57	43	55	51

Fig. 6. Performance total time comparison

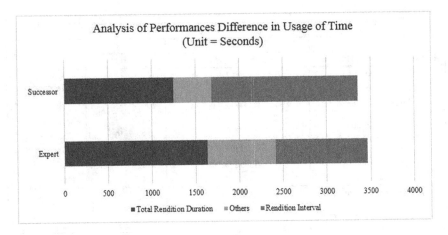

Fig. 7. Comparison in usage of time

4   Conclusion

Our study shows that positive development can be achieved if the performance is well-arranged. This study also implies that paying attention to the core performance requirements and the point of solving ingeniously and adjusting to the audience need while performing is the foundation that results to good performance. Finally, we believe that result of this study can be useful in producing the training video we wish to create.

5   Recommendation

Efficient use of time. Attention is a high priced commodity. Although we did not make a scientific comparison between the effect expert and successor's performance as it goes beyond our objective, we believe that skillful use of the time of the expert played a role in holding the attention span of the audience. We therefore recommend further studies on this matter.

Camera position. Although the front left and right camera captured the general movement of the performer during the actual performance, when we were interview for the process analysis, there were time that the area being pointed out by the performer as the location of the audience that had been the cue of her action and decision was beyond the captured area. In order to resolve this issue on future studies, we recommend of panning the front left and right camera a few degrees to the audiences would best results. An additional camera positioned center-front, set to wide angle could be also an alternative to the latter.

Performer's knowledge of dementia. After this study we feel that there is a necessity to further study if the performer's knowledge of dementia could have an impact on the way he will respond to the needs of the audiences who were suffering from dementia during his performances.

Transfer of expertise. As a result of the current revision of nursing care insurance law in Japan, and the current worsening situation of being short-staffed, more and more pressure are leaning towards the private paid elderly nursing facility on how to be able to deliver quality service to the residents. To be able to minimize the time loss and effectively transfer expertise of different caregiver skills, related studies are recommended.

References

Brotons, M., Koger, S.M.: The impact of music therapy on language functioning in dementia. J. Music Ther. **37**, 183–195 (2000)

Yamamoto, A.: Research on Work Climate at Nursing Home (2015)

Kuwahara, K.: Kaigo Roujin Hoken Shisetsu ni okeru Ongaku Ryouhou to Ongaku wo Riyou Shita Rikuriesyon (in Japanese) (2001)

Noumi, A.: Ongaku Ryouho ni yori BPSD ga keigen shita ninchishou koureisha no 1 rei (in Japanese) (2005)

Takada, H.: Rouken ni okeru ongaku ryouhou ni kansuru kenyuu dai16hou – Ongaku ryouhou no hyouka tsu-ru to shite no bideo kiroku no yuuyousei (in Japanese) (2009)

Mori, K.: Gijutsu•Ginou denshou no tame no ginou bunseki to manyuaru kousei no Houhou (2001)

Nakane, M.: Keido Ninchishou koureisha ni taisuru kobetsu ongaku ryouhou no yuuyousei – Seikatsu Iyoku to ninchi kinou no koujou ga mitomerareta 1 rei (in Japanese) (2013)

Watanabe, T.: Chihousei koureisha ni tai suru ongaku ryouhou ni kansuru systematic review. Aichi Kyouiku Daigaku Kenkyuu Houkoku 54, pp. 57–61 (in Japanese) (2005)

Martin, P.Y., Turner, B.A.: Grounded theory and organizational research. J. Appl. Behav. Sci. **22** (2), 141 (1986)

Faggiolani, C.: Perceived identity: applying grounded theory in libraries. JLIS.it (University of Florence) **2**(1) (2011). doi:10.4403/jlis.it-4592. Accessed 29 June 2013

Grounded Theory, Wikipedia, the free encyclopedia. Accessed 27 February 2015

Glaser and Strauss (1967)

Research of Work Climate at Nursing Home - From Job Separation and Management Capability Point

Akiyoshi Yamamoto[1], Tomoko Ota[4], Akihiko Goto[3], Noriyuki Kida[2],
Hiroyuki Hamada[2], Henry Cereno Barrameda Jr.[1(✉)],
and Tatsunori Azuma[1]

[1] Super Court Co., Ltd, Osaka, Japan
{yamamoto,henrybarramedajr,azuma}@supercourt.co.jp
[2] Kyoto Institute of Technology, Kyoto, Japan
{kida,hhamada}@kit.ac.jp
[3] Osaka Sangyo University, Osaka, Japan
gotoh@ise.osaka-sandai.ac.jp
[4] Chuo Business Group, Osaka, Japan
tomoko.ota@k.vodafone.ne.jp

Abstract. Nursing care insurance system, which was introduced 14 years ago in Japan, helps our life. However, there are some problems such as job separation rate and excess and deficiency of employees at nursing home. "Care Work Foundation (CWF)" investigates about state of care work under name of the investigation "Actual Condition of Care Work" every year. According to the investigation in 2013, Staff Turnover Rate for one year (October 1st, 2012 – September 30th, 2013) was 16.6 % in all. And 56.5 % of the nursing care staff felt that the employee's number was insufficient. (Insufficient = "greatly insufficient" + "insufficient" + "somewhat insufficient") In this research, the work climate at nursing home regarding Staff Turnover Rate and the management capability, which was not analyzed by "Actual Condition of Care Work", was carried out on 44 nursing homes in my company. Specially, analyzed the employee satisfaction, and examined the correlation of the reason and the timing of leaving their job. In addition, there are 6 points as management capability of nursing home; "management principle" "performance capability" "nursing ability" "expressing gratitude to others" "employee satisfaction" "customer satisfaction". Moreover the correlation of Staff Turnover Rate and the management capability on each nursing home was examined as well. These 6 points are based on the screening criterion of a management quality grand-prix. These 6 points are large categories, and there are 20 medium categories inside large category. "Management principle" has a medium category "empathy degree to management principle". "Performance capability" has 5 categories; (1) operating ratio, (2) admission rate, (3) Staff Turnover Rate, (4) labor cost rate, (5) number of nonconformity to ISO. "Nursing ability" has 3 categories; (1) Achievement rate of short-term target, (2) Number of accidents during the care, (3) Number of incident reports. "Expressing gratitude to others"; (1) number of "Thanks" Card, (2) number of "Voice for Super Court Staff" Card. "Employee satisfaction" has 4 categories; (1) satisfaction and fairness to the personnel evaluation, (2) number of interview, (3) Independent and caring

© Springer International Publishing Switzerland 2015
V.G. Duffy (Ed.): DHM 2015, Part II, LNCS 9185, pp. 512–523, 2015.
DOI: 10.1007/978-3-319-21070-4_52

personality, (4) employee satisfaction. In the "customer satisfaction", there are 5 categories; (1) service satisfaction, (2) meal satisfaction, (3) cleaning satisfaction in community area, (4) cleaning satisfaction in the room, (5) total customer satisfaction. The research showed the trend that the lower Staff Turnover Rate at each nursing home becomes, the higher the "operating ratio of nursing home". And the higher Staff Turnover Rate at each nursing home, the higher the "accident frequency rate during nursing care". However, there is no correlation between Staff Turnover Rate and "degree of empathy to management principle", "employee satisfaction" and "total customer satisfaction". The results shows that the nursing home with the maximum number of thanks cards in the 44 nursing home is the least in Staff Turnover Rate.

1 Introduction

Japanese society is becoming a hyper-aging society where the percentage of elderly people is high among its population, making how the elderly people can participate in social activities and enjoy their lives is of at most importance. In order to achieve this, elderly care is a central social policy. If the youth witness misery among the elderly, they could despair of their future and lead to the stagnation of our society's productivity. Therefore, the elderly care in Japan must become the role model for other countries that will become aging societies, which adds another perspective to the importance of elderly care in Japan. Elderly care is a form of service based on human interactions. Even though machines and robot can support the process, manpower will always be in the center. And the care workers learn skills and knowledge through wide-ranging experiences, thus every worker has a different approach and there are thousands of effective methods.

There have not been scientifically valid advices, and these methods only exist as the tacit knowledge among the care workers. This leads to ill health of the workers due to hard works, and they leave the care profession after falling ill. Naturally, an experienced care worker can offer a better care than an inexperienced one. The key question then is how to retain as many experts in the profession of elderly care.

We have always advocated a form of high-grade elderly care where both those being cared and the care workers can retain peace of their mind and can humanely interact while performing their roles. In short, a system where not only the care-receiver but also the care worker can be joyful while engaging in the care work. One method to achieve this is to scientifically systematize the tacit knowledge of the expert care workers and may enable workers to share it. We can basically say that it is how to conduct care without causing back pain. In order to systematize tacit knowledge, we employed every means including movement analysis, eye motion analysis and muscle usage analysis. We have also created structure to utilize our findings at the frontline service. This type of research is certainly helpful in reduce the turnover rate of the care workers. But we also must study the psychological reasons for employees leaving their job. In other words, how to make the care work feel worthwhile.

In this report, we interviewed 1179 employees from the care company that operates 40 elderly care homes in order to determine and analyze the reasons for turnover of care workers. We used data assembled from the 40 care homes including "Index relating to the Performance of the Facility", "Index relating to the Facility", "Employee's Performance Index", "Employee's Self Evaluation Index" and "Index relating to Client's Evaluation".

2 Research Items and Methods

Among the data we used, the response variable was the employee turnover rate (From 2013.9 to 2014.8), and the result of its multiple regression analysis was 0.40 ± 0.23. This is the average of the 40 facilities. The number is higher than common turnover rate due to the inclusion of the part-time staff. The 4 categories of explanatory variables are the "Facility Index", Index relating to Staff Performance, Relating to Employee's Self Evaluation and Relating to Client's Evaluation. We explain each category below.

2.1 Facility Index

We selected these 9 items as index for facility relation.

How long it has been operating (in months), room number, floor number, average care rate, residential style private retirement homes, private retirement homes with in-house nursing care services, conventional style retirement homes, (which has one public kitchen and dining room, not individual as the above two), transportation from the nearest train station, and the time necessary from the nearest train station. The result are shown in the Table 1.

Table 1. Index relating to the facility

Facility type	
Residential	26
Specific	13
Elderly	1
Facility hardware	
Conventional type	31
Unit type	4
Mixed type	5
Transport from the nearest train station	
Walking only	35
Walking and bus	5
Facility Index	$M \pm SD$
Time of operation	60 ± 42.5
Room number	69.7 ± 20.2
Floor number	4.1 ± 1.5
Average care rate	2.5 ± 0.4
Time necessary from the nearest train station (in minutes)	8.1 ± 4.1

Facility Types. "Residential" stands for "Residential style private retirement homes". The definition of this type of facility is that it only provides support in everyday life such as meals, and the care is received in the same way as when the care-receiver is living in his/her own home. In other words, the residents or their family must hire an external care-service provider on their own.

"Specific" stands for "Private retirement homes with in-house nursing care services". This type of facility provides each resident care in bathing, toilet and meal as well as other support in their daily lives and exercises following the care plan. The residents are charged for 10 % of cost (fixed). This type of facility cannot be found in the west.

"Elderly" stands for "Rental housing exclusively for the elderly". This facility type is rental housing built and run by private company and approved by municipality. It mainly accepts residents that require relatively easy or no care. The "Elderly" type facility is decreasing due to the abolishment of the system, and they are shifting towards elderly homes with in-house service.

Facility Hardware. "Conventional" type is the ordinary facility with one centralized canteen.

"Unit" type is the facility with bath and canteen on each floor. In this type, the whole care can be conducted in each floor.

"Mixed" type also has one big canteen just like "Conventional" type. However, the dementia specialized floor has its own canteen and bathroom, which allows it to run complete care within itself.

2.2   Index Relating to Employee Performance

These 5 items are for the Index relating to Employee Performance.

Assessment for short-term target achievement, number of accidents during the care (per 1 resident), number of incident reports (per 1 employee at the end of last month), number of "Thanks" Card (per 1 employee at the end of last month) and number of "Voice for Super Court Staff" (per 1 employee at the end of last month). We explain each item below.

Assessment for Short-Term Target Achievement. "Assessment for short-term target achievement" is calculated as thus: The planning administrator of private retirement homes with charging in-house elderly care services, or the service manager/administrator of charging elderly care visiting residential style private retirement homes produces assessment for short-term care plan target. It is assessed in 4 grades; 1) No effect, 2) effective but not enough, 3) effective, 4) satisfactory. The "assessment for short-term target achievement" is the average of all the plans and clients.

Number of Accidents During Care. The number of accidents during care was assembled according to accident reports. We distinguished between accidents during care and accident occurred outside the care time. In this paper, we calculate the ratio of accident in relation to each facility's number of residents. The type of accidents are: 1.

Fall and fall down, 2. Miss-dosing and dropping of medication, 3. Accidental ingestion, aspiration, 4, Cut, chafing, 5, Bruise, sprain, 6. Damaged or lost property, 7. Unauthorized leave, and 8. Others.

Number of Incident Reports. We believe that it is important to compile the incident reports where care workers realized something that could have resulted in serious accidents. These information are highly valuable in preventing accidents from occurring. If a care worker notes many instances like this, it shows that he/she is attentive and dedicated. We call this "Alarm-Attention-Concern Process". Heinrich's law that shows "for every accident that causes a major injury, there are 29 accidents that cause minor injuries and 300 accidents that cause no injuries" is the basis for this process.

Number of "Thanks" Cards. "Thanks" Card: When a staff felt gratitude toward another staff, he/she writes "who" feels gratitude toward "whom" and "why" in "Thanks" Card and put it in the "Drop BOX". The system is that these cards are gathered weekly and displayed for every staff to see. This way, "Gratitude" is shared by everyone. The purpose of this is to create a corporate culture where people can thank each other easily. It is important to maintain a work environment where the staff can feel satisfied in order to increase the productivity of individuals and organization. We aim for increasing the number of "Company Satisfaction Ratio". We calculate the number of "Thanks" Card in relation to the number of employee. It is deemed that the higher the number of "Thanks" Card, more motivated and attentive the staff.

Number of "Voice for Super Court Staff" Cards. The staff can submit their opinions, requests or comments from the residents to the company through a card called "Voice for Super Court Staff", which is designed to express (1) Complains, (2) Requests and (3) Gratitude. Just like "Thanks" Card, we deem that the higher the number of "Voice for Super Court Staff", more motivated and attentive the staff. Moreover, it can boost the morale of the staff by making the sign of gratitude from the residents and their family readily available. We calculate the number of "Voice for Super Court Staff" in relation to the number of employee.

2.3   Index Relating to Staff Self Evaluation

In order to determine how satisfied the staff are, we gave them this questionnaire with 21 questions. The number of the answers we got was 1179.

Q01:   Do you feel the sense of purpose with the contribution the company makes to the society? (E.g. Elderly care seminar for local residents and businesses, learning experience for students, or presentation of research on elderly care and long life.)

Q02:   Do you think the company follows law strictly?

Q03:   Do you agree with the company policy?

Q04:   Do you think departments and branches are well-coordinated?

Q05:   Do you think the necessary discipline and manners are followed?

Q06:   Are you happy with the Staff Proposal System (Praise for good idea)

Q07:   Do you think the atmosphere of your department is good?

Q08:   Do you think there are many self-sufficient people around you?

Q09:   Do you think your department encourages honest opinions?

Q10:   Do you think the company welfare and facilities are sufficient for this company? (E.g. congratulations and condolences, housing support, support for obtaining new qualifications or self-improvement, the discount tickets for the natural hot spring located in the Super Hotel, Hananoi, Osaka branch, or the free stay tickets at any Super Hotels, etc.)

Q11:   Do you find your current duties worthwhile?

Q12:   Do you feel that your duties and responsibilities are clearly defined at the workplace?

Q13:   Do you think the education and training for improving staff's ability are implemented?

Q14:   Are you happy with the training and education?

Q15:   Can you picture the future in your job?

Q16:   Do you feel that the targets are appropriate?

Q17:   Do you think the evaluation you get is fair?

Q18:   Is the meeting between the staff and their superior based on "Monthly target sheet" held monthly?

Q19:   Do you enjoy working here?

Q20:   Are you interested in this study?

Q21:   Do you find the criteria and method of staff evaluation clear?

2.4   Related to Client's Evaluation

Those related to Client's Evaluation are these 5 items. Satisfaction for customer service (manner and language, average of both the residents and their family), satisfaction for food (taste, only the residents), satisfaction for cleaning of public area (average of both the residents and their family), satisfaction for cleaning of individual rooms (average of both the residents and their family), the total satisfaction rate (average of both the residents and their family). The research method is to collect "questionnaire about life here" from the residents and their family every 6 months.

3   Research Results

3.1   Index Related to Employee Performance

Table 2 shows the result of Index relating to Employee Performance.

3.2   Index Relating to Employee Self Evaluation

Table 3 shows the result of questionnaire relating to Employee Self Evaluation.

We applied factor analysis on these results. Table 4 shows the outcome of this analysis. 2 interpretable factors where eigenvalue is more than 1 were sampled. After

Table 2. Research result of index relating to employee performance

M ± SD
Accident ration during care
(Per 1 resident at the end of this month) (2014.1–2014.8 average) 0.05 ± 0.03
Number of incidents reports
(Per 1 staff at the end of last month) (2014.1–2014.8 average) 1.4 ± 0.5
Number of "Thanks" Card
(Per 1 staff at the end of last month) (2014.1–2014.8 average) 7.8 ± 6.7
Number of "Voice for Super Court Staff"
(Per 1 staff at the end of last month) .7 – July/August average
due to change of index 1.6 ± 0.7
Short-term target achievement ratio (2014.1–2014.8 average) 3.2 ± 0.2

examining the items that constitute the factors, we identified that the first factor related to the employee's satisfaction rate for the job, company and department, and their degree of agreement with the company's management policy and its social contribution activities, and the second factor related to the atmosphere and environment of the workplace including such questions as "Does your department have good atmosphere?" or "Do you think your department encourages honest opinions?" Therefore, we named the first factor "Job Satisfaction Factor" and the second factor "Workplace Atmosphere Factor", and calculated its number in each branch.

3.3   Related to Client's Evaluation

Table 5 shows the result of Client's Evaluation.

3.4   Multiple Regression Analysis

We conducted multiple regression analysis based on the data above. We set Staff Turnover Rate as response variable, we deduced 22 variable from explanatory variable, and conducted the analysis through stepwise method. That result showed R square = .411, F = 9.61, p < .01, the coefficient that has not been standardized are.

Employee Turnover Rate = 0.790 - 0.257 × Facility Hardware Ordinary Type (dummy variable) - 0.002 × Time of operation (in months) - 0.011 × "Thanks" Card coefficient (standardized coefficient).

Facility Hardware Ordinary Type (dummy variable): β = - .466, p < .01, VIF = 1.105.

Time of operation (in months): β = - .329, p < .05, VIF = 1.077.

Number of "Thanks" Card: β = - .310, p < .05, VIF = 1.035.

We will deepen our argument following these results.

Table 3. Result of questionnaire relating to employee self evaluation

	$M \pm SD$
Question 2: On the whole, how satisfied are you with your current job/company/department?	2.8 ± 0.4
Q01: Do you feel the sense of purpose with the contribution the company makes to the society? (E.g. Elderly care seminar for local residents and businesses, learning experience for students, or presentation of research on elderly care and long life.)	1.9 ± 0.2
Q02: Do you think the company follows law strictly?	1.8 ± 0.2
Q03: Do you agree with the company policy?	1.8 ± 0.2
Q04: Do you think departments and branches are well-coordinated?	2.1 ± 0.2
Q05: Do you think the necessary discipline and manners are followed?	1.9 ± 0.2
Q06: Are you happy with the Staff Proposal System (Praise for good idea)	2.0 ± 0.2
Q07: Do you think the atmosphere of your department is good?	1.8 ± 0.2
Q08: Do you think there are many self-sufficient people around you?	2.1 ± 0.2
Q09: Do you think your department encourages honest opinions?	1.9 ± 0.2
Q10: Do you think the company welfare and facilities are sufficient for this company? (E.g. congratulations and condolences, housing support, support for obtaining new qualifications or self-improvement, the discount tickets for the natural hot spring located in the Super Hotel, Hananoi, Osaka branch, or the free stay tickets at any Super Hotels etc.)	2.0 ± 0.2
Q11: Do you find your current duties worthwhile?	1.7 ± 0.2
Q12: Do you feel that your duties and responsibilities are clearly defined at the workplace?	1.8 ± 0.2
Q13: Do you think the education and training for improving staff's ability are implemented?	1.9 ± 0.2
Q14: Are you happy with the training and education?	2.0 ± 0.2
Q15: Can you picture the future in your job?	2.0 ± 0.2
Q16: Do you feel that the targets are appropriate?	1.9 ± 0.2
Q17: Do you think the evaluation you get is fair?	1.9 ± 0.2
Q18: Is the meeting between the staff and their superior based on "Monthly target sheet" held monthly?	2.0 ± 0.3
Q19: Do you enjoy working here?	1.9 ± 0.2
Q20: Are you interested in this study?	2.1 ± 0.2
Q21: Do you find the criteria and method of staff evaluation clear?	2.1 ± 0.2

4 Discussion

Our analysis demonstrated that the employee's turnover rate is related mainly to the type of facility, how long it has been open and the number of "Thanks" Card. Below will present the cause of each factors.

Table 4. Result of factor analysis of questionnaire relating to employee self evaluation relation.

	F1	F2
Q10: Do you think the company welfare and facilities are sufficient for this company? (E.g. congratulations and condolences, housing support, support for obtaining new qualifications or self-improvement, the discount tickets for the natural hot spring located in the Super Hotel, Hananoi, Osaka branch, or the free stay tickets at any Super Hotels, etc.)	.991	−.199
Q03: Do you agree with the company policy?	.973	−.172
Q01: Do you feel the sense of purpose with the contribution the company makes to the society? (E.g. Elderly care seminar for local residents and businesses, learning experience for students, or presentation of research on elderly care and long life.)	.971	−.129
Q21: Do you find the criteria and method of staff evaluation clear?	.874	.038
Q06: Are you happy with the Staff Proposal System (Praise for good idea)	.862	.012
Q02: Do you think the company follows law strictly?	.823	.029
Q20: Are you interested in this study?	.793	.068
Q16: Do you feel that the targets are appropriate?	.763	.094
Q14: Are you happy with the training and education?	.694	.281
Q18: Is the meeting between the staff and their superior based on "Monthly target sheet" held monthly?	.680	.180
Q17: Do you think the evaluation you get is fair?	.665	.261
Q15: Can you picture the future in your job?	.525	.419
Q11: Do you find your current duties worthwhile?	474	.405
Q07: Do you think the atmosphere of your department is good?	−.317	.154
Q09: Do you think your department encourages honest opinions?	−.178	1.031
Q12: Do you feel that your duties and responsibilities are clearly defined at the workplace?	.039	.819
Q08: Do you think there are many self-sufficient people around you?	.165	.683
Q19: Do you enjoy working here?	.249	.647
Q05: Do you think the necessary discipline and manners are followed?	.396	.517
Q04: Do you think departments and branches are well-coordinated?	.438	.501
Q13: Do you think the education and training for improving staff's ability are implemented?	.412	.474

Factor sampling method: Major factor method, Rotation method: Promax rotation

4.1   Employee's Turnover Rate Is Lower When the Facility Is Conventional Type

When the facility is unit type and not conventional type, there are fewer interactions among the care workers and it is not possible to share the responsibilities. The work at unit type is also divided between each floor, meaning there are not many chance to seek advices from one's colleagues, leading to a lack of communication. This influences the turnover rate.

Table 5. Client's evaluation research result

Client's Evaluation (Percentage of high evaluation)	$M \pm SD$
Satisfaction for customer service (manner and language, the residents and their family)	0.78 ± 0.08
Satisfaction for food (taste, only the residents)	0.55 ± 0.20
Satisfaction for cleaning of public area (average of the residents and their family)	0.73 ± 0.11
Satisfaction for cleaning of individual rooms (average of the residents and their family)	0.60 ± 0.10
Total satisfaction rate (average of the residents and their family)	0.69 ± 0.09

4.2   Longer the Facility Has Been Operating, Lower the Turnover Rate

A new facility is operated by staff gathered from different branches. Therefore, there are often not enough communication and many differences of opinions. This leads to some staff leaving due to disagreement in belief. In comparison, a facility that has been operating some time gives staff time to adjust to their colleagues, and those stayed in the job tend to agree with the policy of Super Court leading to lower turnover rate. Also, the administration of the facility stabilizes after some time, which leads to staff having calmer mind and having more time to care for the residents, making them feel more purposeful and influencing the turnover rate.

4.3   Higher the Number of "Thanks" Cards, Lower the Turnover Rate

High number of "Thanks" Card shows that the facility has the culture of expressing gratitude. This can be seen to produce more relaxed work environment, leading to lowering of turnover rate. Also, encouraging the expression of gratitude and notifying every staff about it have an effect of boosting their morale, and make the job feel more worthwhile, leading to the lowering of turnover rate.

4.4   Overview

In order to lower the turnover rate of employee, we learnt from these results that:

1. The fact that turnover rate is lower when the facility is conventional type showed us the importance of communication among the staff.
2. It has been generally considered that the turnover rate is linked to the extent the staff identify with the company policy, and deeper the identification, lower the turnover rate. However, we discovered that how long the facility has been operating is also related to turnover rate. There is statistic that shows the staff of new facility has better understanding of company policy, but this merely reflects the enthusiasm and high self-confidence of new staff and does not necessary prove their better understanding of the company policy. As a result, the discrepancy between their view and management principle lead to higher turnover rate. A new facility is staffed with workers from different branches, which means their different background prevent

them from correct understanding of the company policy. This means the principle is not integrated into their action and leading to discrepancy. Therefore, correct management of a new facility can be considered important.

3. The fact that turnover rate is lower when the number of "Thanks" Card is high showed us that creating a working environment that makes it easier for staff to operate is important.

5 Conclusion

This report held interview with 1179 staff from a care company that operates 40 facilities in order to conduct multiple regression analysis of the factors that leads to high employee turnover rate. We used data collected from the 40 facilities, namely Index relating to the Performance of the Facility, Index relating to the Facility, Index relating to Employee's Performance, Employee's Self Evaluation Index and Index relating to Client's Evaluation. As a result, we gained knowledge that turnover rate is lower when: the facility type is conventional, when the facility is operating for longer time, and when the number of "Thanks" Card and "Voice for Super Court staff" Card.

We will now present how to proceed on each point.

1. We must establish a structure where the staff can communicate with each other no matter whether the facility is Conventional or Unit type. In addition to utilizing IT communication method such as every staff carrying iPad, we will also hold committee for improving the working environment. Also, we are today gradually shifting to the mixed type which uses good aspects of both conventional and unit types.

2. In order to improve staff's understanding of and agreement with the company policy, we are implementing these 4 programs:

   - Hiring people who already share our belief. In order to achieve this, we are constantly improving the questionnaire for interview.
   - Internship
   - Constant improvement of questionnaire during orientation
   - Constant improvement of monthly meeting between staff and their superior (for new recruits the facility manager) based on the monthly target sheet (Q18)

3. In order to reduce the mental pressure of the staff, it is important that they can conduct their duty smoothly and have enough mental space to care about other things. Therefore, an effective training that can reduce their physical hardship is necessary. These are two training for such improvement:

   - We conduct training that can improve the average care skill quality.
   - We conduct their care work movement analysis, for instance during bathing support, in order to standardize the work.

References

1. Kobiyama, N.: Kaigosyoku no Shigoto no Manzokudo to Risyokuikou -Kaigofukushishi shikaku to Sa-bisu ruikei ni Tyumoku shite- Kikan Syakaihosyokenkyu, vol. **45**, No 4 (in Japanese) (2010)
2. Abe, M.: Kaigosyoku no Syokumukeizoku, Risyokuikou to Kanrenyouin ni Kansuru Tyousa. -Kanagawakennai Tokubetsuyougo Roujin Ho-mu no Kaigosyoku wo Taisyou to shita Tyousa kara-, Syakai Ronsyu 17-gou Ronbun (in Japanese) (2014)
3. Nakano S.: Kaigo Fukushi no Risyoku, ISFJ2010 (in Japanese) (2010)
4. Yamato M.: Kaigo Roujin Fukushi Shisetsu ni okeru Kaigo Syokuin no Risyoku Youin, Ningen Fukushigaku Kenkyu, Dai6kan, Dai1gou (in Japanese) (2013)
5. Rosen, J.: Stayers, leavers, and switchers among certified nursing assistants in nursing homes: a longitudinal investigation of turnover intent, staff retention, and turnover. TheGerontologist **51**(5), 597–609 (2011)
6. Leister, D.Z..: The Vanishing Nursing Home Administrator: Stress And Intent To Leave (2009)
7. Tamura, Y.: Risk factors relating to leaving employment in nursing home -A comparison off nurses and non-licensed care assistants-, Ehime Daigaku Kyoiku Gakubu Kiyou Dai60kan 227–233, (2013)

Caregiver's Eye Gaze and Field of View Presumption Method During Bathing Care in Elderly Facility

Akiyoshi Yamamoto[1], Tatsunori Azuma[1],
Henry Cereno Barrameda Jr.[1(✉)], Noriyuki Kida[2],
Akihiko Goto[3], and Tomoko Ota[4]

[1] Super Court Co., Ltd., Osaka, Japan
{yamamoto,azuma,henrybarramedajr}@supercourt.co.jp
[2] Kyoto Institute of Technology, Kyoto, Japan
kida@kit.ac.jp
[3] Osaka Sangyo University, Osaka, Japan
gotoh@ise.osaka-sandai.ac.jp
[4] Chuo Business Group, Osaka, Japan
tomoko.ota@k.vodafone.ne.jp

Abstract. Japan faces a critical need for nursing care as its elderly population continues to grow along with a rise in dementia, the number of elderly people who are bedridden and require extended care. Bathing is one of the most important aspects of daily life in which provision of better quality care can improve quality of life. However, in many elderly facilities, bathing is fraught with dangers, such as falling and drowning in a big bath. Bathroom floors can be slippery and cause residents to fall, and the constant vigilance required can cause caregivers significant mental stress. Advancement in biomechanics along with the development of nursing care devices had reduced the physical stress on the caregivers. However, the efforts to relieve mental burdens are still insufficient, especially when caring with elderly people or those suffering from dementia, whose actions are rather unpredictable. By measuring the caregiver's eye gaze and field of view, we believe we would be able to locate the blind spots during bathing care. With the use of the data gathered we aim to develop a system to improve bathing as a good experience to the customer and a less stressful task to the caregiver. While measurement by video camera was considered optimal, we conducted the experiment using motion sensors due to privacy concerns. We performed four experiments to progress towards our final result set. This paper focuses on the second of these experiments.

Keywords: Caregiver · Elderly facility · Bath care assistance · Presumption method · Blind spot · Motion capture

1 Research Background

Japan faces a critical need for nursing care as its elderly population continues to grow along with a rise in dementia, the number of elderly people who are bedridden and require extended care. According to the 2014 White Paper on the Aging Society, 31.9

© Springer International Publishing Switzerland 2015
V.G. Duffy (Ed.): DHM 2015, Part II, LNCS 9185, pp. 524–532, 2015.
DOI: 10.1007/978-3-319-21070-4_53

million people, or 25.1 % of the entire Japanese population of 127.30 million, are senior citizens over the age of 65 as of October 1, 2013. That number is 14 %, highly above the 7 % threshold that defines a country as an aging society. Japanese society is entering the super aging society. Furthermore, a very high 12.3 % of the population is over the age of 75. Compared to other countries, Japan is facing the super aging society that no country has ever experienced until now. The aging of society has increased demand for nursing care, with 5.49 million people as of October, 2012 qualifying for some type of care in their daily life. This pressing social need necessitated specialized care in the nursing business. In 1987, the Certified Social Workers and Certified Care Workers Act was enacted to provide and maintain quality nursing care, giving specialized nursing care providers with national certification. This also had the effect of directing the spotlight on the overwhelming challenges of the families dealing with nursing care for their elderly, and a growing call for socialized nursing care led to the enactment of the long-term care insurance program in 2000, giving recipients a choice in the type of nursing care they receive. The first article of the long-term care act advocates for socially supported quality welfare services that recognize the right to a dignified life for all individuals. "So that individuals can lead independent lives according to their ability, so that we may grant the necessary medical and welfare services based on the principles of public and mutual solidarity, we put in place a long-term care insurance system, with necessary items applied toward that benefit so that we can provide our citizens with better medical care and welfare."

1.1 Bathing Assistance: Background and Issues

Bathing is indispensable for both hygiene and as part of Activities of Daily Living (ADL). It encourages blood circulation and promotes higher metabolism. It also relaxes the muscles, helps prevent bedsores and infections, regulates bowel movements and supports other such functions of the body. For many elderly people suffering from anxiety and tension, bathing is an important time for them to relax. It has the added mental benefit for the elderly, who consider bathing one of life's pleasures. Furthermore, cleansing the body of dirt and odors helps strengthen interpersonal relationships and encourages active social engagement. Bathing is thereby an extremely significant way to assist in the daily lives of the elderly, and in order to realize quality welfare service, effective bathing assistance is a necessity.

Bathing has many benefits – physiological, mental and social. And yet, it can be risky, fraught with such dangers as falling and drowning. The external causes of bathing accidents include exposure to the cold while dressing/undressing, the warm temperature in the bathtub or bathroom, and the hydrostatic pressure within the bathtub, which is considered to have a negative impact on the bodies of the elderly. In many cases, the elderly tend to suffer from multiple complications, such as high blood pressure and diabetes, as well as arteriosclerotic changes and a deteriorating autonomic nervous system response. Therefore, some of the internal causes of bathing accidents can be attributed to changes in blood pressure, dehydration and blood coagulation. These physiological changes expose the elderly to a higher risk of cardiac arrest, cerebrovascular disorder, dizziness and cataleptic attacks. A complex mix of these factors heightens the risk of falling and injury, drowning or death from drowning. Delivering quality bathing assistance depends on overcoming a variety of issues.

Assisting with bathing is extremely hard work and has been an issue at welfare facilities for the elderly. There have been numerous reports published about the level of burden incurred in the work of bathing assistance (Fujimura 1995). One of them (Nagata 1999) involves a survey of caregivers who work in the nation's 969 nursing facilities for the old. According to the survey, the most physically taxing aspect of care is bathing assistance, followed by diaper change and transfers. The burden incurred by bathing assistance is threefold: physiological, physical and mental. First, the high temperature in the bathroom is demanding on the caregiver's body, and that causes physiological challenges. According to a study by Kawahara and his team (Kawahara 2010), caregivers showed high cortisol levels – a benchmark for stress-response – after assisting with bathing, linking the activity with high physiological stress.

The high stress level can be tied in part to working assembly-line style in a high-temperature bathroom, but also handling a lot of transfers from one place or position to another in that process, namely, supporting the elderly in an upright position while he or she dresses or undresses, transferring from the wheelchair to the bathtub and back, among others. These are all tough on the back. Bathing assistance in a nursing care facility with a large bath involves not only horizontal, but lots of vertical movements that impact and stress the musculoskeletal structure, which in turn invites fatigue. Also, with the progressive bathing system most widely used in care facilities, caregivers end up with five manual transfers of an elderly from one location to another, including the move from the bedroom to the bathroom, which again causes stress to the caregiver.

Because bathroom floors can be slippery and trigger a fall, constant vigilance can cause mental stress to caregivers. According to a survey by Nagata (1999), 18 % of the caregivers cited "fear of a fall" as their biggest mental stress while assisting with bathing. Furthermore, the survey revealed that bathing assistance is the most conducive to feeling negative about nursing care (Kawahara 2010).

As detailed above, bathing assistance is extremely taxing work and is believed to be one of the main reasons why some people leave the job. The turnover rate for care jobs was 18.7 % in 2008, which is high compared against the industry's rate of 14.6 %. With regards to active job-opening ratios, the number declined to 1.34 in September 2009, after peaking at 2.53 in December 2008. To this day, the ratio continues hovering above 1 – a big issue to consider in delivering quality care.

1.2   Research Trends in Bathing Assistance

To tackle the above-mentioned problems, fundamental and practical research is being done, with some of the research showing promise of mitigating the physical toll of bathing on the elderly. For instance, Kanda (1991) published the results of his research involving the physiological burdens of bathing in the winter and in the summer. Nagahiro's research (2006) on the impact of bathroom temperatures on the circulatory system of healthy elderly people shows temperature levels that promote lower blood pressure after bathing.

On the other hand, numerous studies conducted in the areas of sanitary engineering and structural engineering have contributed to the development of comfortable clothing and structural improvements in buildings to reduce the physiological impact of care-giving on care workers.

In terms of dealing with the physical stress, caregivers are provided with ergonomic and biomechanic suggestions and nursing equipment that help reduce back strain. For instance, when comparing the efficiency between the use of a mechanical lift and a manual lift when transferring a fully dependent care receiver to a wheelchair, a Tomioka study (Tomioka 2007) showed that the mechanical lift reduced the work time considerably after a period of training and that the mechanical lift was effective in reducing the caregivers' back strain. Furthermore, after analyzing the burden on the back by studying the angle of the upper body and results of an electromyogram, the Tomioka report (Tomioka 2007) showed that using the mechanical lift to get in and out of the bathtub reduced the caregiver's forward-leaning posture and strain on the muscles – all of which contributed to an overall reduction in work-related stress. The report also pointed to increased back strain that comes from bending forward when the caregiver has to wash a care receiver or help her dress/undress while she remains seated, or when adjusting the footrest on the wheel chair.

1.3   Identifying Problems

There's been a lot of research done for the purpose of lessening the physiological and physical burdens of both the caregivers and the care receivers, many of them outlining specific nursing techniques and new policies.

On the other hand, because bathing assistance is more prone to accidents, the caregiver must be on constant alert, especially when dealing with senior citizens with dementia, who often move and act in unpredictable ways. When it comes to easing the mental burdens, however, basic research doesn't go far enough, and there are as yet no solutions.

Creating a safe way to offer bathing assistance than can prevent falls or drowning accidents is in a way reducing mental stress. This could achieve "peace of mind," and make quality nursing care a reality.

We have identified the main issue in our research as reducing the caregivers' mental stress by preventing accidents, such as falls and drowning.

2   Factors of Occurrence of Falls

Kawamura (2003) pointed out that near-accident occasions surrounding nursing care mostly involve falls. Not just limited to bathing time, falling accidents by elderly people can severely interfere with their health, for instance forcing them to be bed-ridden. A large number of studies have been conducted on the link between fitness levels and falling accidents of an elderly person. Accident-prevention programs based on those findings have been shown to be effective.

There are three factors that can lead to falling accidents care-receivers' physical conditions, these caused by the caregivers, and the environmental factors. The physical factors of care-receivers include there age, diseases and muscle weakness, related to the decline of physical functions. Also some medications such as aceso-dyne, soporific, diuretic, psychotropic medication, may induce dizziness or unsteadiness. The factors relating to caregivers include the lack of awareness to risks and lack of sufficient Understanding in the risk levels. Also this factor is greatly influenced by his/her skill and awareness. The environmental factors include steps, slippery floors, and tripping caused by slippers or dim light. These factors can be prevented by removing dangerous places and objects. More than other industries, nursing care must be done under the appropriate condition where manpower, works, equipments and environments are well coordinated. It also requires flexibility in dealing with care-receivers' sudden movements, making it a difficult field to work. The nursing care field is always short of staff, so the caregivers cannot devote sufficient time to each care-receiver. Also there are many blind spots existing in the elderly care facilities. Some facilities installed security cameras in order to prevent the accidents caused by the seniors' action for research purpose. This research contributes to the elimination of blind spots inside the facilities.

It is desirable for the nursing field that the development of new technology in human engineering is carried out based on its core philosophies, such as supporting independent life, normalization, respect for fundamental human rights and supporting self-realization. Thus, in case of video surveillance for the research purpose of blind spots, we must respect and consider the human rights of care-receivers first, and then quantify the blind spots during the daily nursing cares. The research for quantifying blind spots has just started. Further developments are expected in this filed, including the quantification of blind spot in bathing care and the proposal for optimal positions between care-receiver and caregiver, that does not lead to blind spots.

2.1   Solving Problems

This research recommends that in order to prevent a fall during a bath, a practical system be instituted whereby neither a caregiver's gaze nor the care receiver end up in a blind spot. For that to happen, the caregiver's and care receiver's location in the bathroom or changing room has to be recorded in a timed series. As for the caregivers, tracking their gaze in a timed series can help quantify blind spots, potentially even turning the caregiver's monitoring skill into data.

3   System Outline

In order to solve the above-mentioned problems, we propose the method using the motion sensor. This method enables the approximation of the location and vision of the monitoring targets. The motion sensor has been advance by MEMS technology, and now it has been downsized and made cost efficient. With motion sensors attached to the necessary parts of the target's body, it enables the easy measurement of the rotational movement of physical parts and translational movement. Without using video recording, as this method enables to approximate the location and the vision, it draws high expectation in terms of respecting privacy.

This is a system that uses motion sensors to estimate position and visual field data. Calculating the caregiver and the care receiver's position within 10 cm of accuracy in the bathroom, then making an estimate of the caregiver's visual field data in the direction that the caregiver is facing (front) is thought to be helpful for the caregiver. Position estimation by motion sensors is not new. However, methods for estimating visual fields have yet to be tested and are considered something of a novelty. By dispensing with videos in the process, the system makes no privacy breaches, making it a strong candidate for use in welfare care studies, psychology, ergonomic and other areas of research. Furthermore, the skills caregivers apply during bathing – assisting and monitoring – have always been ambiguous. Quantifying those skills from eye-gaze data offers an unprecedented viewpoint. This research is being used for system development intended as feedback to care sites and has a practical application: reducing mental burden is effective in improving the work environment of care sites.

Using this system will more clearly reveal the difference in bathing assistance and monitoring skills between veteran caregivers and novice caregivers. The system can eventually develop into one that supports skill development and offers assessments that can help with monitoring skills to better assist with bathing. The existence of blind spots in bathing assistance work has been made clear, paving the way for smarter staff appointments. Clarifying policies that promote safe bathing assistance by observing the location and movements of the caregivers and care receivers also contributes to the safe management of care welfare facilities.

3.1   General View of New System Proposal

This study consists of four experiments; experiment 1 and 2 in basic research and experiment 3 and 4 in the applied research. In the previous experiment 1 in the basic research, we established the reliability and validity of motion sensor based on the data obtained from the measuring devices of optical motion and eyes movements.

In the experiment 2 in the basic research of this study, the live bathing care was recorded by a video camera. The 43 min and 58 s long footage which was pre-treated with mosaic effect, the professional technician analyzed the footage and pointed out 8 moments with possible risk. As for the multiple hazard locations that the technician pointed out, we simulated these scenes in the laboratory with actors playing the roles of care-receiver and caregiver. The 3-points reflection markers were attached on the head of the subjects. The optical movement measurement equipment captured the motion data and measured the three-dimensional coordinates of the target's vision, to clarify the validity of the data. The experiment 1 and 2 in the basic research was conducted in the laboratory. (Figure 1).

In the experiment 3 in the applied research, we simulated bathing assistance with a bathtub filled with hot water, to estimate the liability and validity of the range of

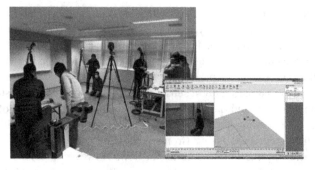

Fig. 1. The experimental scenes in the laboratory

eye-vision information by gathered by motion sensor. In the experiment 4 in the applied research, we estimated the location and visual information of the care-receiver and caregiver in the actual bathing assistance scene. And then evaluated the individual monitoring skills and blind spots quantitatively.

4   Characteristics of Hazard Locations

The Fig. 2 shows the layout of the bathroom in order to showing the schematic diagram of hazard locations. The Fig. 2 shows the image taken by video.

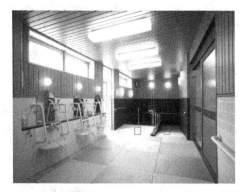

Fig. 2. ① Washing Place ② Bathtub ③ Steps ④ Slope

The Fig. 3 shows the schematic diagrams of the hazard locations identified in the 8 cases. The red dot represents the caregiver and the red arrow shows the line of view of the caregiver. The blue dot represents the care-receiver and the blue arrow shows the line of his view. The black arrow shows the walking directions of both the caregiver and the care-receiver. The yellow mark represents the hazard locations.

(Scene 1) The care-receiver was moving to bathtub alone, but the care-receiver did not watch him. There was high risk of falling accident.

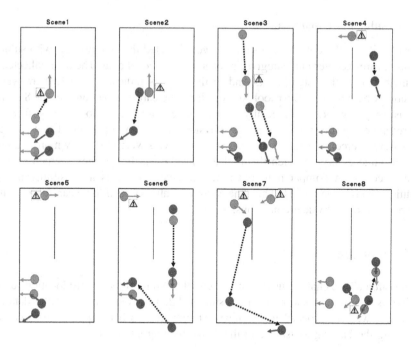

Fig. 3. The schematic diagrams of the hazard locations

(Scene 2) While the caregiver was helping the care-receiver to the bathtub, the caregiver suddenly left the care-receiver because he remembered to do something else.

(Scene 3) The caregiver left the care-receiver alone and helped the other care-receiver to bathtub. While the caregiver was away from him, the first care-receiver tried to get out from the bath tub. Since the floor was wet and slippery, this movement had the high risk causing an accident. Other caregivers in the bathroom also did not notice his movement.

(Scene 4) While the caregiver was watching the safety of care-receivers in the bathroom, he looked away from the care-receivers in order to remove the dust floating in the bathtub.

(Scene 5) Although two caregivers were in the washing place, they did not watch the care-receivers in the bathtub. There was high risk of drowning accidents.

(Scene 6) Although multiple caregivers were in the bathroom, they were looking away from the care-receivers. There was high risk of drowning accidents.

(Scene 7) The caregiver left the two care-receivers in the bathtub for a long time. This increases the risk of drowning accident.

(Scene 8) The caregivers could not switch positions smoothly. This increases the risk of collision accident.

4.1   Results and Discussion

After identifying the dangerous locations, we simulated the care process with subjects playing a care-receiver and caregiver's roles, and collected data. The data collected by this method is highly significant. And in the 8 cases indicated in 4.1, there were 6 occasions where the caregiver looked away from the care-receiver among the 8 scenes. This is very high rate. Especially the caregivers tended to look away from the care-receiver who does not require the physical support. We presumed that the caregivers were overconfident, because these care-receivers were physically more stable, so they felt unnecessary to watch them all the time. Even though they seemed stable in physical condition compared to other care-receivers, there is a possibility of their condition changing suddenly. Thus, the caregivers always need to be careful regardless of care-receiver's physical conditions.

5   Conclusion

The research above enabled us to comprehend the nature of the hazard locations during bathing assistance. As shown in the result of 4.2, with the validity of the data also confirmed, we will proceed to the next experiment step 3 of applied research with simulating the bathing assistance in the actual bathing situation.

References

Fujimura, T.: Roujin Ho-mu ni okeru Kaigo Sagyou no Mondaiten to Youtsuu Taisaku. Roudou no Kagaku **509**, 13–16 (1995). (In Japanese)

Nagata, H.: Tokubetsu Yougo Roujin Ho-mu de no Kaigo Roudou no Jittai Chousa to kongo no Kourei Kaigo Roudou no Kentou. Roudou Kagaku **75**, 459–469 (1999). (In Japanese)

Kawahara, Y.: Current state of bathing care and necessity of new equipment for bathing care institution. J. Hum. Living Environ. **171**, 23–30 (2010)

Kanda, K.: Koureisha no Touki to Kaki ni okeru Nyuuyoku Kankyou to Nyuuyokuji no Seiriteki Futan ni Kansuru Chousa. Bull. Inst. Public Health **40**, 388–390 (1991)

Nagahiro, C.: Effects of room temperature on circulatory dynamics during bathing in the elderly. Jpn. J. Public Health **533**, 178–186 (2006)

Tomioka, K.: Low back load and satisfaction rating of caregivers and care receivers in bathing assistance given in a nursing home for the elderly practicing individual care. San Ei Shi **49**, 54–58 (2007). (In Japanese)

Tomioka, K.: Low back pain among care workers working at newly-built nursing homes for the aged. San Ei Shi **50**, 86–91 (2008). (In Japanese)

Kawamura, H.: Hiyari Hatto: 11,000 Jirei ni yoru Era- mappu Kanzenbon. Igaku shoin 88–91 (2003). (In Japanese)

Author Index

Printed in the United States
By Bookmasters